Treating Children's Psychosocial Problems in Primary Care

Editors: Beth G. Wildman and Terry Stancin
Series Advisor: Stevan E. Hobfoll

Treating Children's Psychosocial Problems in Primary Care

Edited by

Beth G. Wildman

Kent State University

Terry Stancin

MetroHealth Medical Center &
Case Western Reserve University

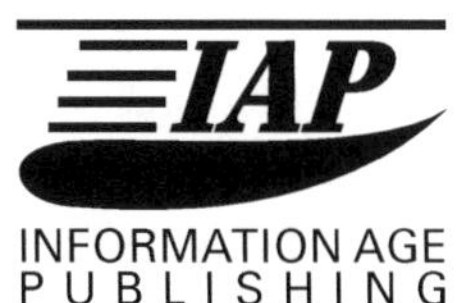

80 Mason Street • Greenwich, Connecticut 06830 • www.infoagepub.com

Library of Congress Cataloging-in-Publication Data

Treating children's psychosocial problems in primary care / edited by
Beth G. Wildman, Terry Stancin.
p. cm.
Includes bibliographical references.
ISBN 1-59311-085-5 (hbk.)—ISBN 1-59311-084-7 (pbk.)
1. Behavior disorders in children. 2. Emotional problems of children.
3. Primary care (Medicine) 4. Pediatrics—Psychological aspects.
I.
Wildman, Beth. II. Stancin, Terry.
RJ506.B44T725 2004
618.92'8914—dc22

2003021885

Printed in the United States of America

CONTENTS

ILLUSTRATIONS

PREFACE

The Forum and this resulting edited volume were among the most professionally exciting and satisfying experiences for the editors. We hope that the participants, both those whose chapters are included in this volume as well those who were invited to contribute to the discussion, found the experience as pleasurable and professionally exciting as we did. We hope that the contents of this book are used to stimulate more attention to behavioral and emotional issues of children within primary care. The issues involved in improving the lives of children are complex and, as reflected in this book, interface with social, economic, political, training, and practice issues. As is apparent from the contributions to this volume, much progress has been made in acknowledging the needs of children, but much more progress is needed if children's mental health needs are going to be met in our society.

The Forum that led to this volume was the thirteenth in an on-going annual series sponsored by the Applied Psychology Center (APC) at Kent State University. The resources and programs of the APC allowed for the prominent clinicians and scholars to attend the meeting and interact informally in the picturesque and relaxing atmosphere of the Inn at Honey Run in the heart of the Amish area of Northeast Ohio. This environment nurtured interaction among the participants for three days and permitted all to leave the Forum with ideas well beyond those presented in the text. We are grateful to the APC for facilitating this endeavor. The editors would especially like to acknowledge the on-going contribution of Kathy Floody, without whose help neither the Forum nor this book would exist. Kathy arranged for every detail of the Forum, from transportation

Treating Children's Psychosocial Problems in Primary Care, ix–x

plans, rooms, food, and drink, to scheduling of papers, discussions, and tours of the local area. Kathy compulsively reviewed all chapters for references, errors, and oversights and maintained a positive disposition and encouraging demeanor throughout the process. The success of the Forum was as much Kathy's doing, as it was the responsibility of the scholars who participated.

In addition to the authors of the chapters, the community experts who participated enriched the discussion of the Forum. These participants included John Duby, Daniel Coury, Liz Thom, Benjamin Newberry, Jeanette Reuter, Michael Little, David Roberts, George Pallotta, Deborah Plate, Ruth Carnes. These individuals represent a variety of disciplines, including pediatrics, family practice, developmental and behavioral pediatrics, clinical psychology, public health nursing, counseling, health psychology, and psychiatry. The graduate students who participated (Meghan Barlow, Courtney Fleisher, Christine Golden, and Tom Yerkey from Kent State University and Chantelle Nobile, from Case Western Reserve University) were wonderful archivists for the Forum and took copious notes about the discussions, which they then summarized. Their summaries appear after each of the chapters in this volume.

Terry Stancin works at MetroHealth Medical Center, a county-funded hospital devoted to providing high-quality care to all residents of Cuyahoga County and beyond. She is particularly grateful for the support of the chair of the Department of Pediatrics, Dr. Robert Cohn, for his support of her work on the Forum and this book. Beth Wildman is on the faculty in the Psychology Department at Kent State University and appreciates the support of the department through the APC for course release and the resources made available for this Forum.

Finally, we appreciate you the reader for your interest in this important topic and hope that the work of the authors leads to improvements in the lives of children through increased attention to mental health issues in primary care medical contexts, improvements in training of primary care physicians, and the stimulation of research to guide improved clinical management. It is the responsibility of all of us interested in the well-being of children to improve the state of the art for their treatment and to advocate for their needs.

Beth G. Wildman
Terry Stancin

INTRODUCTION

Most child health services take place in outpatient or ambulatory medical settings and are provided by pediatricians, family practice physicians, and nurse practitioners. Advances in medical science, especially breakthroughs with immunizations and disease prevention since the 1960s, led to a reformulation of child health care needs with the result being a contemporary focus on primary care services delivered in office settings. Primary care services emphasize health promotion and include prevention (i.e., immunization) and early detection of disease, injury prevention, assessment of family health and safety, and early identification of developmental and behavioral problems (American Academy of Pediatrics [AAP], 1997; Committee on Practice and Ambulatory Medicine, AAP, 2000; Green, 1994). Primary care providers (PCPs) are expected to deliver these services along with taking care of acute medical needs and providing comprehensive care of children with chronic health and developmental conditions.

There are many issues of interest to both PCPs and pediatric or child clinical psychologists, resulting in a growing interest for child mental health services to take place in primary care settings, where most child health services are provided (Perrin, 1999; Stancin, 1999). Both groups are concerned about providing effective and early interventions for child behavior disorders, first by early and accurate identification and screening and then with effective, acceptable, and accessible treatments. There appears to be consensus among PCPs, child mental health professionals, and child development researchers that child behavior problems in primary care settings are common, yet undertreated and underreferred.

Treating Children's Psychosocial Problems in Primary Care, xi–xvii

Examples of primary care settings that incorporate child mental health services have been reported in the literature, but relatively few empirical studies have been conducted to evaluate the impact and effectiveness of interventions (Stancin, 1999).

2001 KENT PSYCHOLOGY FORUM

This text is the product of the 2001 Kent Psychology Forum, an annual think tank hosted by the Applied Psychology Center at Kent State University in northeastern Ohio. The 2001 Forum was held April 22-25 (cochaired by Beth Wildman, Ph.D. and Terry Stancin, Ph.D.) and was entitled "New Directions for Research and Treatment of Pediatric Psychosocial Problems in Primary Care." The overall goal of the Forum was to develop strategies and potential solutions to improve the ability to serve mental health needs of children seen in primary care settings, by developing research strategies to improve identification and treatment of psychosocial problems by primary care physicians, and ways to implement and evaluate the efficacy of prevention interventions and alternative models of care. The Forum was an interdisciplinary effort involving approximately 20 participants, including general and developmental and behavioral pediatricians, a family physician, public health nurses, a child psychiatrist, pediatric and child clinical psychologists and graduate students, a medical economist, and a medical sociologist. The format of the forum included 20-minute presentations followed by discussion. Each forum presentation is included as a chapter in this text.

As the reader will see, all presenters agreed that children with mental health needs are not being adequately served in most primary care settings. Many noted that a PCP is often the first professional to hear about child behavioral concerns, usually from a parent during an ambulatory visit for well-child care. If a concern is raised, the PCP may offer *advice* (parent guidance), *treatment* (parenting skills coaching or prescription for psychotropic medication), or *referral* to a mental health professional for further evaluation and treatment. Epidemiological studies conducted in pediatric primary care settings during the 1980s and 1990s showed that between 10-20% of school-age children may have a diagnosable psychiatric disorder (e.g., Costello, Costello, et al., 1988; Lavigne et al. 1993). Moreover, up to 50% of parents may have behavioral concerns about their child (e.g., Costello & Shugart, 1992; Sharp, Pantell, Murphy, & Lewis, 1992; Starfield & Borkowf, 1969).

PCPs, especially pediatricians, have been the target of criticism for their lack of ability to detect and properly manage (i.e., treat or refer) child behavior problems in primary care settings. Studies comparing pediatrician chart notes with maternal behavior rating scale results have shown that pediatricians identify about half of the children with significant behavior problems and refer only a minority of those identified children to mental health professionals for further evaluation and treatment (Chang, Warner, & Weissman, 1988; Costello, 1986; Costello, Burns, et al.1988). The result of these findings was a call for better screening methods (e.g., Stancin & Palermo, 1997), improved training of PCPs in child behavioral issues (e.g., Coury, Berger, Stancin, & Tanner, 1999), and development of a diagnostic classification system that is better suited for pediatric practices (e.g., *Diagnostic and Statistical Manual for Primary Care (DSM-PC), Child and Adolescent Version*; Wolraich, Felice, & Drotar, 1996). In Chapter 9, Dennis Drotar, Ph.D. (with coauthors Sturner and Nobile) discusses the potential use of the *DSM-PC* for assisting PCPs in making behavioral diagnoses in children. The chapter's description of the tool underscores the collaborative nature of its development and its perceived utility in practice, including potential computerized applications.

Many of the issues discussed during the Forum suggested that mental health issues fail to become a priority for physicians during their encounters with their pediatric patients. One major obstacle facing the PCP is recognition that s/he is unlikely to have the time or expertise to adequately address problems once identified (Perrin & Stancin, 2002). The average length of time physicians spend with children during an encounter is less than 15 minutes. Yet, the physicians explained that if they followed all of the guidelines suggested for health maintenance, as well as required procedures, a visit would have to be 1 hour and 45 minutes. Lack of reimbursement for mental health services provided by PCPs is a frequently cited obstacle to identification and care (Rappo, Chapter 6).

Moreover, referral to a mental health professional is often a difficult process for the primary care practice. In urban areas, long waits are common for appointments with child psychiatrists and psychologists, and in rural areas, these professionals are often not available at all. When referrals are made, feedback and coordination of treatment is rare. As detailed by Douglas Tynan, Ph.D. (Chapter 8), linking mental health services for children can be cumbersome and time consuming, particularly because of the complex "carve out" nature of many insurance policies for mental health services. Lack of control over mental health referrals and subsequent inadequate communication between mental health and primary care clinicians is likely to frustrate and further undermine the motivation of the primary care provider to identify child behavior problems (Perrin & Stancin, 2002).

Pediatricians in attendance at the Forum discussed various attempts at coordinating services between themselves and mental health professionals. Peter Rappo, M.D. (Chapter 6), described issues related to coding and documentation of mental health services. Reimbursement for mental health services in primary care is tied to coding and documentation, and is therefore a critical concern facing PCPs and mental health providers. Joseph Hagan, M.D. (Chapter 4), represented the American Academy of Pediatrics (AAP) at the Forum and described his rural general pediatric practice in Vermont. Dr. Hagan's perspective as the Chair of the Psychosocial Concerns Committee of the AAP demonstrates that the field of pediatrics considers mental health issues to be a critically important component of primary care. Alex Geertsma, M.D., is a developmental-behavioral pediatrician who reported on integrating developmental and behavioral pediatrics into primary care (Chapter 3). As Dr. Geertsma reports, developmental and behavioral pediatrics first emerged as a subspecialty in the wake of the realization that behavior and development were the purview of pediatricians. This group has repeatedly called for greater involvement of practicing pediatricians to address mental health issues in daily primary care practice.

In Chapter 7, Sherry Glied, Ph.D., a medical economist, (along with coauthor Adam Neufeld) presents data suggesting that changing the reimbursement and health care delivery system to allow more time and reimbursement for primary care physicians to spend with their patients would not be sufficient to improve the identification and management of psychosocial problems by primary care physicians. Dr. Glied's data supported the suggestion that primary care physicians need to have effective interventions available to them in order to increase their likelihood of attending to psychosocial issues.

Several models for providing integrated mental health interventions appropriate to primary care were presented by Carolyn Schroeder, Ph.D. (Chapter 1), Terry Stancin, Ph.D. (in Wildman & Stancin, Chapter 11), and Douglas Tynan, Ph.D. (Chapter 8). Although family medicine practices have often incorporated mental health professionals (McDaniel, 1995), most pediatric practices have not (Perrin & Stancin, 2002). Dr. Schroeder, who developed a collaborative care practice in North Carolina in the 1970s, shares her extensive experience and wisdom on integrated services. Dr. Stancin presented data on a behavioral assessment service within an inner city teaching ambulatory clinic. Douglas Tynan, Ph.D., described an alternative clinical model in Chapter 8. The "Triple–P" program is a comprehensive, five-level model of behavioral interventions developed in Australia. The first two levels of the program, which could be readily implemented in primary care settings in the United States, include parent education and prevention, and videotaped presentation of parenting information. The next two levels involve structured interventions with parents, and the fifth level resembles the collaborative practice model.

Because primary care offers a longitudinal perspective that begins in infancy, primary care settings offer a greater opportunity to focus on prevention of child mental health problems. However, Michael Roberts, Ph.D., and Kerrie Brown (Chapter 2) describe a surprisingly limited body of evidence documenting the effectiveness of prevention in primary care settings. Not only is there a lack of data guiding prevention interventions in primary care settings, the authors note that pediatric psychologists often do not receive adequate training in prevention. Development and empirical evaluation of prevention strategies in primary care along with increased training in effective methods are in need.

Robert Johnson, Ph.D., a medical sociologist, and Beth Wildman, Ph.D., a clinical psychologist, presented models addressing how mental health issues come to the attention of primary care physicians, and factors that may influence whether addressing these issues become a priority for both physicians and parents during a child's visit with their primary care physician. Using different models of access to medical care, Dr. Johnson (Chapter 10) emphasized the complexity of the relationship between a person having an illness and receiving care for that illness. Factors that need to be explored, both individually and as interactions, in a model include the nature of the illness, social demographics of the patient, cultural factors, the relationship between the physician and the patient, the physician's clinical training and experience, and the availability of treatment for the disorder. Dr. Wildman (in Wildman & Stancin, Chapter 11) described factors that need to be explored to develop a model specific to understanding what factors are important in making mental health issues a priority during a visit for both the parent and the physician. The factors for this model were divided into parent, child, physician, and system factors.

Political forces in health care services were not overlooked at the Forum. Ted Strickland, Ph.D., is both a psychologist and congressman and was in attendance at the Forum. His perspectives and insights into the national political trends and call for action are included in Chapter 5.

WHAT NEXT?

The result of the Forum was a call for researchers to develop and assess evidence-based interventions for child mental health problems in primary care settings. The participants were unanimous in their call for the evaluation of interventions that could be implemented in primary care. The evaluation of interventions, whether for parents, children, or professionals must include assessment of both the efficacy, as well as the compliance with the intervention. Discussion acknowledged the lack of compliance by physicians with currently effective interventions, such as use of brief screening measures, and lack of compliance by parents with physician recommendations and referrals. Several particular ideas were discussed with regard to research concerning interventions that could be implemented in primary care, including an evaluation of the efficacy of printed materials distributed to parents, compliance and efficacy of advice given during call-in hours, and an evaluation of a program similar to the five-level Triple-P program.

The discussion at the Forum emphasized the need for research to guide practice. The participants expressed concern about the lack of adequate reimbursement for PCPs' time if they address psychosocial problems in their pediatric patients. The physicians also talked about the difficulty they experience in trying to coordinate services for psychosocial problems, and stated that coordinating mental health services tends to be much more difficult than coordinating other specialty medical services. Participants agreed that physicians and mental health professionals both need to develop skills to address behavioral needs in primary care settings. Traditional training experiences for child mental health professionals are not sufficient preparation for the challenges of primary care.

The interdisciplinary panel of national and regional experts present at this forum reached the following consensus: To meet the psychosocial needs of children in primary care settings, empirically-supported treatments must be made available to clinicians (physicians and mental health), and conceptual, theoretical models of prevention, identification, and treatment must be developed to help guide research. It is our hope that the chapters that follow will help other researchers and clinicians in those critical endeavors.

Terry Stancin
Beth Wildman

REFERENCES

American Academy of Pediatrics. (1997). *Guidelines for health supervision III*. Elk Grove Village, IL: Author.

American Academy of Pediatrics, Committee on Practice and Ambulatory Medicine. (2000). Recommendations for preventive pediatric health care. *Pediatrics, 105*, 645.

Chang, G., Warner, V., & Weissman, M. M. (1988). Physician recognition of psychiatric disorders in children and adolescents. *American Journal of Disease Control, 142*, 736-739.

Costello, E. J. (1986). Primary care pediatrics and child psychopathology: A review of diagnostic, treatment, and referral practices. *Pediatrics, 78,* 1044-1051.

Costello, E. J., Burns, B. J., Costello, A. J., Edelbrock, C., Dulcan, M., & Brent, D. (1988). Service utilization and psychiatric diagnosis in pediatric primary care: The role of the gatekeeper. *Pediatrics, 82,* 435-441.

Costello, E. J., Costello, A. J., Edelbrock, C., Burns, B. J., Dulcan, M. K., Brent, D., & Janiszewski, S. (1988). Psychiatric disorders in pediatric primary care: Prevalence and risk factors. *Archives of General Psychiatry, 45,* 1107-1116.

Costello, E. J., & Shugart, M. A. (1992). Above and below the threshold: Severity of psychiatric symptoms and functional impairment in a pediatric sample. *Pediatrics, 90,* 359-368.

Coury, D., Berger, S., Stancin, T., & Tanner, L. (1999). Curricular guidelines for residency training in developmental and behavioral pediatrics. *Journal of Developmental and Behavioral Pediatrics, 20,* S1-S38.

Green, M. (Ed.). (1994). *Bright futures: Guidelines for health supervision of infants, children and adolescents.* Arlington, VA: National Center for Education in Maternal and Child Health.

Lavigne, J. V., Binns, H. J., Christoffel, K. K., Rosenbaum, D., Arend, R., Smith, K., Hayford, J. R., McGuire, P. A., et al. (1993). Behavioral and emotional problems among preschool children in pediatric primary care: prevalence and pediatricians' recognition. *Pediatrics, 91,* 649-655.

McDaniel, S. H. (1995). Collaboration between psychologists and family physicians: implementing the biopsychosocial model. *Professional Psychology, 26,* 117-122.

Perrin, E. C. (1999). The promise of collaborative care. *Journal of Developmental and Behavioral Pediatrics 20,* 57-62.

Perrin, E,. & Stancin, T. (2002). A continuing dilemma: Whether and how and to screen for concerns about children's behavior in primary care settings. *Pediatrics in Review, 23,* 264-282.

Sharp, L., Pantell, R. H., Murphy, L. O., & Lewis, C. C. (1992). Psychosocial problems during child health supervision visits: Eliciting, then what? *Pediatrics, 89,* 619-623.

Stancin, T. (1999). Introduction to the special issue on pediatric mental health services in primary care settings. *Journal of Pediatric Psychology, 24,* 367-368.

Stancin, T., & Palermo, T. M. (1997). A review of behavioral screening practices in pediatric settings: Do they pass the test? *Journal of Developmental Behavioral Pediatrics, 18,* 183-194.

Starfield, B., & Borkowf, S. (1969). Physicians' recognition of complaints made by parents about their children's health. *Pediatrics, 43,* 168-172.

Wolraich, M. L., Felice, M. E., & Drotar, D. (Eds.) (1996). The classification of child and adolescent mental diagnoses in primary care. *Diagnostic & Statistical Manual for Primary Care (DSM-PC), Child and Adolescent Version.* Elk Grove, IL: American Academy of Pediatrics.

CHAPTER 1

A COLLABORATIVE PRACTICE IN PRIMARY CARE

Lessons Learned

Carolyn S. Schroeder
University of Kansas

Pediatricians and child psychologists would appear to form a natural collaborative team in primary care settings given their many common interests in the health and development of children. Even before the establishment of the American Academy of Pediatrics in 1930 and the Society of Pediatric Psychology in 1968, there were early reports of these two professions working together.

Jean McFarlane, a developmental psychologist, worked in a children's hospital as early as 1917-1918 and Arnold Gesell, a medical doctor, interested in pediatrics and a PhD psychologist, wrote in 1919 about the important role for clinical psychology in medical settings working with children (Drotar, 1995; Gesell, 1919; Routh, 1994). It seems that pediatricians were initially more aware of the potential benefits of collaborating with psychologists, or at least wrote more about this team approach, than psychologists. For example in his presidential address to the American Academy of Pediatrics, Wilson (1964) stated: "one of the things I would do

Treating Children's Psychosocial Problems in Primary Care, 1–34

if I could control the practice of pediatrics would be to encourage groups of pediatricians to employ their own clinical psychologists" (p. 988).

By the mid 1960s and early 1970s psychologists seemed to take the idea of collaborating with pediatricians more seriously. Jerome Kagan (1965), for example, described the pediatrician-psychologist relationship as a "new marriage" and others described a new breed of psychologists, "pediatric psychologists", and their role in nonpsychiatric medical settings (Wright, 1967; Salk, 1970). Logan Wright outlined a number of important issues that pediatric psychologists would have to address in order to make their work viable. These included formal ways to communicate and work together, the development of formal training for this new profession, and the development of a base of scientific knowledge that would be unique to pediatric psychology. He also exhorted psychologists to become "card carrying members of a militant group set out to destroy inappropriateness and inefficiency in psychological services, as well as the dearth of behavioral information, in pediatric settings" (p. 325). In the years since, pediatric psychology has become a viable specialty with the founding of the Society of Pediatric Psychology (American Psychological Association, Division 54), the publication of the scholarly *Journal of Pediatric Psychology*, and the development of training programs at the graduate, internship and postdoctoral level. It is also safe to say that the psychological needs of children suffering from chronic diseases or who are hospitalized are well recognized and that more appropriate and effective psychological services are being offered to them. To date, however, the majority of pediatric psychology research, practice and teaching continues to focus on children who are physically ill and to be carried out in large university medical centers versus community primary care settings (Kelleher, 1999). It appears that now is the time to be more militant in our efforts to include psychology in pediatric primary care.

The need for pediatric psychologists to move beyond medical hospitals and educational settings to the front lines of community-based primary care is clearly illustrated by prevalence studies. It is estimated that 11-20% of children seen in primary care settings have significant developmental, emotional, or behavioral problems (Costello, 1989; Briggs-Gowan, Horowitz, Schwab-Stone, Leventhal, & Leaf, 2000). Lavigne and colleagues (1999) indicate that the percentages are much higher, especially during the preschool years. In addition to children with significant mental health problems, half of the parents of children seen for well-child visits are reported to bring up psychosocial concerns, the majority of which go unanswered (Briggs-Gowan et al., 2000; Sharp, Pantell, Murphy, & Lewis, 1992). Leaders in the field of pediatrics have acknowledged the importance of physicians being able to identify psychosocial problems and to be more responsive to these needs (e.g., Haggerty, 1986; Steinberg, Gadomski, & Wilson, 1999). Attempts have been made to improve pediatricians' ability to identify and treat psychosocial problems through such methods as interdisciplinary training, the development of the specialty of behavioral and developmental pediatrics, and the anticipatory guidelines and prevention-related strategies provided by the American Academy of Pediatrics. Nonetheless, these attempts, as well as psychologists' attempts to find better ways to help pediatricians identify, treat, and refer these children, have not always been successful (Kelleher, 1999; Perrin, 1999). The reality is that pediatricians rarely have the training or time to deal with both the physical and psychosocial needs of even a small percentage of the children in their practices. Further, the goal of pediatric psychologists' providing the needed preventive and mental health services to children and families in the primary care setting has met with limited success. Family medicine with its biopsychosocial approach to training and practice appears to have been more successful integrating mental health services into primary care practices (American Academy of Family Physicians, 1994). This may be due, in part, to a long history in which residency programs in family medicine are required to have a psychosocial professional on the faculty.

Although there are some early publications describing psychologists and pediatricians working together in community pediatric primary care settings (Fischer & Engeln, 1972; Smith, Rome, & Friedheim, 1967; Schroeder, 1979, 1994, 1996a) and a 1983 article in the *American Psychologist* highlighting the value of this work (Routh, Schroeder & Koocher, 1983), few psychologists are practicing in these settings. Interest in working with primary care physicians, however, is on the rise and the time seems ripe for psychologists to be as much a part of pediatric primary care practices as nurses or nurse practitioners. Health care reforms are making traditional private practice for psychologists less appealing and pediatricians have even less time to devote to mental health issues. There is also a greater awareness of the importance of providing comprehensive and coordinated educational, psychological, and medical care for children and families (American Psychological Association, 1994; Steinberg et al., 1999). Through the excellent publications of Dennis Drotar (1995) and others (e.g., Haley et al., 1998; Seaburn, Lorenz, Gunn, Gawiski, & Mauksch, 1996), psychologists entering the arena of primary care have timely information and research to help guide their work. In addition, the recent development of guidelines for training psychologists in primary care (McDaniel, Behar, Schroeder, Hargrove & Freeman, 2002; Spirito, 2000) as well as predoctoral and doctoral training programs located in the primary care setting (Anderson & Lovejoy, 2000; Hunter & Peterson, 2001) will provide properly trained psychologists to do this work. The special issues of the *Journal of Pediatric Psychology* focusing on research in primary care (Drotar & Lemanek, 2001; Stancin, 1999), and the Kent Forum on new directions for research and treatment of pediatric psychosocial problems in primary care (Wildman & Stancin, 2001) further set the stage for increasing our efforts to be more effective in community primary care settings.

This chapter will describe a collaborative pediatric-psychology practice spanning 28 years. Serendipity often plays a part in many successful endeavors and this was true for the pediatric psychology program at Chapel Hill Pediatrics. In the 1970 and 1980s the presence of influential public health professionals and forward looking pediatricians at the University of North Carolina provided an atmosphere that encouraged trying innovative ways to meet the needs of children and families in their communities. People such as Dr. Arden Miller in the School of Public Health, Dr. Floyd Denny, Chair of Pediatrics, Dr. Harrie Chamberlin, director of a university affiliated program and a champion of interdisciplinary work, and Drs. Frank Loda and Michael Sharp in ambulatory pediatrics, along with many others were influential in setting the stage for this work. Also, the pediatricians at Chapel Hill Pediatrics were forward looking and their encouragement and support over the years allowed pediatric psychologists to become an integral part of their pediatric practice. The psychologists at Chapel Hill Pediatrics were able to engage in service, professional training and research as well as collaborate with other community agencies that serve children. These activities have been described, in part, in other publications (e.g., Hawk, Schroeder, & Martin, 1987; Kanoy & Schroeder, 1985; Mesibov, Schroeder, & Wesson, 1977; Routh et al., 1983; Schroeder, 1996a, 1996b, 1979 ; Schroeder & Gordon, 1991; Schroeder, Gordon, Kanoy, & Routh, 1983). A brief description of several models for psychology-pediatric collaboration in primary care will be followed by a focus on the model used at Chapel Hill Pediatrics. After a brief description of the practice, lessons learned from this collaborative work will be presented.

CHAPEL HILL PEDIATRICS/ CHAPEL HILL PEDIATRIC PSYCHOLOGY

Psychologists have used a number of models to establish collaborative relationships with pediatricians (Drotar, 1995; Hamlett & Stabler, 1995). The most common approach involves the psychologist acting as an independent specialist who receives referrals from pediatricians and provides direct services to children and families. Psychologists and pediatricians have also acted as educational consultants to each other. In this model they provide information and advice to each other about particular families and children but they do not provide direct service. A third, more collegial, model involves the psychologist and pediatrician sharing their unique skills in the care of particular children and families. This is often the approach taken with children who have chronic illnesses. A fourth model moves beyond the individual child and family to collaborating at the practice level where the focus is on the needs of the children in the community and working together to find appropriate ways to meet them (Perrin, 1999). This usually involves the psychologist and pediatrician sharing the same space, defining common goals, and contributing their unique skills and knowledge to meeting the needs in their joint practice. In this model, patients could be seen alone by a pediatrician, psychologist, or both to varying degrees. The activities or services offered will depend on the particular setting including the needs of the parents and children, the interests of the pediatricians, the interests and skills of the psychologist, time constraints, the available space and economic factors. Although the various models of collaboration can be effective, this fourth model has the greatest potential to effect changes in the lives of children and is the most challenging to accomplish. Often, pediatricians and psychologists begin their relationship with a referral or educative model and move into a more collaborative one.

The work at Chapel Hill Pediatrics began in 1973 as a result of an interest in early intervention and prevention on the part of a public health nurse, a social worker, and a psychologist who worked in a training clinic serving children with developmental disabilities at the University of North Carolina (Schroeder, Goolsby, & Stangler, 1975). Chapel Hill Pediatrics was the only community pediatric group in this small university town and four pediatricians served 8,000-10,000 children. At the time, the pediatricians had an early morning call hour to handle questions about health issues and to schedule children who were sick. Many of the calls, however, focused on developmental and management issues which took considerable time to answer and kept the parents with more pressing health issues "on hold." The pediatricians were, therefore, interested in finding a better way to handle these concerns. To further explore this need, as well as to determine how best to meet the need, a randomly selected group of 100 parents with preschool-age children from the pediatric office were surveyed by telephone. As a result of the survey, the following psychosocial services were offered: (1) a "Call-In Hour" twice a week, when parents could ask questions about child development and behavior; (2) weekly evening parent groups, which focused on different ages and stages of development; (3) half-hour "Come-In" times 2-4 hours a week, to give parents an opportunity to discuss their child-related concerns in greater depth; and (4) developmental screening. These services as well as consultation to the pediatricians were offered free of charge in exchange for allowing graduate students in psychology, medicine, nursing, and social work to participate. All services were carried out in the primary care setting.

In 1982, as a result of increased requests from both the parents and pediatricians to provide more in-depth assessment and treatment, as well as a desire to demonstrate the viability of a fee-for-service mental health practice in primary care, the author left the university for a full-time position in the pediatric practice. At the advice of lawyers a separate psychological corporation was established, Chapel Hill Pediatric Psychology. The psychologist was included on the pediatricians' letterhead and in their informational material. The pediatricians covered overhead costs for the first two years of this collaborative practice; when additional mental heath staff were added to the practice, space and administrative support were paid by the pediatric psychology group. Over the years the practice grew. The number of pediatricians increased to six and the mental health staff increased to four and a half full-time psychologists, one and a half full-time psychiatrists, and a master's level marriage and family therapist. Space was an ongoing problem and in 1994, the mental health professionals moved to an adjacent building. One office in the primary care facility was kept for on-site consultation with parents, the Call-In Hour and for research. In 1998 the author retired from the practice. Although Chapel Hill Pediatrics and Chapel Hill Pediatric Psychology continue to collaborate and many of the same services exist, this chapter examines services offered from 1973 to 1998. Currently the two professional groups are planning to move to a new building where the practices can once again occupy the same space.

Although parents and children receiving psychological services were primarily from the pediatric practice, anyone in the community could use the services, and a referral from a pediatrician was not necessary. The population served was primarily well educated, middle class, and Caucasian. Contracts with the Department of Social Services and other community agencies provided opportunities to work with more diverse cultural, ethnic, and economic population.

The following section will present the clinical services, community collaboration, training, and research activities carried out in the pediatric office.

Clinical Services

The primary care setting requires a shift in the way mental health services have been traditionally offered: (1) More clients are seen; (2) less time is spent with each client; and (3) clients generally present with less debilitating disorders (Wright & Burns, 1986). Thus, there is a greater focus on prevention and early intervention than on treatment of severe psychopathology. A developmental-behavioral approach that targets specific behaviors or problems, is solution based, and takes into account the child and family's development is imperative. The clinical services offered by Chapel Hill Pediatric Psychology focused on prevention, early intervention, assessment, and treatment.

Prevention/Early Intervention

The Call-In Hour, offered twice a week, was a time when parents could ask questions about child development and behavior management concerns. Parents routinely call pediatricians for information and we found this to be an excellent way to make contact with parents when they have an initial concern. Reports on the types and frequency of problems, as well as the effectiveness of the advice given, have been published in a number of sources (Kanoy & Schroeder, 1985; Mesibov et al., 1977; Schroeder et al., 1983). Over the years, approximately 17% of the parents using the Call-In Hour were referred for further assessment/treatment. Those parents who followed through with the referral rated the suggestion very highly, but one study (Kanoy & Schroeder, 1985) found that 33% of the parents who had been referred did not follow through with the referral suggestion. In 1982 when more clinical services became readily available in the pediatric setting, it was rare that a parent did not follow through with the recommendation for referral.

The psychologists offered the Call-In Hour at no cost to the parents or pediatricians. It was, however, one of the best ways to demonstrate the importance of psychologists in the pediatric setting and, as such, was great publicity. The Call-In Hour was advertised in the general information about the pediatric practice as well as in newspapers as one of the services offered by the practice. Anyone in the community could use the service.

Parent education groups were a popular way to provide information to parents about development and management. The pediatricians offered prenatal parent groups that focused on health, development and safety issues. A member of the mental health staff with a license in marriage and family therapy as well as a masters in child development offered weekly group meetings for parents of newborn to 6-month-olds and for parents of 7-month to 24-month olds. These groups were free to the parents with the pediatricians paying the psychology group to do them. Another parent group was held for 90 minutes one evening a week on age-specific topics. For example, a month of sessions might focus on toddlers with the following topics: Ages and Stages; Toilet Training; Preventing Power Struggles; Survival Tactics: Dinner Through Bedtime. For adolescence the topics might be Adolescence: What to Expect; Balancing Their Needs: Independence and Rules; and Tips for Parenting During the Adolescent Years. The sessions were limited to 20 parents each and organized to include a didactic presentation of material and an opportunity for questions and answers. For the first 10 years, there was no charge for these groups; the decision to charge a fee did not decrease the number of parents attending the groups (Schroeder, 1996a).

Written material is another way used to provide prevention services to parents and children. Parents' first choice of an information source is books or reading material (Clarke-Stewart, 1978), although there is little empirical evidence on the effectiveness of books in preventing problems. A parent library was developed in response to the continual requests of parents for reading material on child-related issues. These books were widely used by the general pediatric clientele, in addition to being used as adjuncts to treatment. The psychology practice bought and maintained the books as well as operated the library. In addition, the public library was periodically given an update on recommended books so that they would be available to the general community.

Parent handouts provide quick information or anticipatory guidance and typically are produced by drug companies for use in pediatric offices. The pediatric psychologists developed a set of handouts about common problems to use as follow-up material for parents who used the Call-In Hour, as well as to give to parents at well-child physical examinations. We discovered, however, that it was difficult to develop a system in which the age-specific handout was routinely given at the appropriate office visit. Handouts were most often given at a parent's request for information.

Developmental screening is often a routine part of a well-baby checkup for children up to age 3 years. This, however, was not a routine service at Chapel Hill Pediatrics, but as a result of the number of parents who called in with concerns regarding developmental delays, the Denver Developmental Screening Test (Frankenburg & Dodds, 1967) was given to all children at their 3-year-old checkup. Calls about developmental delays decreased accordingly. Several years later the age for screening was changed to 24 months to permit earlier intervention. Although the pediatric psychologists were involved in training the nurses to do the screening, it was also important to have ongoing contact with the nurses to monitor test results, provide up-to-date information on stimulation, offer referral sources in the community, and determine when to refer to psychology for a more extensive evaluation. Unfortunately, no data were kept on the effectiveness of the formal screening and after several years it was discontinued.

Direct Clinical Service

Referrals for Direct Intervention

Over time the number of new referrals for direct psychological services increased. An early survey (Hawk et al., 1987) indicated that 681 new referrals were received in a five-year period. In a two-year period from 1989-1990 the number of new referrals were 714 (Schroeder, 1992). In 1996 new referrals averaged 37 per month or approximately 444 in a year. In a review of 714 new referrals over a two-year period (1989-1990), Schroeder (1992) found 54% were boys and 46% were girls, with an age distribution as follows: birth to 5 years, 22%; 6 to 10 years, 44%; 11 to 15 years, 21%; and 16 years and older, 13%. The most frequent problems were negative behavior (18%); anxiety (15%); Attention-deficit Hyperactivity Disorder (ADHD) (12%); learning problems and school problems (17%); divorce and separation (9%); peer/self-esteem (7%); depression (6%); child abuse (6%); and developmental or medical problems (3%). Although we initially expected to see a significant number of children with physically related problems, we learned that most children in community primary care do not present with major medical or developmental problems. The children who had serious physical problems were usually followed in tertiary settings which have their own psychologists. Other psychologists working in pediatric primary care settings have reported similar findings (Schroeder, 1994).

The length of time children and families were seen remained fairly stable over time, with 13% seen for only one session and the mean number of sessions being five (Schroeder, 1992). Although the focus was on problems requiring short-term treatment, the reality is that in a population of 20,000 pediatric patients one would expect that approximately 200 children will have significant emotional or behavioral problems at any given point in time. The parents and pediatricians did not want to refer these cases out of the clinic, arguing for continuity of care and working with people they have come to trust (Schroeder & Gordon, 1991). The dilemma was how to meet the extensive needs of these children with significant psychosocial problems while continuing to serve the large number of children with less significant problems. Eventually the mental health staff was increased to meet these needs but this also increased the need to coordinate with more people within and across disciplines as well as find more space to carry out the work.

In addition to seeing "new" cases, we discovered that certain children are psychologically more vulnerable and benefit from brief intervention from time to time. Some examples include: an increase in environmental stresses (e.g., dealing with a parent with psychopathology); a particular stage of development exacerbating a preexisting problem (e.g., the child with a chronic illness or developmental problem or the child who has been sexually abused); or persistent emotional or behavioral problems at a subclinical level that are exacerbated by a certain developmental stage or transition. Gordon and Jens (1988) describe this as the "moving-risk model" wherein these vulnerable children appear to need help at different points in their lives, but not necessarily ongoing treatment. We discovered that successful treatment did not necessarily mean a cure for these children (Schroeder, 1996b). Rather, with periodic help children and families learned to cope with the stresses of life. Thus, the psychologists, like the pediatricians, had the opportunity to follow children over the course of their development and help make the trajectory of that development more successful. This was perhaps one of the most rewarding aspects of working in a pediatric primary care setting.

Although the number of direct referrals increased over time (and continues to increase with an average of 50 or more new referrals per month for the year 2000), there was a shift in the percentage of referrals for younger children. For example, in the five-year period from 1982 to 1987 the percentage of referrals from birth to 5 years was 34% (Hawk et al., 1987). From 1989 to 1990 the percentage of referrals for these young children dropped to 22% (Schroeder, 1992), and in a five-month period from January to May 1997 the percentage dropped to 7%. Thus, it appeared that the early identification and treatment of children with psychosocial problems during the crucial early years of development were no longer a major focus of the pediatric psychologists' work. Part of the drop could have been due to the pediatricians giving more information to parents, or to the introduction of the parent groups for infants and toddlers. But the drop also could have been influenced by other factors such as the increasing influence of managed care, the psychologists' move to an adjacent building, or a decreased interest in serving this population. Although managed care appears to serve young families well, the reimbursement for psychological services is often so low that psychologists choose not to be service providers for many insurance plans. This was true for the psychologists in Chapel Hill Pediatric Psychology. Regardless of the reason, the population receiving direct services had shifted to prepuberty/adolescent children with significant mental health needs and adults (primarily for marital problems). Although these data require further analysis, it is clear that early intervention, which would appear to be the hallmark of psychological work in primary care settings, was no longer the norm for the Chapel Hill Pediatric Psychology services by 1997.

Assessment Services

Assessment was an integral part of every contact, whether it was having a phone consult with a parent about a specific problem, consulting with the pediatrician about a child, helping a nurse deal with a fearful child, determining the need for treatment, or doing an evaluation that involved collaborating with a number of community agencies. Both the parents and the pediatricians presented a wide range of questions and problems that often demanded concise, rapid and "on target" answers (e.g., "How do I tell my child his mother just died?" "What can I do to calm a 14-year-old girl who is having a panic attack in the exam room?", "How do I help a 5-year-old answer questions about a birth mark on her face?"). There were also the more complex questions that demanded in-depth assessment (e.g., "I think my ex-husband is sexually abusing our daughter", "The teacher thinks this child has a learning disability and is hyperactive", "Should I be concerned that my 6-year-old has developed a number of motor and verbal tics?")

We used a behaviorally-oriented system for assessment that is based on Rutter's (1975) work and which we call a Comprehensive Assessment-to-Intervention System (CAIS). The CAIS is described in detail in Schroeder and Gordon (1991, 2002). The CAIS was developed initially as a framework to systematically and quickly assess a problem and offer suggestions to parents who used the Call-In Hour. It allows the clinician to get an understanding of the dimensions of the problem without having to attach a label to the problem with a system such as *DSM-IV* (American Psychiatric Association, 1994). This is particularly important in the primary care setting, since many of the referral problems would not be considered clinically significant or pathological although they may significantly impact the child or family's life (Schroeder, 1996b). The CAIS system clusters information in six areas: the referral question, the social context of the referral, information on general child development and characteristics of the family, specifics of the concern including a functional analysis, the effects of the problem, and areas for intervention. We found that it is often not necessary to have all of this information to assess and plan intervention for a specific problem but the format alerts the clinician to important factors. In our experience with the Call-In Hour, much of the necessary information was shared in the first 5 to 10 minutes of contact with the parent. The CAIS framework allowed us to gather and process information efficiently, resulting in a quick understanding of the problem and how it should be handled, including the necessity for a referral for further evaluation.

The diagnosis of ADHD and the appropriateness of treating the disorder with stimulant medication were frequent questions in the primary care setting. Although the pediatrician is the professional most often asked to diagnose this disorder and treat the child with stimulant medication, they are not always in the best position to make these decisions. Their contact with the child is often limited and gathering systematic information from the school and parents is often outside their area of expertise and made difficult by time constraints. Through working with the psychologists, the pediatricians in the practice came to appreciate the complexity of diagnosing and treating ADHD and refused to prescribe medication without some formal assessment of the problem. Thus, if a child was suspected of having ADHD, the psychologist worked with the child's pediatrician, the parents, the child, and school to assess the behavior through formal psychometric testing, direct behavioral observations, parent and teacher questionnaires, and daily observational data (Schroeder, 1996b). If the child received a diagnosis of ADHD, a trial of medication was often prescribed along with recommendations for behavior management in the school and home. A trial of medication involved a double-blind, placebo-controlled assessment of the effects of high and low doses of medication carried out over a three-week period and included teacher and parent questionnaires, laboratory measures of attention, and academic analog tasks. This practice-based clinical protocol was based on a research protocol developed by Barkley (1990). This approach proved to be clinically effective in determining the child's response to medication and was very positively received by the children and parents. They felt that the structured assessment gave them a better understanding of the effects of the medication. It also presented the opportunity for long-term follow-up on the cognitive functioning of children on stimulant medication.

Child abuse and neglect, another frequent concern in primary care settings, involved close collaboration among the medical, social services, mental health, and legal systems. The primary care setting was an optimal place for the coordination of assessment for this difficult and complex problem. For example, as part of the state-funded Child Medical Evaluation program, the pediatricians provided physical examinations for abused children and the psychologist assisted the social service agencies in the investigation process. Dr. Charles Sheaffer, a pediatrician in the practice, was responsible for developing many of the services for physically and sexually abused children in North Carolina. Further, through weekly collaborative meetings with professionals from the community's social service agency, the police department, and mental health system, he encouraged coordination of services in the best interest of the child. For example, in the 1970s, the number of times a child was interviewed was greatly decreased by having the initial interview observed through a one-way window by the other involved professionals. Tape-recording the session became an established procedure. Dr. Sheaffer was also instrumental in getting the state to fund psychological evaluations for children for whom abuse or neglect was suspected or had been substantiated. The psychologists became part of a statewide Child Mental Health Evaluation

Program, which involved answering a wide range of referral questions, including: "Has the child been abused?" "What are the effects of the abuse?" "Is the mother or father capable of protecting the child?" "Does the child need treatment?" "How will the child be effected by going to court?"

Intervention/Treatment

Although we use the word "treatment," psychologists in primary care are most often "consultants" to pediatricians, parents or teachers who carry out the necessary program for behavioral or emotional change. The many roles that a pediatric psychologist can assume include:

1. Educator: This involves verbally sharing information in either individual or group meetings or providing written sources of information to help parents, teachers, and other significant people understand the child's needs.
2. Advocate: This can involve a variety of tasks including alerting the community to children's needs (e.g., through speaking engagements, the newspaper), speaking for the child in court, helping parents negotiate the educational system, or advocating for the child's needs within the family system.
3. Treatment provider: This can involve providing direct treatment to the child or family, consulting with significant people in the child's life and/or supervising others to carry out the intervention.
4. Case manager: Coordinating the services or service agencies involved in helping a child is often the task of the pediatric psychologist.

The role of case manager is particularly pertinent to the primary care setting. This involves networking the often fragmented and specialized services of the community in order to meet the individual needs of the child and family. This approach, as described by Hobbs (1975), involves looking for unique ways to use the available services and seeking creative ways to develop services that are needed but unavailable. It requires the clinician to be very familiar with the resources in the community and to become skilled in negotiating cooperation between agencies (Schroeder, 1996b). It takes time to learn about a community and to develop relationships with people in day-care settings, schools, recreational facilities, social services, and the legal system (police, lawyers, judges). While these relationships usually begin around a particular child, they can also be developed by presenting or sharing material, attending meetings and being an active citizen and professional in the community.

Chapel Hill Pediatric Psychology offered individual treatment for children and parents, as well as couple and family therapy. Although each child and family is unique, the time spent in treatment was cut significantly by the development of protocols for treating common childhood problems such as enuresis, encopresis, sleep, negative behavior, bad habits, anxiety, and for stressful events such as death, divorce, and sexual abuse. These protocols were published in a book by Schroeder and Gordon (1991, 2002), *Assessment and Treatment of Childhood Problems: A Clinician's Guide*. Handouts for parents on these problems as well as other commonly used material such as behavior diaries, were also developed to use in treatment.

The empirical literature indicates that, through groups, we should be able to meet the needs of parents and children in a more cost-effective and efficient manner. This would appear to be particularly true in the primary care setting. We offered group treatment for both parents and children focused on specific problem areas or life events such as ADHD, divorce, social skills, sexual abuse, and step parenting. However, scheduling difficulties—finding the right mix and number of children or parents at the right time—made it very difficult to provide a variety of treatment groups on an ongoing basis. A treatment group that was very successful, however, was for parents of children with ADHD. This was probably due to the significant number of children who were evaluated in the practice for this problem. The parents in the ADHD group met for four consecutive sessions and then attended a monthly support group. A member of the psychology staff also became very involved in the local Children with Attention Deficit Disorders group and many services that would have normally been provided in the clinic occurred in that setting.

The primary care setting is also a good place to develop treatment programs in coordination with other agencies. In the Chapel Hill community, for example, children who were sexually abused and their parents were not always able to access services or the available services were limited (Schroeder & Gordon, 1991). The pediatric psychologists joined with the local social service agency to get funding for group treatment for these children and their parents. The service agency provided a facility for the treatment as well as transportation for the families; the pediatric psychology staff were funded to do the treatment. Although the pre- and post-data plus the consumer satisfaction questionnaires indicated that the program was effective in treating these children and their families, the funding for the program was discontinued. In general, finding funding for prevention, assessment, and treatment programs is an ongoing task for professionals in primary care settings. In addition, the advent of managed care and the consequent decreased financial resources made it increasingly difficult to offer pro bono services to those families and children who are often in the greatest need.

Community Collaboration

Being in a primary care setting gives the professional a great deal of visibility in the community, and also a great deal of responsibility to advocate for children. We discovered that when the newspaper wanted information about a particular issue (e.g., "Is it morally right to tell children there is a Santa Claus?") or the court system wanted information on a particular problem ("Can 5-year-olds accurately report what happened to them?"), they were likely to call the pediatric office for this information or advice. The pediatric psychology staff soon found themselves interacting with the community on a number of levels and being given the opportunity to effect the lives of the children in the community. Much of this work was made possible by interacting with a community group around a particular child or family, which identified problems and solutions that could then be applied to the benefit of other children in the community. For example, we participated in an ongoing coordinated community effort on behalf of children who had been neglected or abused (Schroeder & Gordon, 1991). Further, this work led to more than a decade of research carried out in the primary care setting regarding children's knowledge of sexuality and children's memory. Moreover, we were able to provide formal training for the North Carolina Guardian Ad Litem program, district judges, district attorneys, the Department of Social Services, and the Rape Crisis Center.

Another example of community involvement grew out of the concern that children in the community were not receiving sex education or sex abuse prevention training in any systematic or coordinated manner. After a number of meetings, the local school system agreed to provide this information to children in the 5th grade. The pediatric psychologists advocated beginning the training in kindergarten but this was felt to be unnecessary and inappropriate. The psychologists were, however, asked to consult on training materials and to provide training for the teachers. This initial effort was well received by the parents and children. Then, within a period of six months, two 7-year-old girls were sexually abused and brutally murdered. The importance of helping children understand and cope with sexual abuse was brought to the forefront of the community. Parents and teachers not only wanted sex education and sex abuse prevention taught at the kindergarten level in the schools, they demanded it, and we helped them accomplish it. Daycare centers also joined in this effort to provide prevention information to parents and children.

Another tragedy gave us the opportunity to educate the community (and ourselves) about suicide. After a 9-year-old committed suicide we were asked to talk with the child's parents and siblings, consult with parents and teachers at the child's school, give information on suicide prevention to the child's minister for use in the funeral service, and field questions from other professionals in the community.

Training

Training professionals in a busy private clinic takes patience, time, and effort. But the investment can be recouped, in part, by the trainees' work in the community or with families who cannot afford the full fee for service. The ultimate benefit is having more mental health professionals trained to work in primary care settings and having pediatricians who become more aware of mental health issues and the desirability of having psychologists practice with them (Schroeder, 1996b). In reality, however, not many physicians or psychologists working in primary care settings are in a position to provide professional training. The mental health services at Chapel Hill Pediatrics began, in part, due to a training need and the willingness of a university to support training in that setting. A brief description of what kind of training can take place in primary care is worthwhile in the hopes that more university training programs will find ways to support this work.

As previously stated, from 1973 to 1982 graduate students, interns, and postdoctoral fellows in psychology; graduate students in social work; and medical students and residents participated in all aspects of the mental health services offered in Chapel Hill Pediatrics. The practice also participated in a training program developed by the Division of Community Pediatrics at the University of North Carolina at Chapel Hill Medical School (Sharp & Lorch, 1988). In 1982, all first-year pediatric residents (and fourth-year medical students who were taking an ambulatory pediatrics elective) began a training program designed to increase their knowledge of child development and the factors that can effect it. This was done by having them spend time in community agencies serving children. This was a unique approach to training pediatricians in the biopsychosocial aspects of development, and in 1984 the program won the prestigious American Academy of Ambulatory Pediatrics Excellence in Teaching Award. The pediatric psychology practice was one of 25 community agencies involved in this training. Each resident or medical student spent one day a week for a month with a psychologist in the primary care setting.

They learned about the types of developmental and behavioral problems parents bring to the pediatric office, were trained to interview parents and develop intervention strategies for common problems, and learned when children should be referred for mental health services. Although there are plans to survey the more than 160 graduates of this program to determine how they now interface with psychologists, we already know that a number of them (three in our area alone) have psychologists in their practices. This program was unique in a number of ways including the university paying the psychologist to train the pediatrician. As is often the case, in 1992, the funds for this training program were cut and the formal training stopped. Residents, however, continued to spend time with the psychologists on a more informal basis.

Other training that occurred over the years included a two-year postdoctoral fellow in psychology, jointly sponsored by our practice and the University of North Carolina Medical School Department of Pediatrics. Psychology interns spent up to two days a week for a year in the practice and clinical psychology graduate students participated in the Call-In Hour and provided treatment one afternoon a week. The majority of this training was without monetary compensation and, thus, fluctuated over time.

Research

The primary health care setting is a fertile ground for psychological research (Wright & Burns, 1986). The sheer number of children who are developing along a normal continuum offers opportunities for interesting developmental research. Moreover, the smaller number of children who have chronic physical and behavioral or emotional disorders encourages research on treatment effectiveness as well as longitudinal research on these problems (Schroeder & Gordon, 1991). The primary health care setting also offers the opportunity to evaluate the effectiveness of primary and secondary prevention programs. However, time constraints, funding, and support services make it difficult to do research in primary care settings. In addition, the parents and pediatricians have to be convinced that the research will benefit them in some way. Major research studies or even most minor ones must have some type of outside support, given the financial and time constraints of the practicing psychologist. Program evaluation, however, can and should be an ongoing part of any psychology practice and can be done in the primary care setting. Indeed, if psychologists want to practice in primary care settings they will have to demonstrate the need for and the effectiveness of their services. Pediatricians will expect this and reimbursement by insurance companies will require it. For example, the discontinuation of the developmental screening program was, in part, due to the lack of data on its effectiveness.

Being close to several universities and medical schools has afforded numerous opportunities for both the pediatricians and the psychologists in the Chapel Hill practice to be part of research studies. For the most part, research evolved out of clinical questions and the pediatric psychologists' participation in the research focused on helping to formulate questions, developing credible and viable treatment or research protocols to be used in primary care settings, providing space, and supporting parents and children to participate in the research. For example, work with children who were sexually abused raised questions from the legal system for which there were no answers: "Can we believe what young children tell us about what has happened to them? Can children remember and report events as completely and as accurately as adults, especially when events may have been traumatic? Are children particularly vulnerable to suggestive and leading questions? What are the effects of repeated questioning on children's abilities to remember particular events?" (Schroeder & Gordon, 1991). To answer these questions the pediatric psychologists and pediatricians collaborated with developmental and clinical psychologists from the university in a series of funded and unfunded studies.

The study of children's knowledge of sexuality is one example of research done at Chapel Hill Pediatrics. A common belief among professionals who testify in court on behalf of abused preschoolers is that young children's knowledge of sexuality is limited, and therefore that these children cannot describe sexual acts unless they have actually experienced them. To provide empirical evidence for this belief, 192 nonabused children (ages 2-7) were studied in the pediatric office to determine their knowledge of gender identity, body parts and functioning, pregnancy and birth, adult sexual behavior, private parts, and personal safety skills (Gordon, Schroeder, & Abrams, 1990a). There were significant age differences in children's knowledge of all areas of sexuality, but under the age of 6 or 7 years, children had little knowledge of adult sexual behavior. The children's sexual knowledge was directly related to their parents' attitudes about sexuality: Parents with more restrictive attitudes had children who knew less about sexuality than parents who had more liberal attitudes. A second study examined sexual knowledge of children for whom sexual abuse had been substantiated and these results were compared with an age-matched control group of nonabused children (Gordon, Schroeder, & Abrams, 1990b). This study indicated that sexually abused children do not necessarily have greater knowledge of sexuality than nonabused children of the same age. The children who were sexually abused, however, gave qualitatively unusual responses to the stimulus materials. For example, a 3-year-old withdrew in fright when presented with a picture of a child being put to bed by an adult. Carrying out this work in the primary care setting tested our credibility with parents and children alike! Introducing the studies to parents actually gave us an opportunity to inform them about sexuality, sexual abuse, the importance of educating children, and the importance of learning more about children's development in this area. Very few parents refused to participate and most were eager to receive the results of the studies.

A second line of investigation carried out in the practice was more basic research and focused on factors that influence the accuracy of children's testimony. This research was initially supported by a National Institute of Mental Health (NIMH) grant and examined children's memory for a personally experienced event, a physical examination (an analog to sexual abuse). The purpose of this research was to establish baseline data for children's memory over varying periods of time, and to examine factors that influence children's memory (e.g. repeated interviews, use of props in interviews, reinstatement, prior knowledge of visits to the doctor, painful procedures, and traumatic injuries). This research has been presented and published extensively (e.g; Baker-Ward, Gordon, Ornstein, & Clubb, 1993; Baker-Ward, Hess, & Flanagan, 1990; Gordon, Baker-Ward, & Ornstein, 2001; Gordon et al., 1993; Ornstein, Gordon, & Larus, 1992; Principe, Ornstein, Gordon, & Baker-Ward, 2000). The clinical implications of this work are important and guidelines for interviewing young children and evaluating their responses were developed (Gordon & Schroeder, 1995; Gordon, Schroeder, Ornstein, & Baker-Ward, 1995). This basic research, born out of clinical work and carried out by necessity in the primary care setting, is an excellent example of the type of research that can be done in natural settings (Schroeder & Gordon, 1991). However, it could not have been done without the collaborative relationship with the pediatricians and staff and the support of the children and families we served.

Other research looked at treatment effectiveness. For example, Martin (1988), as a doctoral dissertation in the University of North Carolina School of Public Health Department of Epidemiology, compared a group of 2 to 7-year old children who had received Parent-Child Interaction Training (Eyberg & Boggs, 1998) for noncompliance with a control group matched for age and level of noncompliance. The research questions focused on whether the treatment would be effective and (given the age of the children) whether the behavior of the untreated control group would improve without intervention. Martin found that at a three-month follow-up, the 31 children in the treatment group showed clinically and statistically significant decreases in both the number and frequency of behavior problems. The behavior of the 22 untreated control children did not improve over the same time period. Although a longer follow-up period would have been desirable and is possible in a primary care setting, this information gave support for our continuing to provide this treatment. Other research on the effectiveness of the Call-In Hour (Kanoy & Schroeder, 1985; Mesibov et al., 1977) gave credibility to continuing this unique way of helping parents and children. Data were also used to improve specific services. For example, the clinical data of over 100 children who underwent the assessment process for stimulant medication were analyzed with a focus on its effectiveness and ways to streamline the protocol to make it more cost effective (Riddle, 1993).

Doing any type of research in the primary setting presents obstacles. There are often time constraints on physicians, nurses, and patients to collect extensive data. Getting representative subject samples usually requires gathering data from several offices in several communities. Instruments that focus on the kinds of concerns reflected in a primary care setting are often not available. Developing collaborative relationships with the physicians takes time. There is often little time and no money to support the psychologist to do the research. The importance of doing this work, however, is reflected in NIMH and the Agency for Health Care Prevention and Research funding research on mental health services in primary health care settings. With the increased interest in providing mental health services for children and parents in this arena, data driven approaches should be forthcoming. Further, the *Diagnostic and Statistical Manual–Primary Care* (*DSM-PC*; Drotar, 1999) should help identify emotional and behavioral problems in primary care settings that are distinct from the psychiatric disorders, such as, *DSM-IV* (American Psychiatric Association, 1994). These types of activities will, hopefully, generate further training, clinical services, and research in the primary care setting. The reader is referred to Drotar & Lemanek (2001) for a further discussion of barriers and solutions to research in primary care settings.

Lessons Learned from the Chapel Hill Pediatric Psychology Practice

Logan Wright's advice for the developing field of pediatric psychology in 1967 seems to be true today for pediatric psychology in community pediatric settings. Promoting pediatric psychology in primary care will require the development of formalized training experiences, a research foundation for the field, and a method of communication between professionals working in primary care. Some of the lessons learned from practicing 28 years in a primary care setting will be outlined.

1. Determining the needs and resources of the primary care setting is imperative before beginning a collaborative practice and should continue as an on-going process.

Each primary care setting is unique in terms of the patient population, the medical team, and the community support network. Preconceived ideas of what is wanted/needed rarely match up to the reality of the situation. It is important to take the time to determine what the medical team wants, how they operate, their resources, and their referral network. It is also important to understand the patient population, what the parents expect from the psychology practice, and how they would like those expectations to be met. One should, thus, approach a primary care practice much as a consultant would approach a review of an agency or a clinician would approach a new referral. To do otherwise is very likely to result in providing unneeded or unwanted services, losing credibility, and generally being frustrated that the work is not going "as expected."

2. Setting explicit personal and professional goals is important.

It is important to know what you want to accomplish professionally and how those goals fit with your personal goals. Long-term goals should be set and interim steps developed to meet the long-term goals. For example, in the Chapel Hill Pediatric Psychology practice, clinical services, training and research were viewed as essential activities of the practice and each activity was seen as interacting and enhancing the other activities. The first five years of full-time work at Chapel Hill Pediatrics was devoted to developing clinical services with a plan to devote the second five years to developing research activities. Thanks to the proximity to the University of North Carolina and their medical school, trainees from psychology, medicine, pediatrics, social work, and nursing were able to be an integral part of the practice. Steps for accomplishing goals were set on a yearly basis with periodic review and discussion with the pediatricians. As staff were added, they also were expected to determine their professional and personal goals (including writing them down!) and to share these goals with the staff as a whole. Goals also have to be prioritized so that thoughtful decisions can be made regarding the use of time and resources. For example, if a top priority is to make a certain amount of money or only work three, eight-hour days then those priorities will effect other priorities. If setting up an assessment clinic for children with seizure disorders is a high priority, then plans to develop more services for children with asthma, may have to have a later target date.

3. Data should guide the process.

Systematic data collection on important practice variables helps guide the development of the practice. Developing a data collection system that can become part of the clinical routine is particularly important in the primary care setting. With the pressures of clinical work important information can be lost and, at the same time, there is no time to collect unnecessary information. For example, if a goal is to increase referrals, then on the initial contact, one could keep data on the number of new referrals and source of referrals on a monthly basis. Further, keeping a tabulation of new referrals by the month gives information on seasonal fluctuations so staffing needs can be better determined. However, if one is interested in increasing or tracking particular types of referrals, then more specific data are needed, such as, age, sex, problem, and so forth. The data systems do not have to be elaborate, they just have to contain the desired information which is collected in a systematic manner. Examples of practice data collected at Chapel Hill Pediatrics are the Call-In Hour data, consumer satisfaction questionnaires, and effectiveness of treatment.

4. Pediatric psychology is practiced at many levels.

Consultation with the health care providers, parents, and community, providing direct clinical services, case management, forensic work, training, business, and developing services in the community are all part of the pediatric psychology role in primary care. Carrying out these varied tasks requires a support network which must be developed both within the office and the community. Setting explicit goals and ways to meet them allows one to develop the necessary skills and expertise over time. To meet the needs of the children in our practice we found ourselves going beyond the MD/PhD relationship and collaborating with a range of health care workers (e.g., occupational therapist, physcial therapist, nutritionists) as well as other professionals or agencies dealing with children (e.g., social services, rape crisis center, the school). This takes time but the reality is many people and factors impinge on the lives of children and practicing in primary care requires one to reach beyond traditional professional boundaries to meet their needs.

5. Formal supervised training in the primary care setting is important.

We found that staff who were most effective in dealing with the many roles in primary care had experience in working with other disciplines as well as supervised experience in the primary care setting. There are increasing opportunities at the graduate level to receive both formal and practicum training in pediatric psychology, but experience in community pediatric settings is imperative if pediatric psychology is to move beyond the hospital setting. The clinical challenges in primary care are often unique and it requires a flexibility and creativity that is best learned by experience. Prompt effective responses are required for questions such as "How do I tell my 2-year-old that her mother died last evening in childbirth?" or "How do I deal with a teacher who is overly punitive with my child" or "How do I help my child deal with a birthmark on his face that looks like a bruise? " or "How do I get my teenager, who is diabetic, to eat properly when he is with his friends?"

6. Communication and visibility lead to creativity and flexibility.

Working in a primary care setting is a humbling experience. No amount of training can prepare you for all of the difficult situations you will be asked to help resolve. Communication and visibility allows you to become more aware of the available resources, allows you to learn what works and does not work, and provides opportunities for creative solutions. For example, we had a number of parents who were overwhelmed with the care of their difficult newborn, particularly at night. We included the nurses in the discussion of how to help these families and they came up with the idea of giving the mothers respite by offering to care for the infant. The nurses not only provided much needed respite for the parents but they also were able to provide support and reinforce appropriate care in the natural environment. Likewise, the weekly meetings of community agencies involved with children who had been sexually abused provided an opportunity for interdisciplinary training and the development of unique approaches to the problem.

7. Individual cases can lead to public health initiatives.

Problems that children face are rarely unique but dealing with an individual child and family can raise the awareness of particular problems and provide an opportunity to deal with the problem in a broader context. For example, the 9-year-old who committed suicide gave us the opportunity to deal with childhood suicide on a community-wide basis with churches, schools, and so forth. Another example of moving beyond the individual child was working with community agencies dealing with children who were sexually abused and developing sex education programs in the schools, training attorneys, law enforcement officers, and so forth.

8. Sharing physical space does not mean that you have a collaborative practice.

Although it would appear that a collaborative pediatric/psychology practice is best carried out in the same physical space, it does not always mean that sharing space equals collaboration. We discovered that psychologists who had not had previous experience or training in primary care settings did not know how to establish a collaborative relationship and/or did not want to put the extra time or effort into the challenges presented by such a relationship. This leads to limiting their practice to more traditional therapeutic approaches with almost a resentment to having their time requested for "nonpaying" activities or activities that did not fit into the "expected" model of psychological practice. In this instance, although the ease of referral is appreciated, joint goals or concerns are not articulated and ease of referral is the primary goal. This is not to say that all pediatrician/psychologist encounters are welcome, even in a collaborative practice. In our practice, for example, it was sometimes the case that the psychologist literally hid from the approaching pediatrician! One could be sure that at 6:30 on a Friday night the request that was about to be made would take the weekend to resolve. The point of this lesson is that it takes more than sharing space to share a practice. Sharing responsibility for patients, at times, can be overwhelming but also provides better patient care and greater professional satisfaction.

9. Dealing with economic issues is part of the job.

Fee-for-service is the usual payment method for professionals working in primary care but that does not cover all of the time and services that are required to have an effective practice. The decrease in the number of preschool children seen in the Chapel Hill Pediatric Psychology practice over the past 10 years aptly illustrates the problem of fee-for-service. To provide the array of services that are often needed in primary care, the psychologist will most likely have to look for a variety of funding sources. Developing consultation or funded collaboration with other community agencies, grants for training, and research grants are some of the ways to help support the needed but unfunded or low-reimbursement services.

Using clinic data to get reimbursement from insurance companies is difficult but possible. For example, sharing the average and maximum number of visits for different problems with a major insurance carrier led to their approval of up to seven visits without prior approval. This greatly cut down on paperwork for both the administrative and professional staff which, in effect, decreased costs. With the help (insistence) of the pediatricians we were also able to get insurance coverage for the

Ritalin trials. Having the data readily available and demonstrating the value of the service were key to these negotiations

10. It is important to plan for the neediest clients who have the fewest resources and require the greatest effort to meet their needs.

Planning for clients who have multiple or complex needs involves learning about the community resources and developing relationships with the people in charge of delivering them. Communities often have free hearing clinics, dental services, developmental evaluations, and schools evaluations, but it often difficult for parents to access the services or understand the requirements to receive the services. Working with the agencies to meet the needs of the family can ensure that the needed services are provided in the most effective and efficient manner. Being aware of the community resources can also lead to identifying needed services and finding ways to fund them. For example, there were no funds for initial psychological evaluations for children who had been sexually abused but the pediatrician in the clinic who was the county medical examiner was able to work with the state to fund these psychological evaluations.

The primary care setting is often a place where pro bono work is the norm versus the exception. By recognizing that this is the case one can often plan to deliver the services in a cost-effective way. For example, a low-income housing project was within walking distance from the clinic and mothers would often show up wanting care for a child. To meet this need one of the pediatricians offered a "free" evening clinic once a week for this particular housing project. This allowed these patient's needs to be met in a more systematic manner, decreased the number of daily interruptions and allowed aspiring nursing and medical students to volunteer to help with the clinic.

11. Traditional clinical services continue to be needed but they may be delivered in nontraditional ways.

It is often difficult for psychologists to move beyond the 50-minute appointment or doing an extensive evaluation before offering any type of treatment. The primary care setting, however, offers the opportunity to do short, timely interventions yet be able to follow the client over a long period of time. Examples of time-sensitive interventions at Chapel Hill Pediatrics were the Call-In Hour, scheduled 15-minute phone consults, half-hour appointments, consultation with the pediatricians or nurse who carried out the intervention, and groups for different stages of development. The primary care setting allows relationships over a long period of time with a number of health care professionals so you can more readily determine if something is not working and provide more intensive intervention as needed. Likewise, clients who know you over a period of time are more likely to use you on a "as needed" basis as well as seek help before a crisis occurs.

12. Providing an effective and well-received service does not mean it will be continued.

Effective and well-received services may not continue if funding is no longer available or if there is not appropriate staff to provide the service. For example, the successful groups for children who had been sexually abused and their parents were discontinued when funds were no longer available. Likewise, Parent-Child Interaction Training was decreased as the number of preschoolers decreased due to the psychologists not being on certain insurance panels. In addition, new staff brought new interests and areas of expertise and there was often simply no one willing or able to provide particular services. Although this is reality, it is not easily accepted in a clinic where the pediatricians and parents have come to depend on specific services. Needless to say, it is important to work together to find solutions for these problems.

13. Practicing in an ethical manner is imperative but it might not be according to the published standards.

Psychologists are used to sharing only the most minimal information while physicians want and expect to receive detailed information about their clients. Determining ways in which sensitive information can be shared while still protecting the client's confidentiality is tricky and takes some learning on the psychologists part and understanding on the pediatricians part. It is also important to have written permission to receive and share information with the pediatrician's even though they are in the same clinic and may have referred the client. In our clinic we routinely ask parents for this permission on the Intake Form.

Given the size of the client population in primary care it is very likely that you will know the clients in other contexts, especially if you practice in a small community. In fact, in our clinic the pediatricians provided medical care for the psychologists children and if the pediatricians had questions regarding their children they insisted that we see them. Other physicians in the community with whom we worked also referred their children to us. Referring to known professionals is often the norm in medicine while it is discouraged in psychology. Handling these dual professional and therapy relationships with known people in the community can be potentially difficult and it is imperative that the psychologist determine from the outset if they can separate their various roles and keep them separate in the therapy process. If there is any doubt, seeking consultation from a colleague is important. Interestingly, we have found that keeping relationships separate is not as difficult in reality as it is in theory, but it does involve constant monitoring. A greater problem is the psychologist's visibility in the community and keeping their private and professional lives separate. Many professionals choose to live in another town but even then one has to recognize that if you are in a primary care setting you are going to be a "known" person in the community. This is certainly not all negative, but one has to act accordingly.

14. Clinical questions lead to the most feasible research in primary care.

At best it is difficult to incorporate research into the clinical setting and if the research does not appear to have relevance to the other health professionals and the parents then it is not likely to be well received. We also found it very difficult for the psychologist to carry out the research without some major assistance from colleagues and/or students from the university. In essence, we found that the psychologist could formulate important research questions and facilitate the research but it had to be funded with a coprincipal investigator. Research protocols should be developed with the realities of space and time, a high priority, and doing pilot work to determine the feasibility of the protocol fitting into the clinic routine. If the staff understand what you want to do and why, they can be very helpful in developing a reasonable plan. It is not only important to share information about the research and its importance but it is also important to give periodic feedback to the clinic as a whole (all parents and staff) regarding the findings. Placing flyers regarding the study in the waiting room, having open forums, and presenting at staff meetings can provide the necessary feedback for the time-consuming studies on children's memory for personally experienced events that were done over a number of years, we hung a plaque in the waiting room thanking the parents and staff for their participation in each completed study. As the number of plaques increased the comments and interest in the work also appeared to increase.

SUMMARY

This chapter was in essence a story of a collaborative psychology-pediatric practice that spanned 28 years. Although there were certainly struggles, obstacles, and disappointments during those years, for the most part it was a very positive personal and professional experience for the pediatricians, nurses and psychologists. This story was told with the goal of encouraging other psychologists and pediatricians to enter into integrated practices that take a biopsychosocial approach to caring for children's physical, social, and mental health needs. The primary care setting offers an opportunity for prevention, early identification and treatment of children who present with behavioral, emotional, and social problems or who must deal with life events that could interfere significantly with their development. It is also a setting that offers an opportunity to track mental health problems and their outcomes with a variety of treatments and without treatment. This is particularly relevant with the increase of psychotropic drug prescriptions for children for which there are few efficacy studies let alone effectiveness research.

Although there is an increased awareness of the need to provide integrated services for children and a trend for more integrated training in primary care, there continue to be many obstacles to this approach. A major obstacle is our health care financing system that does not support the integration of mental and physical health care. Changing this will involve more than demonstrations that collaborative practices are feasible. The recent report of the Children's Mental Health Alliance Project (Steinberg, Gadomski, & Wilson, 1999) points out, among a number of cogent recommendations, that there must be more research-based evidence that increased communication between the primary care physician and the psychologist or other specialist actually improves the quality of patient care. Other important questions focus on what is the ideal primary care-behavioral relationship and does the continuity of care and quality of care improve when services are under one roof? Answering these important questions will require not only the training of medical and psychological professionals to work collaboratively in primary care settings but also the systematic collection of information that will evaluate the outcomes of this work as compared to other models of care. Many of the chapters in this book focus on these questions and/or the process needed to answer them. It is this work that will ultimately determine the value of collaborative relationships in primary care settings and, thus, provide the sequel to the story told in this chapter.

REFERENCES

American Academy of Family Physicians, Commission on Health Care Services. (1994). *White paper on the provision of mental health services by family physicians* (AAFT Order # 714). Kansas City, MO: Author.

American Psychiatric Association. (1994). *Diagnostic and statistical manual of mental disorders* (4th ed.). Washington, DC: Author

American Psychological Association, Task Force on Comprehensive and Coordinated Psychological Services for Children: Ages 0–10. (1994). *Comprehensive and coordinated psychological services for children: A call for service integration.* Washington, DC: American Psychological Association.

Anderson, G. L., & Lovejoy, D. W. (2000). Predoctoral training in collaborative primary care: An exam room built for two. *Professional Psychology: Practice and Research, 31*, 692-697.

Baker-Ward, L. E., Gordon, B. N., Ornstein, P. A., & Clubb, P. A. (1993). Young children's long-term retention of a pediatric examination. *Child Development, 64*, 1519-1533.

Baker-Ward, L. E., Hess, T. M., & Flanagan, D. A. (1990). The effects of children's involvement on children's memory for events. *Cognitive Development, 4*, 393-407.

Barkley, R. A. (1990). *Attention deficit hyperactivity disorder: A handbook for diagnosis and treatment*. New York: Guilford Press.

Briggs-Gowan, M. J., Horowitz, S. M., Schwab-Stone, M. E., Leventhal, J. M., & Leaf, P. J. (2000). Mental health in pediatric settings: Distribution of disorders and factors related to service use. *Journal of American Academy of Child and Adolescent Psychiatry, 39*, 841-849.

Clarke-Stewart, K. A. (1978). Popular primers for parents. *American Psychologist, 33*, 359-369.

Costello, E. J. (1989). Child psychiatric disorders and their correlates: A primary care sample. *Journal of the American Academy of Child and Adolescent Psychiatry, 28*, 851-855.

Drotar, D. (1995). *Consulting with pediatricians: Psychological perspectives*. New York: Plenum Press.

Drotar, D. (1999). The diagnostic and statistical manual for primary care (DSM-PC), child and adolescent version: What pediatric psychologists need to know. *Journal of Pediatric Psychology, 24*, 369-380.

Drotar, D. & Lemanek, K. (2001). Steps toward a clinically relevant science of interventions in pediatric settings: Introduction to the special issue. *Journal of Pediatric Psychology, 26*, 385-394.

Eyberg, S. M., & Boggs, S. R. (1998). Parent-child interaction therapy: A psychosocial intervention for the treatment of young conduct-disordered children. In J. M. Briesmeister & C. E. Schaeffer (Eds.), *Handbook of parent training: Parents as co-therapists for children's behavior problems* (2nd ed., pp. 61-97). New York: Wiley.

Fischer, H. D., & Engeln, R. G. (1972). How goes the marriage? *Professional Psychology, 3*, 73-79.

Frankenburg, W. K., & Dodds, J. B. (1967). The Denver Developmental Screening Test. *Journal of Pediatrics, 71*, 181-191.

Gessell, A. (1919). The field of clinical psychology as an applied science: A symposium. *Journal of Applied Psychology, 3*, 81-84.

Gordon, B. N., Baker-Ward, L., & Ornstein, P. A. (2001). Children's testimony: A review of research on memory for past experiences. *Clinical Child and Family Psychology Review, 4*, 157-181.

Gordon, B. N., & Jens, K. G. (1988). A conceptual model for tracking high-risk infants and making service decisions. *Developmental and Behavioral Pediatrics, 9*, 279-286.

Gordon, B. N., Ornstein, P. A., Nida, R. E., Follmer, A., Crenshaw, M. C., & Albert, G. (1993). Does the use of dolls facilitate children's memory of visits to the doctor? *Applied Cognitive Psychology, 7*, 1-16.

Gordon, B. N., & Schroeder, C. S. (1995). *Sexuality: A developmental approach to problems*. New York: Plenum Press.

Gordon, B. N., Schroeder, C. S., & Abrams, J. M. (1990a). Children's knowledge of sexuality: Age and social class differences. *Journal of Clinical Child psychology, 19*, 33-43.

Gordon, B. N., Schroeder, C. S., & Abrams, J. M. (1990b). Children's knowledge of sexuality: A comparison of sexually abused and nonabused children. *American Journal of Orthopsychiatry, 60*, 250-257.

Gordon, B. N., Schroeder, C. S., Ornstein, P. A., & Baker-Ward, L. E. (1995). Clinical implications of research in memory development. In T. Ney (Ed.), *True and false allegations of child sexual abuse: Assessment and case management* (pp. 99-124). New York: Brunner/Mazel.

Haggerty, R. J. (1986). The changing nature of pediatrics. In N. A. Krasnegor, J. D. Arasteh, & M. F. Cataldo (Eds.), *Child health behavior: A behavioral pediatrics perspective* (pp. 9-16). New York: Wiley & Sons.

Haley, E. E., McDaniel, S. H., Bray, J. H., Frank, R. G., Heldring, M., Johnson, S. B., Lu, E. G., Reed, G. M., & Wiggins, J. G. (1998). Psychological practice in primary care settings: Practical tips for clinicians. *Professional Psychology: Research and Practice, 29*, 237-244.

Hamlett, K. W., & Stabler, B. (1995). The developmental progress of pediatric psychology consultation. In M. C. Roberts (Ed.), *Handbook of pediatric psychology* (pp. 39-54). New York: Guilford Press.

Hawk, B. A., Schroeder, C. S., & Martin, S. (1987). Pediatric psychology in a primary care setting. *Newsletter of the Society of Pediatric Psychology, 11*, 13-18.

Hobbs, N. (1975). *The futures of children*. San Francisco: Jossey-Bass.

Hunter, C. L., & Peterson, A. L. (2001). Primary care psychology training at Wilford Hall Medical Center. *The Behavior Therapist, 24*, 220-222.

Kagan, J. (1965). The new marriage: Pediatrics and psychology. *American Journal of Diseases of Childhood, 110*, 272-278.

Kanoy, K., & Schroeder, C. S. (1985). Suggestions to parents about common behavior problems in a pediatric primary care office: Five years of follow-up. *Journal of Pediatric Psychology, 10*, 15-30.

Kelleher, K. J. (1999). Commentary: Pediatric psychologist as investigator in primary care. *Journal of Pediatric Psychology, 24*, 459-462.

Lavigne, J. V., Gibbons, R. D., Arend, R., Rosenbaum, D., Binns, H. J., & Christoffel, K. K. (1999). Rational service planning in pediatric primary care: Continuity and change in psychopathology among children enrolled in pediatric practices. *Journal of Pediatric Psychology, 24*, 393-403.

Martin, S. L. (1988). *The effectiveness of a multidisciplinary primary health care model in the prevention of children's mental health problems.* Unpublished doctoral dissertation, University of North Carolina–Chapel Hill.

McDaniel, S. H., Belar, C. B., Schroeder, C. S., Hargrove, D. S., & Freeman, E. L. (2002). Recommendations for education and training in primary care psychology. *Professional Psychology: Research and Practice, 33*, 65-72.

Mesibov, G. B., Schroeder, C. S., & Wesson, L. (1977). Parental concerns about their children. *Journal of Pediatric Psychology, 2*, 13-17.

Ornstein, P. A., Gordon, B. N., & Larus, D. M. (1992). Children's memory for a personally experienced event: Implications for testimony. *Applied Cognitive Psychology, 6*, 49-60.

Perrin, E. C. (1999). Commentary: Collaboration in pediatric primary care: A pediatrician's view. *Journal of Pediatric Psychology, 24*, 453-458.

Principe, G. F., Ornstein, P. A., Gordon, B. N., & Baker-Ward, L. (2000). The effects of intervening experiences on children's memory for a physical examination. *Applied Cognitive Psychology, 14*, 59-80.

Riddle, D. B. (1993, August). *Double-blind protocol research within a pediatric practice.* Paper presented at the meeting of the 101th Annual Convention of the American Psychological Association, Toronto, Canada.

Routh, D. K. (1994). *Clinical psychology since 1917: Science, practice and organization.* New York: Plenum Press.

Routh, D. K., Schroeder, C. S., & Koocher, G. P. (1983). Psychology and primary health care for children. *American Psychologist, 38*, 95-98.

Rutter, M. (1975). *Helping troubled children.* New York: Plenum Press.

Salk, L. (1970). Psychologist in a pediatric setting. *Professional Psychology, 1*, 395-396.

Schroeder, C. S. (1979). Psychologist in a private pediatric office. *Journal of Pediatric Psychology, 1*, 5-18.

Schroeder, C. S. (1992, August). *Psychologists working with pediatricians.* Paper presented at the 100th Annual Convention of the American Psychological Association, Washington, DC.

Schroeder, C. S. (1994). Models of practice. *Progress Notes, 18*, 4-7.

Schroeder, C. S. (1996a). Mental health services in pediatric primary care. In M. C. Roberts (Ed.), *Model programs in service delivery in child and family mental health* (pp. 265-284). Mahwah, NJ: Lawrence Erlbaum Associates.

Schroeder, C. S. (1996b). Collaborative practice: Psychologists and pediatricians. In R. J. Resnick & R. H. Rozensky (Eds.), *Health psychology through the life span: Practice and research opportunities* (pp. 109-131). Washington, DC: American Psychological Association.

Schroeder, C. S., Goolsby, E., & Strangler, S. (1975). Preventive services in a private pediatric practice. *Journal of Clinical Child Psychology, 4*, 32-33.

Schroeder, C. S., & Gordon, B. N. (1991). *Assessment and treatment of childhood problems: A clinician's guide.* New York: Guilford.

Schroeder, C. S., & Gordon, B. N. (2002). *Assessment and treatment of childhood problems: A clinician's guide* (2nd ed.). New York: Guilford.

Schroeder, C. S., Gordon, B. N., Kanoy, K., & Routh, D. K. (1983). Managing children's behavior problems in pediatric practice. In M. Wolraich & D. K. Routh

(Eds.), *Advances in developmental and behavioral pediatrics* (Vol. 4, pp. 25-86). Greenwich, CT: JAI Press.

Seaburn, D. B., Lorenz, A. D., Gunn, W. B., Gawiski, B. A., & Mauksch, L. B. (1966). *Models of collaboration: A guide for mental health professionals working with health care practitioners*. New York: Basic Books.

Sharp, M. C., & Lorch, S. C. (1988). A community outreach training program for pediatric residents and medical students. *Journal of Medical Education, 63,* 316-322.

Sharpe, L., Pantell, R. H., Murphy, L. O., & Lewis, C. C. (1992). Psychosocial problems during child health supervision visits: Eliciting, then what? *Pediatrics, 89*, 619-623.

Smith, E. E., Rome, L. P., & Freidheim, D. K. (1967). The clinical psychologist in the pediatric office. *Journal of Pediatrics, 21*, 48-51.

Spirito, A. (2000, August). *Symposium: Training issues for pediatric psychology in the 21st century.* Presented at the 108th Annual Convention of the American Psychological Association, Washington, DC.

Stancin, T. (1999). Introduction to special issue on pediatric mental health services in primary care settings. *Journal of Pediatric Psychology, 24*, 367-368.

Steinberg, A. G., Gadomski, A., & Wilson, M. D. (1999). Children's mental health: The challenging interface between primary and specialty care. A report of the Children's Mental Health Alliance Project, Philadelphia, PA. Available from A.G. Steinberg, Children's Seashore House of Children's Hospital of Philadelphia, 3405 Civic Center Boulevard, Philadelphia, PA 19104.

Wildman, B., & Stancin, T. (2001, April 22-25). *New directions for research and treatment of pediatric psychosocial problems in primary care.* The Thirteenth Annual Kent State Psychology Forum, Millersburg, OH.

Wilson, J. L. (1964). Growth and development in pediatrics. *Journal of Pediatrics, 65*, 984-991.

Wright, L. (1967). The pediatric psychologist: A role model. *American Psychologist, 22*, 323-325.

Wright, L., & Burns, B. J. (1986). Primary mental health care: A "find" for psychology. *Professional Psychology: Research and Practice, 17*, 560-564.

DISCUSSION SUMMARY
written by Christine Golden

The importance and impressiveness of Dr. Schroeder's work was clear to all those present at the Forum. Many individuals commented following the completion of her presentation and then throughout the conference, that they wished that they were a part of a collaborative primary care practice. Both physicians and psychologists agreed that the model she presented was ideal and something for all of them to aspire to.

Dr. Schroeder began her presentation by placing the collaborative care model within a historical context. She aptly pointed out that this model has existed on a conceptual basis since as early as 1917-1918. Although familiar with the collaborative care model, forum participants appeared surprised to learn how long this model has existed. It seemed that they were intrigued to hear Dr. Schroeder discuss how such a useful model has existed for so long and yet has so rarely been implemented.

Chapel Hill Pediatrics represented the ultimate goal of both the physicians and psychologists present at the Forum. Dr. Schroeder illustrated that the collaborative primary care practice can and does exist. As she pointed out, this type of model "has the greatest potential to effect changes in the lives of children and is the most challenging to accomplish." These words struck a cord with Forum participants as each in their own way has experienced the challenges of implementing this model within their work. As Dr. Schroeder moved through her discussion of Chapel Hill Pediatrics the uniqueness of her practice became clear. Primary care settings present a wide range of questions and problems that often demand concise, rapid and on target answers. In a collaborative primary care practice this burden will fall upon both the physician and psychologist in terms of questions and problems raised by parents and children, as well as each other.

Dr. Schroeder discussed the many roles that a pediatric psychologist can assume. She pointed out that psychologists in primary care are most often "consultants" to pediatricians, parents, or teachers who carry out the necessary program for behavioral or emotional change. She highlighted that pediatric psychologists can assume the role of educator, advocate, treatment provider, and/or case manager in their primary care work. These distinctive roles available to pediatric psychologists working in primary care require special training. Dr. Schroeder discussed the many challenges of training issues specific to work in a collaborative care practice such as the patience, time, and effort that are required to train professionals in a busy primary care clinic. She emphasized however, that the benefits of this investment are recouped by the trainees' work in the community or with families who cannot afford the full fee for service. As Dr. Schroeder stated, "the ultimate benefit is having more mental health professionals trained to work in primary care settings and having pediatricians who become more aware of mental health issues and the desirability of having psychologists practice with them."

Forum participants both wondered and asked how such a model can be established within the managed care context. Dr. Schroeder was realistic in her treatment of these issues as she honestly stated that several programs that were begun at Chapel Hill Pediatrics have not continued due to financial constraints. However she motivated participants to work around these issues in creative ways, suggesting the importance and utility of research within the primary care setting. Research, she suggested is a way for psychologists in primary care settings to demonstrate the need for and the effectiveness of their services. She stated that "pediatricians will expect this and reimbursement by insurance companies will require it." Dr. Schroeder advocated for pursuit of training grants, research grants, and collaboration with community resources as possible means for attaining funding. She also highlighted the fact that while research in primary care is difficult, the importance of it is reflected in NIMH and the Agency for Health Care Policy and Research funding research on mental health services in primary care settings.

Dr. Schroeder concluded her presentation by discussing the lessons that she has learned from practicing 28 years in a primary care setting. The wisdom of these years was evident as Forum participants listened intently to Dr. Schroeder's experiences and advice. As she went through each of the "lessons learned," participants took notes and attempted to integrate the information for use in their own lives and work. She discussed such things as determining the needs and resources of the primary care setting prior to establishing a collaborative practice, the importance of setting both personal and professional goals, the value of having data guide the process of a collaborative practice, the significance of formal supervised training in the primary care setting, and the fact that dealing with economic issues is part of the job.

As Dr. Schroeder concluded her presentation, it was clear that she had accomplished the task of being the initial presenter at the Forum. She had intrigued, taught, and motivated the Forum participants. Dr. Schroeder's presentation successfully served to set the tone for a productive conference weekend that is evidenced within the chapters of this text.

CHAPTER 2

PRIMARY CARE, PREVENTION, AND PEDIATRIC PSYCHOLOGY

Challenges and Opportunities

Michael C. Roberts and Keri J. Brown
University of Kansas

Prevention is taking action to avoid development of a problem or identifying problems early enough to minimize the potential negative outcomes. As Russell (1993) pointed out, "the primary reason to invest in prevention, as in other medical care, is to promote health—to extend life, improve functioning, and prevent suffering" (p. 354). Although often seen for remediation of immediate medical problems, the primary care provider is frequently the first professional encountered by children and families who might intervene to prevent the development of behavioral and emotional problems. The primary care provider's office is an ideal arena for discussion and referral of behavioral problems in part because children are seen regularly for inoculations and various well-child visits from birth to the entry of grade school. As children age, such appointments as physicals for various extracurricular activities provide additional opportunities for parent/physician/patient interaction. Lynch, Wildman, and Smucker (1997) found that 40-80% of parents have psychosocial

Treating Children's Psychosocial Problems in Primary Care, 35–60

questions to ask the primary care provider (although these questions do not necessarily get asked during an appointment). This venue provides an accessible, trusting, and confidential arrangement where parents can address their concerns regarding their child's development and behavior. These "is it normal" types of questions can be more casually mentioned in the office setting of the pediatrician or family physician without the hassle or stigma that might be associated with making a separate appointment to talk with a pediatric/clinical child psychologist or child psychiatrist.

Primary care providers are also in a position to identify issues and events that may affect a child's development. Multiple appointments with one or more children in a family provide opportunities to identify potential stressors such as parental divorce, child or parent physical illness, violence, or poverty. Guiding parents to appropriate community and psychological supports may head-off subsequent development of psychosocial problems as a result of these family stressors. Potentially one in five children who visit their primary care provider could have a clinical-level *Diagnostic Statistical Manual* (*DSM*) disorder (Costello & Shugart, 1992). Early identification is of instrumental importance in the treatment for a number of childhood difficulties including attention deficit disorder, oppositional defiant disorder, and depression. The primary care provider can refer the child to appropriate professionals to aid in the management of current psychological sequelae, as well as to potentially prevent development of further psychopathology. Thus, the health care provider in the primary care setting may be the right person in the right place for prevention of psychosocial problems. Indeed, as Schroeder (1999) asserted "the potential is greatest for prevention, early identification, and intervention of psychosocial problems" (p. 448) because primary care providers are where more children are seen most often.

Durlak (1997) stated that prevention of psychological problems of children and adolescents can be conceptualized, implemented, and evaluated successfully in a variety of settings. This prevention implementation can easily occur in the practices of primary care physicians (and psychologists). Indeed, the definition of primary care providers includes the professional disciplines of pediatricians, family practitioners, pediatric psychologists, and other mental health professionals whose interests are in these settings. The primary care provider has certain assets, such as building long-term relationships with the same patients for continuity of care, trust, knowledge, and familiarity. This longitudinal relationship can develop whether the provider is a physician or a psychologist (Schroeder, 1999). Prevention of psychosocial problems can include a wide array of problems presenting, not just severe psychopathology, but problems on a continuum. In this chapter, we will examine the challenges and the opportunities facing health care providers in primary care settings related to prevention of psychosocial problems.

CHALLENGES

We raise five questions of concern regarding the prevention of psychosocial problems in primary care settings by pediatricians, family physicians, and psychologists.

1. Do the disciplines have an adequate conceptual framework for *prevention of psychosocial problems* in psychology, pediatrics, and family practice for primary care settings?

The concept of psychosocial care in pediatric primary care settings has been around for a long time for both psychologists and pediatricians (e.g., Roberts & Wright, 1982; Schroeder, 1979; Schroeder, Goolsby, & Stangler, 1975; Wright, 1967, 1978, 1985; Wright & Burns, 1986). Yet, comprehensive models for both disciplines do not fully exist, especially for prevention. Pediatrics and family medicine have been more prevention oriented than psychology, and overall more developmentally focussed. Still, an overarching model of psychosocial care is lacking—with implementation sporadic and dependent on individual differences of the physician (e.g., Wissow, Roter, & Wilson, 1994). When studies are conducted into psychosocial care in primary care settings, they focus on such issues as screening and identification of psychological/behavioral problems, provision of counseling/guidance for identified existing problems, and may generally give more guidance to assessing more easily recognized externalizing problems such as Attention-deficit Hyperactivity Disorder (ADHD) (Holden & Schuman, 1995; McCain, Kelley, & Fishbein, 1999; Riekert, Stancin, Palermo, & Drotar, 1999; Stancin & Palermo, 1997; Wildman, Kinsman, Logue, Dickey, & Smucker, 1997). Rarely do these studies examine prevention issues. In fact, pediatricians report some wariness in their attitudes toward mental illness prevention (Yager et al., 1989). That is, although "favorable," pediatricians raise a number of questions involving barriers to prevention interventions for mental health problems in their own practices.

The concept of anticipatory guidance approaches prevention (Brazelton, 1975), yet this too falls short as a conceptual/guiding framework, because it does not typically rise above relatively minor difficulties faced by parents, and lacks solid evidence of implementation and effectiveness. Although given much lip service (Prazar, 1990), rarely is a systematic approach to anticipatory guidance for parents defined in the literature.

When programs are defined, empirical research evaluating effectiveness is rare. For example, Pierre the Pelican is a series of 28 pamphlets for first-time parents on topics such as working mothers and teenage pregnancies. In addition, the series provides nine keys to improving mental health (Rowland, 1989). We were unable to determine if the effectiveness of this series has been established. When anticipatory interventions are evaluated, parental attitudes and knowledge of behavioral expectations have been addressed with some effectiveness (Showers, 1989). Extending these research lines to measure changes in actual behavior due to anticipatory intervention would be much more valuable. Pediatrics has a little better track record in injury prevention—both in terms of a guiding model (TIPP—The Injury Prevention Program) and in partially evaluating its effectiveness. Unfortunately, the results of the evaluation have been equivocal as to whether these primary care efforts are effective (Miller & Galbraith, 1995; Pless & Arsenault, 1987).

Consequently, prevention of psychosocial problems gets neglected in pediatric and family medicine. This is true also in psychology (Roberts, 1991, 1992, 1994; Roberts & Brown, 2000; Roberts & Peterson, 1984a). Psychologists generally do not think preventively. At the interface of psychology and medicine, the lack of adequate conceptualization hinders collaboration and comprehensive action. Simply, insufficient models lead directly to insufficient implementation. This is the first challenge to prevention of problems for psychosocial problems in primary care settings.

2. Do the professional disciplines have an adequate body of research on primary care, especially on prevention of psychosocial problems?

As others have pointed out (e.g., Stancin, 1999), there is an underdeveloped research examination of primary care and psychosocial problems within pediatrics, family medicine, and psychology. Pediatricians probably have the largest research base, largely developed through the Pediatric Research in Office Settings network (see www.aap.org/pros) and a few other studies. Some of these have dealt with psychosocial care, but rarely on prevention of psychosocial problems. Family medicine has less on psychosocial care. While this seems to be increasing, there is still much less on prevention so far. In psychology primary care, for example, there are reports such as by Schroeder (1996), Evers-Szostak (1997) and Sobel, Roberts, Rayfield, Barnard, and Rapoff (2001). These few reports did not fully examine prevention of psychosocial problems, although some aspects of Carolyn Schroeder's clinic and practice certainly relate to prevention (e.g., parenting classes, come in/call in service, consultation). This type of activity is excellent, but not enough to demonstrate convincingly that prevention is effective. In most reports of psychologists in primary care settings, the focus is on psychological therapeutic treatments. These could only be called secondary/tertiary prevention at best.

As another example of the dearth of research on prevention, the outstanding series of articles in the *Journal of Pediatric Psychology* on empirically-supported treatments in pediatric psychology (Spirito, 1999) has no article reviewing preventive interventions, yet articles covered enuresis, encopresis, headaches, abdominal pain, procedural pain, severe feeding disorders, obesity, disease related symptoms, asthma, and sleep disorders (*Journal of Pediatric Psychology*: Vols. 24(2), 24(3), 24(4), 24(6), 25(4)). The judgment of the task force selecting the topics appears to be that insufficient research has been conducted to justify the inclusion of prevention. Indeed, Roberts (1992) noted that only 3.8% of articles published in the *Journal of Pediatric Psychology* were on topics of prevention whereas 74.7% were on chronic illness issues. Nonetheless, there is a strong and growing literature on prevention in other areas of psychology such as in community psychology and some in clinical child psychology (Durlak, 1997).

The lack of research stems largely from the lack of a conceptual model, but even sporadic attempts would be welcomed as groundbreaking. There are likely many prevention efforts taking place in primary care settings that have not been evaluated and published, but these may be too dependent on the proclivities of the health care provider to be generalizable demonstrations. As Yager et al. (1989) determined in their survey of pediatricians, "there was considerable uncertainty and disagreement about whether the efficacy of prevention had been substantiated by research evidence" (p. 1088). For many pediatric psychologists, prevention is simply an unknown concept in daily practice. Brown and Roberts (2000) found a moderately high endorsement for prevention in a Delphic poll of researchers and clinicians in pediatric psychology. However, their day-to-day activities likely do not include much preventive work (Kaufman, Holden, & Walker, 1989).

All too often, primary care providers may be engaging in ineffectual prevention (a) unknowing about the effectiveness, (b) because it is intuitively correct, comfortable, or familiar, or (c) because of the perception that something needs to be done, regardless of proven effectiveness. Pediatric textbooks describe pamphlets and brochures as essential to medical practice. Nonetheless, there is little or no evidence that, for example, handing out a pamphlet, probably the most frequent preventively-oriented action, is going to change parent or child behavior and prevent later problems. The pamphlets prepared by the American Academy of Pediatrics contain, on average, 750 words with titles such as: "Your Child's Growth: Developmental Milestones; Sleep Problems in Children"; "Bed-wetting"; "Alcohol: Your Child and Drugs"; "Marijuana: Your Child and

Drugs"; "Substance Abuse Prevention: What Every Parents Needs to Know"; "Television and the Family; Understanding the Impact of Media on Children and Teens"; "Healthy Communication With Your Child: A Guide for Parents," and many others. More lengthy pamphlets written by psychologists for their own practices might be more effective because more information is conveyed. These are favorably received by parents. The research evidence, however, is slim to none for effectiveness in changing behavior or improving preventive outcomes. For example, Nicholas Long has prepared parent handouts on such topics as Children's Development: Fifteen to Eighteen Months; Eighteen to Twenty-four Months; Two to Three Years"; "Helping Children Cope with Stress"; "Time Out as a Discipline Technique." Carolyn Schroeder has handouts on "Toilet Training"; "Negative Behavior: How to Manage It"; "The New Baby: Helping Older Children Adjust"; "Managing Children's Anxieties"; "Divorce: Helping Your Children Adjust." Ed Christophersen (1994) has published his extensive number of handouts in a book including such topics as "Separation Anxiety"; "Toilet Training Resistance"; "Peer Interaction Skills, Discipline for Toddlers"; "Time Out"; "Attention-Deficit Disorder". Relatively few of these have been empirically scrutinized. Most of the time, these handouts are used in conjunction with psychologist/physician counseling. Accordingly, few studies have demonstrated that primary care physicians' individual attention and feedback are more useful than media or other communication channels in changing patient knowledge and behavior (Mullen, Green, & Persinger, 1985).

As Durlak (1997) and others have pointed out, however, unfortunately information-only prevention campaigns are not going to be sufficient for prevention. He notes:

> Programs that rely on information strategies to change behavior have not been effective in any area of prevention in which they have been tried. In fact, the evidence is overwhelming that such programs do not significantly change behavior. The use of information-only programs in prevention should be abandoned. These types of programs are still used because they are brief, easy to administer, and thus relatively inexpensive to operate, and their existence might serve to satisfy administrative or social pressure to do something about prevention. However, information programs provide a false sense of security that prevention is being accomplished when it is not. (pp. 192-193)

We could not identify any published research on the effectiveness of these types of interventions in psychosocial prevention in primary care settings. However, Schultz and Vaughn (1999), in their survey of parents in a primary care clinic, found a high endorsement of written materials to take home on developmental-behavioral topics.

There has been some study of these forms of health promotion and education in the area of injury prevention (e.g., Christophersen & Gyulay, 1981; Roberts & Layfield, 1987). TIPP has some evidence for positive effects, but also has some contradictory evidence for these types of pamphlet/information provision interventions (Miller & Galbraith, 1995; Pless & Arsenault, 1987; Roberts, Fanurik, & Layfield, 1987). Yet, this intervention of information provision through pampleteering and counseling is likely the largest consistent prevention effort made in primary care settings. However, given the amount of time available for anticipatory guidance and counseling, it is unclear whether primary care providers are actually doing this or other preventive work of this type (Bradbury, Janicke, Riley, & Finney, 1999). Current practices may be the beginning point for further prevention work with every activity needing further empirical support. In doing so, pamphlets plus counseling, plus behavioral follow-up seems more likely to be successful (Roberts et al., 1987).

All in all, there does not appear to be an adequate body of knowledge about effective prevention interventions for psychosocial problems in primary care settings, despite increasing evidence that prevention can be successfully implemented in other settings (Durlak, 1997; Roberts & Peterson, 1984a).

3. Do the professional disciplines have adequate training in prevention of psychosocial problems in primary care in pediatrics, family practice, and psychology?

Kelleher and Long (1994) suggest that there is not enough attention in training to these issues. For example, in pediatrics, relatively very little time is devoted in the residency curriculum to prevention in general let alone to prevention of psychosocial problems (Wolraich, 1999). According to the Accreditation Council for Graduate Medical Education (ACGME) preventive healthcare should be a part of each pediatric resident rotation. However, the majority of training in the area of psychosocial issues is during a one-month block rotation in behavioral and developmental pediatrics. Truly gaining an understanding of children and adolescents' behavioral needs in such a short period of time seems unreasonable, as residents are expected to obtain formal instruction in the following areas: normal and abnormal child behavior/development in cognitive, language, motor, social and emotional; family structure, adoption, family care; interviewing techniques; psychosocial screening tests; behavioral counseling and referrals; strategies to help children with special needs management; needs of children at risk; and impact of chronic disease or death. The formal training appears to address current behavioral difficulties with no specific attention to the prevention of psychosocial problems (other than screening tests) for a program to be accredited. Even in the residency curriculum for developmental-behavioral pediatrics, there is only scant space devoted to prevention such as on anticipatory guidance (Coury, Berger, Stancin, & Tanner, 1999). In family medicine training, even less is mentioned about prevention/health promotion activities. (See www.acgme.org for the basic curriculum requirements for accreditation of most residency programs, including pediatrics and family practice.) Of course, these formal training components cannot convey what is likely happening in training: in prevention of health and psychosocial problems through well-child care visits with physicians in their continuity care clinics, for example. These may be unsystematic, but important experiences advancing the physicians' understanding of and clinical functioning related to prevention.

Regardless of what is suggested as vague curricular goals, Pace, Mullins, Chaney, and Olson (1995) asserted that, "although primary care physicians are now being trained in behavioral sciences, this training may often be somewhat narrow and idiosyncratic" (p. 125) such that knowledge will differ across physicians and the skills will be variable.

Within psychology, prevention receives no mention in the accreditation guidelines and principles (American Psychological Association, 1996) with the result that very few programs devote any time at all to the topic. Current accreditation in psychology is very conservative and traditional. The belief abounds that "clinical psychology" means psychotherapy with psychopathology, that adult work is "basic" for a clinical psychologist to be trained in "broad and general psychology," and that child work is added-on. Although ostensibly written to foster innovation, the actual implementation of the psychology accreditation guidelines and principles restricts innovation and a much stronger focus on prevention in any great way would likely be punished. (School psychology and counseling psychology may actually have more affinity for prevention than clinical given their traditions and focus.) Even in our own training program in clinical child psychology (Roberts, 1998), prevention is given 1/16 attention relative to other topics in a course on therapeutic interventions with children. The pediatric psychology emphasis similarly lacks a preventive focus (Roberts & Steele, 2003). Community psychology programs have a tradition inherent in prevention (Durlak, 1997), but these graduates rarely venture into primary care settings.

Despite its ostensible importance in the panoply of health care, prevention is inadequately trained. Thus, health care professionals should not expect any more thorough implementation than what well-intentioned people might intuitively devise. With a conceptual model and stronger research support, the training might follow. Beliefs in prevention interventions and corresponding behavioral action by practitioners, both medical and psychological, will increase.

4. Is there time and energy available in primary care to accomplish prevention of psychosocial problems?

There are many pressing problems in primary care settings requiring immediate attention. Primary care providers are pushed and pulled to implement a vast array of treatment recommendations and practice parameters. All of these in combination could never be fully implemented by the diligent physician (e.g., in terms of taking a media history, monitoring immunization, monitoring diet/exercise, growth). Even if primary care physicians could implement everything their academies tell them to do, they would have much less time for a lengthy list of risk factors for psychosocial problems psychologists might devise, especially when there might not necessarily be any issues of concern at the time. In addition, patients and their families come in for reasons of their own (not just for the provider's reasons) and these presenting issues require attention. In the few minutes available to the primary care provider, what is going to be given the most attention? Prevention will get short shrift in the press of time. Indeed, the survey of Yager et al. (1989) found the pediatricians divided in attitudes about whether they had "sufficient time to be concerned about the mental health of patients" (p. 1088). Similarly, Cheng, DeWitt, Savageau, and O'Connor (1999) found that only 53% felt they had adequate time for preventive work.

Psychologists, having focussed on the acquisition of assessment and therapeutic skills of existing psychopathology (not predicted problems), correspondingly provide services immediately called for, for which he or she has been trained (e.g., assessment for ADHD/learning disabled; behavioral management of oppositional defiant disorder, conduct disorder, and ADHD), and for which are likely to be reimbursed. Prevention will be gotten to, only if time allows, and it rarely does. There is just too much to do under the current system, too many current needs not getting filled as it is, to anticipate psychosocial problems. Some primary care providers may get involved outside their practice in community-based intervention programs, such as injury prevention or parenting programs, sometimes for altruistic reasons, sometimes for practice-marketing purposes (or both). However, these interventions are not conducted within the primary care setting.

What is typically ignored in discussions of prevention of psychosocial problems is that it requires greater effort in order to be effective than can be easily accomplished in the primary care setting time frame. This effort requirement is true for most psychosocial interventions. There is no psychosocial equivalent to immunizations, antibiotics, or bronchodilators. Effective prevention requires much time and energy on the part of the physician or psychologist and more coordination with other professionals and agencies outside the practice. There are simply too many demands for primary care providers competing for precious little time within the practice to devote to prevention of psychosocial problems.

5. Is reimbursement adequate in primary care for pediatricians, family practitioners, and psychologists for prevention of psychosocial problems?

This challenge might be the most difficult obstacle to providing psychosocial care and prevention in primary care settings. As one preventionist wrote many years ago in the title of an article, "who pays when nobody's sick?" (Baxter, 1977). Indeed, the pediatric respondents in the survey of Yager et al. (1989) indicated their belief "that neither patients nor third-party payers were willing or likely to pay for preventive mental health services" (p. 1088). The reimbursement issue has always been a problem for prevention (Roberts & Peterson, 1984a, 1984b). Health maintenance organizations might have earlier endorsed an orientation to health promotion and problem prevention, because of a financial return over the life of an enrollee (Roberts & Brown, 2000). Unfortunately, current managed care plans do not have much investment in prevention (Jellinek, 1997). Primary care physicians are feeling the effects of the lack of funding for prevention efforts because only 17% of primary care physicians reported believing that they received adequate reimbursement for preventive activities (Cheng et al., 1999).

If prevention efforts were properly supported financially, at least to the degree that are other efforts to improve physical and psychological conditions, then attention would be devoted to it. Primary care providers would find a way. Of course, the professional disciplines should not expect reimbursement for intervention with insufficient evidence to support its effectiveness (Skulstad, 1985). Nonetheless, the preventive effort should be compensated if a value is placed on preventing problems in a variety of areas. Green (1985) noted that "remuneration can obviously be either a major reinforcer or a deterrent to change" (p. 193).

SUMMARY TO CHALLENGES

These five challenges are posed to primary care providers in the prevention of psychosocial problems. There are other questions and challenges hindering the development of prevention in primary care settings, including primary care providers' reluctance to label children, negative stigma associated with psychiatric problems and seeking help, families not recognizing that the physician is a potential source of assistance, and limited availability of qualified mental health professionals to whom to refer and to collaborate in prevention efforts (Drotar, 1999; Wolraich, 1999). These issues are similar to the other obstacles requiring professional attention.

OPPORTUNITIES

For every challenge there exist opportunities for resourceful professionals to find ways to overcome the obstacles. What do health care professionals need to do? Paralleling the challenges, we now outline five opportunities for further work by psychologists, pediatricians and family physicians in primary care settings in order to advance the case for preventing psychosocial problems in primary care settings.

1. The professions need to develop conceptual models for prevention in primary care.

It is simple enough to assert that a conceptual model needs to be developed in order to guide interventions and research. Much more difficult would be actually designing that model to cover the range of issues covering prevention in addition to designing the part associated with the identification and intervention for psychosocial and cognitive-development problems. In some ways, the *DSM-PC* can serve as a conceptual model (Drotar, 1999; Wolraich, 1997). Any beginning framework for prevention would have to rely somewhat on the ability to identify early and predict later problems. To think preventively, the concepts of the three levels of prevention can be adopted as utilized by the National Institute of Mental Health (1998) and the Institute of Medicine (see Muñoz, Mrazek, & Haggerty, 1996). These include universal prevention approaches, selective prevention approaches, and indicated prevention strategies. *Universal prevention* is provided to all children and families, including those that are considered well-functioning. In other domains, such actions as immunizations for all children, fluoride in the water, and safer cars would be considered universal, because all children benefit from the prevention effort, not just those who might have greater need for it. *Selective prevention* would be provided to those who have indicated several factors that might be related to greater risk for the child or the family. A greater than average number of stressors or risk factors, or a decrease in coping ability or supports, might constitute higher risk. Prevention interventions would be provided only to those who exhibit the indicated risk factors. *Indicated prevention* services would be provided for those who have much greater or intense risk factors. Children and families may already be demonstrating considerable difficulties and intervention is clearly necessary to return them to regular developmental pathways in addition to helping them to avoid future difficulties. Indicated prevention may involve more therapeutic interventions than preventive ones. These issues are discussed in Durlak (1997) and Domitrovich and Greenberg (2000).

Mental health and other primary care disciplines need to ascertain what are the risk factors associated with certain psychosocial problems and which ones relate to each of these prevention intervention strategies. At its simplest, prevention assumes a developmental stance and additive/multiplicative algebra regarding emergence of psychosocial problems:

$$X_1 \rightarrow X_2 \rightarrow X_3 \rightarrow X_4 \Rightarrow \textit{problems}$$

Each of the *X*s would symbolize preemergent signs or risk factors leading to the eventual development of a psychosocial problem (see Roberts, 1991). If one can assume knowledge of this sequence or at least parts of the sequence, health care professionals can preventively intervene at X_1, or X_2 , or X_3 , or elsewhere to break the chain of stressors, risk factors, and events and behaviors leading to the psychosocial problems.

In order to get to that framework/conceptual model to frame prevention efforts, the professional disciplines would need to do three things:

(a) *Identify the risk factors associated with psychosocial problems.* In order to know the *X*s (and interaction thereof), health care professionals would need to have solid criteria for identifying the risk factors in psychosocial problem development. A review of the literature and everyday practice would result in a list of such risk factors including: marital separation/divorce, aggressive behavior, teen pregnancy, school difficulties, physical punishment by parents, family death, poor family cohesion, low social support, genetic risk factors, and parental impairments, including psychopathology. Although increasingly research is investigating developmental risk factors, these risk factors (or others, e.g., see Sanders, Markie-Dadds, Tully, & Bor, 2000) require much more empirical support before these can be solidified in the approaches by primary care providers. Professionals need to be careful not to construct screening lists of factors for which there is scant evidence for the relationship to outcomes and development of psychosocial problems.

(b) *Develop decision rules for these risk factors to assign action on the part of the primary care provider.* Once risk factors are identified, the associated preventive action needs to be identified for the professional to undertake. These might include: (i) "watch" for further development; (ii) preventively intervene within the practice; and (iii) consult or refer to a mental health professional for more intensive interventions. These action-decision rules are needed to organize assessment, identification, and follow-through by the primary care provider.

(c) *Develop effective prevention interventions tied to the identified risk factors and the decision rules*. Currently, there is an underdeveloped literature on prevention interventions that can be implemented in primary care settings in relation to specific factors of risk. What are the preventive interventions that can be conducted in these settings if the risk factor of maternal psychopathology is determined to be a valid one and is detected with a patient's mother? What are the psychosocial/preventive interventions to be implemented if the risk factor of impending divorce (after being empirically supported as a major element) is ascertained in a family? The professions do not have all that is needed to identify and act.

The parenting intervention models documented by Matthew Sanders in Australia can be suggestive of what needs to occur (but have not been definitively demonstrated in typical primary care settings). For example, Sanders (1999) described the Triple P–Positive Parenting Program. Level 1 involves a media-based parenting information campaign on a universal basis. Level 2 is a selected parenting program conducted in one to two sessions through brief consultation during well-child visits. Level 3 is a primary care integration of brief consultation in four sessions for implementation in pediatric and family medicine settings. Additional levels are more intense for indicated problems (see Tynan, this volume, for more information about Triple P). Sanders et al. (2000) stated the ultimate goal of their clinical research effort was to develop an "entire multilevel system of parenting and family support as a universal, accessible, high quality, low cost, multidisciplinary prevention strategy to enhance competent parenting" (p. 639). In the United States, Tynan and his enterprising colleagues have demonstrated implementation of parenting training in a managed care environment of a medical setting (Tynan, Chew, & Algermissen, in press; Tynan, Schuman, & Lampert, 1999). Domitrovich and Greenberg (2000) outlined some prevention programs that are considered effective, but are not yet integrated into primary care types of settings or practice including adolescent transitions, anger coping, children of divorce, social skills training, family bereavement, interpersonal cognitive problem-solving, and peer coping.

2. The professions need to develop a research agenda for prevention in primary care.

The primary care professions need to develop evidence-based practice parameters and guidelines for effective prevention-oriented screening, early identification, preventive intervention, and referral for psychosocial problems. These cannot be done with the more focussed research that has been conducted to this point. In order to resolve the problems associated with the lack of empirical support for prevention in psychosocial problems presenting in primary care settings, we propose to mount a large scale, multisite investigation to (a) gather information to identify what is happening in primary care settings with regard to prevention, and (b) determine what short- and long-term outcomes are associated when certain services are provided (preventively). This type of study would be similar to or a part of the Pediatric Research in Office Settings network or the Ambulatory Sentinel Practice Network.

The purpose of this project would be to demonstrate the relationship of prevention and outcomes, including behavioral improvements, improved quality of life, and possible cost savings. The latter would not be the only criterion for success because overall savings may not be reached. Prevention should not be held to a higher standard beyond other services. The study would have to be large scale and longitudinal to prove the worth of a comprehensive commitment to prevention and promotion in primary care. Both intermediate and proxy variables would be useful to assess progress, but there needs to be a long-term commitment to funding in order to ascertain full prevention-related outcomes. In design, this project might be similar to the Fort Bragg demonstration project in approach to continuum of care and multimethod assessment (Bickman et al., 1995). This approach requires funding of model clinical services and a comprehensive research evaluation component. If the theory and premise of prevention holds true, and the promise of primary care access is attained, then improved physical health and mental health outcomes would be expected (but not necessarily resulting in no problems at all). Additional outcomes would include some cost savings over long-term (medical cost offsets may be obtained, but even if not, still the improvements can be worthwhile), increases in longevity (which may wash out cost savings), and enhanced quality of life. (Notably, similar to the Fort Bragg demonstration, professionals must be willing to accept, up-front, that psychosocial preventive services may turn out not to be effective.)

Part of the needs for empirical support can be met with an examination of prevention in the same way it has been conducted for injury prevention through physician interventions. Miller and Galbraith (1995) evaluated The Injury Prevention Program (TIPP) by analyzing other studies that implemented portions of what TIPP did. They found that for each dollar spent on TIPP, there was an annual savings of $13. Bass et al. (1993) did a similar analysis of research on effectiveness of counseling to prevent childhood injuries based in primary care. This type of research could be done for psychosocial prevention and counseling, if a comprehensive demonstration cannot be mounted.

Research Agenda

Reflecting the findings of this previous research, the new research agenda would need to investigate how to break down the barriers from the perspective of the parents. Those who may most benefit from psychosocial guidance may be the least likely to seek it. Although most parents report that it is acceptable to talk with a pediatrician about psychosocial problems (81.1%), only 40.9% actually did discuss hypothetical situations with a physician (Horwitz, Leaf, & Leventhal, 1998). Briggs-Gowan, Horwitz, Schwab-Stone, Leventhal, and Leaf (2000) also noted that most parents do not discuss behavioral/emotional issues with their pediatrician. Parents who are more highly educated and earn more money, are Euro-American, older, married, and those with medical insurance are more likely to solicit the advice of their pediatrician (Horwitz et al., 1998). Mothers who are of lower socioeconomic status have been found more likely to think that the physical aspects of health should be the focus of pediatric visits and were less interested in addressing psychosocial issues (Cheng, Savageau, DeWitt, Bigelow, & Charney, 1996).

Research might consider whether computerization allows better monitoring and surveillance of psychosocial problems. Computers assist monitoring and prompting for immunizations, does it help other preventive care? Protocols that pop out at particular times according to the child's lifestage, or entered risk factors, could be developed for the physician, psychologist, or preventionists to implement. Of course, any mechanization of primary care is not a substitute for the providers recognizing and intervening. Indeed, continuity of care seems to be the best predictor of a child's problem getting detected by physicians (Holden & Schuman, 1995).

To conduct adequate investigations, the barriers to research would need to be overcome in these settings as outlined by Kelleher and Long (1994). These barriers include the diversity of primary care settings, problems with sampling, data collection, assessment, and problems with methodology and design. Nonetheless, Kelleher and Long found "no studies of the outcomes of current practices by primary care providers have been published" (p. 139). While these authors assert that there is a need for medical outcome research in children with mental health problems, we argue the same for preventive efforts.

The well-child visit is, in essence, a surveillance opportunity, where screening and universal prevention can take place. Additionally, if budding externalizing disorders are identified, then early intervention and selective prevention could take place in pediatric practice, as suggested by Costello and Shugart (1992). Lavigne et al. (1999) raised basic research questions of importance for screening, early identification, prevention and intervention: "Is there a particular age at which screening for a disruptive behavior disorder could best be done? At what age would it be most appropriate to screen for anxiety or affective disorders? Or, if we wanted to develop an intervention program for a particular set of disorders, what age group should we target to reach the most children with that problem?" (p. 395).

This research agenda may find that primary care versus specialty mental health care is not effective, or is only effective with a limited range of problems whether preventively or therapeutically, or is effective for a wide array of problems and situations. Cost effectiveness needs to be comparatively investigated in terms of short- and long-term costs versus prevention services provided through other systems (e.g., schools, communities, or faith-based organizations).

3. The professions need to change training models to enhance prevention in primary care.

The ways in which pediatricians, family practitioners, and psychologists are currently trained fail to adequately educate and practice prevention concepts and actions. The model of training psychologists to provide services for children and adolescents (Roberts et al., 1998) seems quite applicable to changing the training models for all primary care disciplines (not just psychologists):

> *Prevention, Family Support, and Health Promotion.* Professional psychologists working with children, adolescents, and families should have the ability to provide different levels of intervention, not just with individuals and not just with already well-entrenched problems. Prevention, health promotion, and family support represent psychological interventions fundamental to improving quality of life and avoiding serious problems before they arise. Training in this topical area should include, for example, enhancing social and problem-solving skills, promoting positive attachments, increasing positive experiences, teaching safety and health practices, and increasing the responsiveness of the community and service systems to the needs of children, adolescents, and families.

> *Justification.* Given the human and economic cost of emotional and behavioral disorders, it is essential to reduce their incidence and prevalence by strengthening the protective variables, reducing the risk variables, and supporting families in their development. (p. 298)

The report of the Task Force on Training Pediatric Psychologists (Spirito et al., 2003), follows the above recommendations and states:

> Pediatric psychologists often work in primary care settings, and therefore may have greater opportunities than other psychologists to conduct disease prevention and health promotional activities. An important role for pediatric psychologists is promoting healthy lifestyles and preventing the development of health-risk behaviors in both healthy and chronically ill children. Particularly important in primary care is the promotion of exercise and a healthy diet to prevent childhood obesity and associated sequelae such as hypertension and type 2 diabetes. For adolescents, prevention efforts are geared toward health-risk behaviors such as unprotected sex, smoking, substance abuse and other high-risk health behaviors including those that may result in unintentional injuries. Pediatric psychologists should be knowledgeable of physical and familial factors that may place children and adolescents at risk for disease later in adulthood and take steps to mitigate these risk factors in childhood.
>
> Given the increased risks of psychosocial problems in children with chronic illness, pediatric psychologists should employ preventive interventions whenever possible to diminish the potential development of negative emotional sequelae in these children. Pediatric psychologists should work in conjunction with pediatric healthcare providers to identify and intervene with families at risk for domestic violence, child abuse, or neglect.
>
> Pediatric psychology trainees should receive didactic coursework, formal readings, or seminars on the science of prevention and principles of behavioral change pertinent to healthy development and prevention of disease in adulthood. Coursework and lectures on healthy behavior and health-risk behavior should be offered, as well as seminars on screening and how to identify children in primary care who are at-risk for or experiencing abuse and neglect. Finally, trainees should have supervised experience in addressing multiple behavioral health issues that include the promotion of health lifestyles and disease prevention; safety, nutrition, weight management, and exercise; and how to address family risk factors such as family violence, sexual and physical abuse, and individual risk factors such as substance use (including nicotine). (Spirito et al., 2003, p. 94)

Training in primary care psychology would need to become preventively focussed first and employ therapeutic interventions only when prevention fails. To achieve this, changes will have to occur in coursework, with a reconceptualization of core courses such as psychopathology and psychotherapy/interventions. Students would participate in required prevention practica and need to learn case conceptualization in preventive terms. Opportunities for clinical experiences in the primary care setting early in training are essential. Of course, to achieve this, there needs to be a change in faculty orientation and a corresponding change in accreditation attitudes and behavior.

Curricula in pediatric and family medicine (as well as developmental-behavioral pediatrics) needs to be more inclusive of prevention concepts and activities. Whereas current curricula are merely suggestive, a greater emphasis is needed on prevention of psychosocial problems in an enhanced program of training. Of course, in both professions of psychology and medicine, development of conceptual models and empirical evidence will guide practice parameters and recommendations as well as training. There is some evidence that training does seem to help in mental health problem detection and intervention. For example, Holden and Schuman (1995) reviewed several studies indicating that newer trained physicians conducted more psychosocial management than earlier trained physicians.

4. The professions need to adapt focus to allow more time for prevention in primary care.

There is too much to do in a brief period of time in primary care settings, so the addition of prevention may be just too much more (similar to the recommendations and practice parameters that have proliferated). The contact time may need to be expanded and more practitioners may be needed to see fewer patients per day with energies focussed on the most important issues. For example, Lavigne et al. (1999) evaluated studies that suggested that focus should be given to problems with high intraindividual stability, such as, disruptive disorders. However, other problems may be amenable as well with proper attention devoted to them.

Wright and Burns (1986) questioned the overall effectiveness and efficiency of having primary care physicians providing mental health care. Of course, given the obstacles to physicians handling much of the psychosocial problems presenting in primary care, the role of the properly trained psychologist may be enhanced. Psychologists need to be consultants and coproviders, acting as preventionists. As described by Drotar (1995), collaboration and consultation activities can meet the needs more fully, certainly for prevention as much as for existing psychosocial problems. However, not all prevention requires a doctoral level psychologist to implement (Hanley, 1994). Thus, professional extenders can be employed for specialized prevention (and intervention) under the supervision of the physician or psychologist. Nurses, physician's assistants, social workers, child life specialists, and master's level psychologists may be proven as effective when implementing manualized, empirically-supported prevention and treatments. The field is never going to graduate enough properly trained psychologists to fill the need, it must be acknowledged, and the situation may not always require doctoral level psychologists or physicians. Once devised and tested, preventive interventions could be implemented by these prevention specialists.

5. The professions need to innovate for funding for prevention in primary care.

The poor reimbursement for prevention deters its development and implementation. In order to enhance prevention work, the professions should first seek to demonstrate the effectiveness and prove the worth of prevention activities, not only in human outcomes, but also in financial terms. For both the research agenda and later implementation of evidence-based prevention activities in primary care settings, professionals need to seek funding support from (a) foundations with prevention orientations, (b) health maintenance organizations (develop contracts for prevention efforts, in the manner of Tynan et al., 1999), (c) affected business and their organizations (e.g., chambers of commerce, SAS in North Carolina), (d) government programs such as Medicaid and SCHIP, and (e) tax dollars. For the latter, some states have dedicated tax revenues for children's services councils, including prevention and early intervention activities. Meyers (1994) described the example of Florida in obtaining tax dollars for these activities. Other governmental programs may incorporate primary care if the linkages can be demonstrated. For example, the U.S. Department of Agriculture has ventured into support for childhood obesity prevention through the Supplemental Food Program for Women, Infants, and Children (WIC) program (e.g., Cincinnati Children's Hospital Medical Center). Tobacco settlement money may be used for prevention efforts in some states, depending on the orientation of the panels set up to distribute the money. (Of course, "guilt"/"feel-good" money might be obtained from the tobacco industry directly if ethical concerns can be overcome, e.g., from Philip Morris.) Nobody is going to pay for anything in prevention or psychosocial services unless they can be demonstrated to be effective and can be implemented in the manner under which they were tested.

Concluding Remarks: Final Question on A Good Idea

The concept of the pediatrician or family physician serving more roles in the primary care setting for psychosocial problems (what was called in the late 1970s as "the new morbidity") has been around for a long time.

The Task Force on Pediatric Education (1978), for example, promulgated what seemed to be a novel idea at the time which would gain children better access to prevention, early identification, and treatment for these problems than they had previously (and would likely open up more roles for pediatric psychologists as well, Roberts & Wright, 1982). Over a short period of time, some professionals' enthusiasm seemed to wane (e.g., Wright & Burns, 1986). Reflecting back over 20-plus years, we have to wonder why a good idea, if it is so good, has not taken hold? Why has the promise not been fully fulfilled? At this point, where is the evidence that this idea has any worth? Why are the disciplines continuing to struggle over conceptualization and implementation? Perhaps pediatricians and family physicians should do what they have the most interest in and where proven their worth to be in terms of preventing and treating medical problems. Instead, maybe another profession (not necessarily psychologists) should be found who can do the psychosocial work needing to be done in both prevention and remediation.

Through all of this work in meeting the challenges and fulfilling the opportunities, of course, there needs to be determinations made regarding what are appropriate prevention interventions (or any psychosocial intervention) to be conducted by pediatricians and family physicians versus those to be made in the setting by psychologists and other mental health professionals. Although the medical professions have a stronger presence in and focus on primary care, psychology in primary care is still developing. There are insufficient numbers of psychologists in such settings to perceive anything more than suggestions of what can be accomplished. This setting needs to be seen as different from the traditional private practice models. Importantly to the point of this chapter, the focus on prevention should certainly be greater in primary care psychology than it is in traditional models of mental health delivery.

REFERENCES

American Psychological Association. (1996). *Guidelines and procedures for accreditation*. Washington, DC: Author.

Bass, J. L., Christoffel, K. K., Widome, M., Boyle, W., Scheidt, P., Stanwick, R., & Roberts, K. (1993). Childhood injury prevention counseling in primary care settings: A critical review of the literature. *Pediatrics, 92*, 544-550.

Baxter, F. Z. (1977). Funding—who pays when nobody's sick. In D. C. Klein & S. E. Goldstein (Eds.), *Primary prevention: An idea whose time has come* (DHEW ADM Publication No. 77-447). Washington, DC: US Government Printing Office.

Bickman, L., Guthrie, P. R., Foster, E. M., Lambert, E. W., Summerfelt, W. T., Breda, C. A., & Helflinger, C. A. (1995). *Evaluating managed mental health services: The Fort Bragg experiment*. New York: Plenum Press.

Bradbury, K., Janicke, D. M., Riley, A. W., & Finney, J. W. (1999). Predictors of unintentional injuries to school-age children seen in pediatric primary care. *Journal of Pediatric Psychology, 24,* 423-433.

Brazelton, T. B. (1975). Anticipatory guidance. *Pediatric Clinics of North America, 22,* 533-544.

Briggs-Gowan, M. J., Horwitz, S. M., Schwab-Stone, M. E., Leventhal, J. M., & Leaf, P. J. (2000). Mental health in pediatric settings: Distribution of disorders and factors related to service use. *Journal of the American Academy of Child and Adolescent Psychiatry, 39,* 841-849.

Brown, K. J., & Roberts, M. C. (2000). Future issues in pediatric psychology: Delphic survey. *Journal of Clinical Psychology in Medical Settings, 7,* 5-15.

Cheng, T. L., DeWitt, T. G., Savageau, J. A., & O'Connor, K. G. (1999). Determinants of counseling in primary care pediatric practice: Physician attitudes about time, money, and health issues. *Archives of Pediatrics and Adolescent Medicine, 153,* 629-635.

Cheng, T. L., Savageau, J. A., DeWitt, T. G., Bigelow, C., & Charney, E. (1996). Expectations, goals, and perceived effectiveness of child health supervision: A study of mothers in a pediatric practice. *Clinical Pediatrics, 35,* 129-137.

Christophersen, E. R. (1994). *Pediatric compliance: A guide for the primary care physician.* New York: Plenum Medical Book.

Christophersen, E. R., & Gyulay, J. (1981). Parental compliance with car seat usage: A positive approach with long-term follow-up. *Journal of Pediatric Psychology, 6,* 301-312.

Coury, D. L., Berger, S. P., Stancin, T., & Tanner, J. L. (1999). Curricular guidelines for residency training in developmental-behavioral pediatrics. *Developmental and Behavioral Pediatrics, 20,* S1-S38.

Costello, E. J., & Shugart, M. A. (1992). Above and below the threshold: Severity of psychiatric symptoms and functional impairment in a pediatric sample. *Pediatrics, 90,* 359-368.

Domitrovich, C. E., & Greenberg, M. T. (2000). The study of implementation: Current findings from effective programs that prevent mental disorders in school-aged children. *Journal of Educational and Psychological Consultation, 11,* 193-221.

Drotar, D. (1995). *Consulting with pediatricians: Psychological perspectives.* New York: Plenum Press.

Drotar, D. (1999). The *Diagnostic and Statistical Manual for Primary Care* (*DSM-PC*), child and adolescent version: What pediatric psychologists need to know. *Journal of Pediatric Psychology, 24,* 369-380.

Durlak, J. A. (1997). *Successful prevention programs for children and adolescents.* New York: Plenum Press.

Evers-Szostak, M. (1997). Psychological practice in pediatric primary care settings. In L. Vandecreek, S. Knapp, & T. L. Jackson (Eds.), *Innovations in clinical practice: A source book* (Vol. 16, pp. 325-333). Sarasota, FL: Professional Resources Press.

Green, M. (1985). The role of the pediatrician in the delivery of behavioral services. *Developmental and Behavioral Pediatrics, 6,* 190-201.

Hanley, J. H. (1994). Use of bachelor-level psychology majors in the provision of mental health services to children, adolescents, and their families. *Journal of Clinical Child Psychology, 23*(Suppl.), 55-58.

Holden, E. W., & Schuman, W. B. (1995). The detection and management of mental health disorders in pediatric primary care. *Journal of Clinical Psychology in Medical Settings, 2,* 71-87.

Horwitz, S. M., Leaf, P. J., & Leventhal, J. M. (1998). Identification of psychosocial problems in pediatric primary care: Do family attitudes make a difference? *Archives of Pediatric and Adolescent Medicine, 152,* 367-371.

Jellinek, M. S. (1997). Bridging pediatric primary care and mental health services. *Journal of Developmental and Behavioral Pediatrics, 18,* 173-174.

Kaufman, K. L., Holden, E. W., & Walker, C. E. (1989). Future directions in pediatric and clinical child psychology. *Professional Psychology: Research and Practice, 20,* 148-152.

Kelleher, K., & Long, N. (1994). Barriers and new directions in mental health services research in the primary care setting. *Journal of Clinical Child Psychology, 23,* 133-142.

Lavigne, J. V., Gibbons, R. D., Arend, R., Rosenbaum, D., Binns, H. J., & Cristoffel, K. K. (1999). Rational service planning in pediatric primary care: Continuity and change in psychopathology among children enrolled in pediatric practices. *Journal of Pediatric Psychology, 24,* 393-403.

Lynch, T. L., Wildman, B. G., & Smucker, W. D. (1997). Parental disclosure of child psychosocial concerns: Relationship to physician identification and management. *Journal of Family Practice, 44,* 273-280.

McCain, A. P., Kelley, M. L., & Fishbein, J. (1999). Behavioral screening in well-child care: Validation of the Toddler Behavior Screening Inventory. *Journal of Pediatric Psychology 24,* 415-422.

Meyers, J. C. (1994). Financing strategies to support innovations in service delivery to children. *Journal of Clinical Child Psychology, 23(*Suppl.), 48-54.

Miller, T. R., & Galbraith, M. (1995). Injury prevention counseling by pediatricians: A benefit-cost comparison. *Pediatrics, 96,* 1-4.

Mullen P. D., Green L. W., & Persinger, G. (1985). Clinical trials of patient education for chronic conditions: A comparative analysis of intervention types. *Preventative Medicine, 14,* 753-781.

Muñoz, R. F., Mrazek, P. J., & Haggerty, R. J. (1996). Institute of medicine report on prevention of mental disorders: Summary and commentary. *American Psychologist, 51,* 1116-1122.

National Institute of Mental Health. (1998). *Priorities for prevention research at NIMH: A national advisory health council workshop on mental disorders prevention research.* Washington, DC: Author.

Pace, T. M., Mullins, L. L., Chaney, J. M., & Olson, R. A. (1995). Psychological consultaiton with primary care physicians: Obstacles and opportunities in the medical setting. *Professional Psychology: Research and Practice, 26,* 23-131.

Pless, I. B., & Arsenault, L. (1987). The role of health education in the prevention of injuries to children. *Journal of Social Issues, 43,* 87-103.

Prazar, G. (1990). Psychosocial risk factors in childhood. What can the pediatrician in practice do? *Journal of Developmental and Behavioral Pediatrics, 11,* 210-211.

Riekert, K. A., Stancin, T., Palermo, T. M., & Drotar, D. (1999). A psychological behavioral screening service: Use, feasibility, and impact in a primary care setting. *Journal of Pediatric Psychology, 24,* 405-414.

Roberts, M. C. (1991). Overview to prevention research: Where's the cat? Where's the cradle? In J. H. Johnson & S. B. Johnson (Eds.), *Advances in child health psychology* (pp. 95-107). Gainesville, FL: University of Florida Press.

Roberts, M. C. (1992). Vale dictum: An editor's view of the field of pediatric psychology and its journal. *Journal of Pediatric Psychology, 17,* 785-805.

Roberts, M. C. (1994). Prevention/promotion in America: Still spitting on the sidewalk. *Journal of Pediatric Psychology, 19,* 267-281.

Roberts, M. C. (1998). Innovations in specialty training: The Clinical Child Psychology Program at the University of Kansas. *Professional Psychology: Research and Practice, 29,* 394-397.

Roberts, M. C., & Brown, K. J. (2000). Overcoming obstacles to prevention in pediatric psychology. *SPP Progress Notes, 24*(3), 11-14.

Roberts, M. C., Carlson, C. I., Erickson, M. T., Friedman, R. M., La Greca, A. M., Lemanek, K. L., Russ, S. W., Schroeder, C. S., Vargas, L. A., & Wohlford, P. F. (1998). A model for training psychologists to provide services for children and adolescents. *Professional Psychology: Research and Practice, 29,* 293-299.

Roberts, M. C., Fanurik, D., & Layfield, D. A. (1987). Behavioral approaches to prevention of childhood injuries. *Journal of Social Issues, 43,* 105-118.

Roberts, M. C., & Layfield, D. A. (1987). Promoting child passenger safety: A comparison of two positive methods. *Journal of Pediatric Psychology, 12,* 257-271.

Roberts, M. C., & Peterson, L. (Eds.). (1984a). Prevention models: Theoretical and practical implications. In Roberts & L. Peterson (Eds.), *Prevention of problems in childhood: Psychological research and applications* (pp. 1-39). New York: Wiley.

Roberts, M. C., & Peterson, L. (1984b). *Prevention of problems in childhood: Psychological research and applications.* New York: John Wiley & Sons.

Roberts, M. C., & Steele, R. (2003). Predoctoral training in pediatric psychology at the University of Kansas Clinical Child Psychology Program. *Journal of Pediatric Psychology, 28,* 99-103.

Roberts, M. C., & Wright, L. (1982). The role of the pediatric psychologist as consultant to pediatricians. In J. M. Tuma (Ed.), *Handbook for the practice of pediatric psychology* (pp. 251-289). New York: Wiley.

Rowland, L. (1989). Pierre the pelican. *Prevention in Human Services, 6,* 117-122.

Russell, L. B. (1993). The role of prevention in health reform. *The New England Journal of Medicine, 329,* 352-354.

Sanders, M. (1999). Triple P-Positive Parenting Program: Towards an empirically validated multilevel parenitng and family support strategy for the prevention of behavior and emotional problems in children. *Clinical Child and Family Psychology Review, 2,* 71-90.

Sanders, M., Markie-Dadds, C., Tully, L. A., & Bor, W. (2000). The Triple-P Positive Parenting Program: A comparison of enhanced, standard, and self-directed behavioral family intervention for parents of children with early onset conduct problems. *Journal of Consulting and Clinical Psychology, 68,* 624-640.

Schroeder, C. S. (1979). Psychologist in a private pediatrics office. *Journal of Pediatric Psychology, 1*, 5-18.

Schroeder, C. S. (1996). Mental health services in pediatric primary care. In M. C. Roberts (Ed.), *Model programs in child and family mental health* (pp. 265-284). Mahwah, NJ: Lawrence Erlbaum Associates.

Schroeder. C. S. (1999). Commentary: A view from the past and a look to the future. *Journal of Pediatric Psychology, 24*, 447-452.

Schroeder, C. S., Goolsby, E., & Stangler, S. (1975). Preventive services in a private pediatric practice. *Journal of Clinical Child Psychology, 4*, 32-33.

Schultz, J. R., & Vaughn, L. M. (1999). Brief report: Learning to parent: A survey of parents in an urban pediatric primary care clinic. *Journal of Pediatric Psychology, 24*, 441-445.

Showers, J. (1989). Behaviour management cards as a method of anticipatory guidance for parents. *Child Care, Health and Development, 15*, 401-415.

Skulstad, J. R. (1985). Responses to Dr. Green: Discussants' remarks and small group summaries. *Journal of Developmental and Behavioral Pediatrics, 6*, 194-195.

Sobel, A. B., Roberts, M. C., Rayfield, A., Barnard, M. U., & Rapoff, M. A. (2001). Evaluating outpatient pediatric psychology services in a primary care setting. *Journal of Pediatric Psychology, 26*, 395-405.

Spirito, A. (1999). Introduction to special series on empirically supported treatments in pediatric psychology. *Journal of Pediatric Psychology, 24*, 87-90.

Spirito, A., Brown, R. T., D'Angelo, E., Delamater, A., Rodrigue, J., & Siegel, L. (2003). Society of Pediatric Psychology Task Force Report: Recommendations for the training of pediatric psychologists. *Journal of Pediatric Psychology, 28*, 85-98.

Stancin, T. (1999). Introduction to special issues: Pediatric mental health services in primary care settings. *Journal of Pediatric Psychology, 24*, 367-368.

Stancin, T., & Palermo, T. M. (1997). A review of behavioral screening practices in pediatric settings: Do they pass the test? *Journal of Developmental and Behavioral Pediatrics, 18*, 183-193.

Task Force on Pediatric Education. (1978). *The future of pediatric education*. Evanston, IL: American Academy of Pediatrics.

Tynan, W. D., Chew, C., & Algermissen, M. (in press). Concurrent parent and child therapy groups for externalizing disorders: The rural replication. *Cognitive and Behavioral Practice*.

Tynan, W. D., Schuman, W., & Lampert, N. (1999). Concurrent parent and child therapy groups for externalizing disorders: From the laboratory to the world of managed care. *Cognitive and Behavioral Practice, 6*, 3-9.

Wildman, B. G., Kinsman, A. M., Logue, E., Dickey, D. J., & Smucker, W. D. (1997). Presentation and management of childhood psychosocial problems. *The Journal of Family Practice, 44*, 77-84.

Wissow, L. S., Roter, D. L., & Wilson, M. E. H. (1994). Pediatrician interview style and mothers' disclosure of psychosocial issues. *Pediatrics, 93*, 289-295.

Wolraich, M. L. (1997). *Diagnostic and Statistical Manual for Primary Care (DSM-PC)* child and adolescent version: Design, intent, and hopes for the future. *Journal of Developmental and Behavioral Pediatrics, 18*, 171-172.

Wolraich, M. L. (1999). The referral process: The pediatrician as gatekeeper. In R. T. Brown (Ed.), *Cognitive aspects of chronic illness in children* (pp. 15-22). New York: Guilford Press.

Wright, L. (1967). The pediatric psychologist: A role model. *American Psychologist, 22*, 323-325.

Wright, L. (1978). Group consultation and bibliotherapeutic aids. *Feelings and Their Medical Significance, 20*, 21-24.

Wright, L. (1985). Psychology and pediatrics: Prospects for cooperative efforts to promote child health: A discussion with Morris Green. *American Psychologist, 40*, 949-952.

Wright, L., & Burns, B. J. (1986). Primary mental health care: A "find" for psychology? *Professional Psychology: Research and Practice, 17*, 560-564.

Yager, J., Linn, L., Leake, R. B., Goldston, S., Heinicke, C., & Pynoos, R. (1989). Attitudes toward mental illness prevention in routine pediatric practice. *American Journal of Diseases of Children,143*, 1087-1090.

DISCUSSION SUMMARY
written by Meghan Barlow

In keeping with his reputation, Dr. Michael Roberts presented on the role of prevention in primary care and pediatric psychology. Dr. Roberts' talk focused on the issue that prevention was introduced as an intervention in 1978 however, to date, there is very little research on prevention as an effective intervention and there is a great deal of struggle relating to the conceptualization and implementation of preventive interventions. He outlined several challenges that impede the research and practice of preventive interventions as well as the opportunities for improving prevention as an intervention. The discussion following Dr. Roberts' talk developed around several questions that he raised.

Dr. Roberts offered as an obstacle to prevention that physicians have little time to devote to current problems their child patients may be experiencing, much less the problems that they have yet to develop and, as a result, prevention suffers. He raised the question: Is the psychological training that physicians undergo adequate? Physicians spend, on average, one month of their residency in psychiatry, with a total of five hours spent on psychological training and the remainder of the month spent in psychiatric medicine. Many of the physicians present agreed that time is a major obstacle to overcome, especially in terms of practicing preventive interventions. The majority of physicians present also agreed that psychological training may be inadequate. One physician recalled that the month of psychiatry is often the month that students take their vacations.

Physician and psychological training became the focus of discussion not only in the time immediately following Dr. Roberts' presentation, but throughout the course of the forum. Dr. Roberts suggested the possibility of changing training models. Instead of training in therapy first, he suggested training students in prevention and then how to treat the problem if the prevention is ineffective. Additionally, research should focus on identifying various risk factors that physicians can be trained to recognize in order to target preventions more appropriately for each patient. Many of the physicians who were present are responsible for training medical students. In general, they expressed a desire to understand how training can be adapted in order to more effectively address issues in prevention. The majority agreed that the standard pamphlets and anticipatory guidance is often not enough to be considered prevention within primary care. Further, they seemed to agree that research determining risk factors and effective prevention tools is greatly needed to help train their students in the specifics of prevention.

Another question resulting from Dr. Roberts' talk was: Which professionals are the appropriate people to make which interventions for which children? The forum participants agreed that more research, particularly focusing on developmentally normal children and their outcomes, is needed to begin to answer this question. Additionally, it was agreed that those answers could potentially impact reimbursement and training issues as well.

An example of an early intervention program in action was provided by a public health nurse from Minnesota. She reported that in Minnesota, all pregnant mothers have the opportunity to be visited by a public health nurse twice during pregnancy and twice postpartum.

Dr. Roberts' talk clearly led to much discussion concerning the consensus that prevention was both very important and very neglected. Participants agreed that research addressing which children were most at risk for specific problems would aid in making prevention efforts time effective. In addition, participants left the forum with the realization that prevention is often not addressed in either medical or psychology training programs.

CHAPTER 3

THE INTEGRATION OF DEVELOPMENT AND BEHAVIOR IN PEDIATRIC PRACTICE

History, Present Status, Current Challenges

M. Alex Geertsma
St. Mary's Hospital, Waterbury, CT

INTRODUCTION

I have been assured by a very knowing American of my acquaintance in London, that a healthy child well Nursed is at a year Old a most delicious, nourishing, and wholesome Food, whether Stewed, Roasted, Baked, or Boyled, and I make no doubt that it will equally serve in a Fricasie, or a Ragoust.

—Jonathan Swift (A Modest Proposal, 1729)
(Kessen, 1965)

Jonathan Swift's 1729 satirical "proposal" was a vehicle to express his outrage at the failure of his government to make adequate provision for the needs of children. The state of affairs for children's mental health in this

Treating Children's Psychosocial Problems in Primary Care, 61–92

country may begin to approach that of Irish children in the early eighteenth century if significant action is not taken. (Author)

Perhaps the most cogent argument for pediatric practitioner involvement with children's behavior and development has been our nation's expanding crisis in children's mental health. There is growing recognition, as outlined in the U.S. Surgeon General's report on children's mental health (U.S. Public Health Service Report of the Surgeon General's Conference on Children's Mental Health, 2000), that the scope and degree of emotional difficulty facing the nation's children cannot be addressed without the aid of the country's close to 60,000 pediatricians. In addition, the Carnegie Foundation's report (Carnegie Task Force on Meeting the Needs of Young Children, 1994), and more recently the National Academy of Sciences' (NAS) comprehensive summary (Committee on Integrating the Science of Early Childhood Development, Board on Children, Youth, and Families, National Academy of Sciences, 2000), have both publicized the critical importance of early detection of children at developmental and behavioral risk.

The Carnegie report taken with the NAS' extensive scientific reinforcement, have documented the relative "explosion" of neurobiological, behavioral, and social science research documenting the critical effects of early life experience. The NAS summary emphasizes the inseparable and interactive effects of genetics and the environment on early brain development and human behavior. Both documents emphasize our capacity to increase the odds of optimal developmental and emotional outcome through planned early intervention. Also central to the conclusions of both documents is the role that health care providers, particularly pediatricians and family physicians could play in the process of early involvement.

However, despite strong recommendations by the 1978 Task Force on Pediatric Education (American Academy of Pediatrics, 1978), there is evidence that over 20 years of concerted educational effort has not appreciably increased the amount of consistent and collaborative involvement with, screening for, and identification of developmental and behavioral difficulties by pediatricians. Even less certain has been the degree to which pediatricians provide useful and valid preventive behavioral advice in everyday practice (Schuster, Duan, Regalado, & Klein, 2000).

Although pediatrics as a formal discipline has only existed since the turn of the twentieth century, the integration of development and behavior into pediatric practice has been a central issue from the beginning. The early writings and work of pediatricians such as Milton Senn (1977), and child psychiatrists such as Leon Eisenberg (1988), have consistently argued for a balanced and integrated clinical approach that neither excludes consideration of the emotional nor the somatic from the care of children. Despite this consistent theme, other proponents of integration such as Haggerty (1982) and Green (1993), have continued to reflect on a lack of attention and actual resistance to an integrated approach.

Another common rationale for an integrated approach has been the assumption by the public that pediatricians should be able to answer common parental concerns about children's behavior and development. Formal surveys (Young, Davis, Schoen, & Parker, 1998) have not only confirmed that expectation, but informal surveys also share a degree of parental disappointment with the typical general pediatrician's response to those concerns. Furthermore, an extensive body of research literature has reinforced the importance of consideration of behavioral, emotional, and developmental factors in chronic disease outcome. Despite such persuasive evidence, the all too common lack of integration of considerations developmental and behavioral in everyday pediatric practice remains an enigma, at least on the surface (Eisenberg, 1988; Haggerty, 1982; Green, 1993).

Reasons for this are complex. Potential contributions include a lack of emphasis on development and behavior in undergraduate and postgraduate medical education, the personality characteristics of practicing pediatricians, economic limitations, lack of efficacious models of practice integration, and current patterns of pediatric primary care practice. An initial review of the histories of the fields of pediatrics and of developmental and behavioral pediatrics will help to provide an important foundation for understanding the complexity of the issues. Succeeding sections will explore specific causes, implications for changing and shifting the emphasis toward a more integrated approach, and potential solutions. This will, in turn, help to define what critical research and public policy questions remain.

HISTORY OF PEDIATRICS AND DEVELOPMENTAL AND BEHAVIORAL PEDIATRICS—IMPLICATIONS FOR AN INTEGRATED MODEL OF PEDIATRIC PRACTICE

The History of Pediatrics—Evolution of a Subculture

One could realistically argue that the field of pediatrics had its origins with the very beginnings of medicine. This is reflected by the content of ancient treatises on the medical care of children. As Mahnke (2000) notes in a recent history of pediatrics, the Roman physician Celsus was apparently the first to formally write of the need to treat children differently than adults, somewhere around 50 AD. While writing on pediatric medical topics continued sporadically over the centuries, pediatrics as a truly recognized specialty did not actually spring forth until around the beginning of the twentieth century.

Predating the development of pediatrics as a formal specialty was the evolution of a major public health challenge whose origins reflected significant sociocultural changes of the times and also foretold of future pervasive pediatric professional leanings. The mid-1800s were characterized by a growth in urban city populations and increasing infant mortality. The horrifying infant death rate of the times was largely attributable to infectious diseases such as tetanus, diphtheria, and tuberculosis. Other life threatening diseases related to nutritional deprivation, such as rickets, also became prevalent. Similarly, a shift away from breast-feeding and toward artificial formula feeding led to malnutrition and often fatal infections secondary to contaminated sources of water and cow's milk. This shift, ironically, came from the lower/working class need for women to enter into the labor market in cities, and the upper class view of the "rural-peasant" process of breast-feeding as out of fashion.

For these reasons, increasing numbers of dedicated physicians took up the call of curing prevalent infectious diseases, and developing methods of preventing the other causes of infant mortality. This led to the coalescing of groups of physicians exclusively treating children. The immortal "Father of Pediatrics," Abraham Jacobi, and his less well-known pioneering pediatric colleague, Job Lewis Smith, published extensively in the area of preventive physical health and helped establish the "Pediatric Section" of the American Medical Association, the forerunner of the present day American Academy of Pediatrics.

This public health focus on organic disease in children fortuitously paralleled the changing nature of medicine at the turn of the twentieth. Medicine up to that point was literally a guild of primitive practitioners using not much more than medieval incantations and procedures as barbaric and scientifically unfounded as blood letting, blistering, or purging. While the application of the scientific method was utilized to make decisions about medical practice by some, it was not part of the medical mainstream of the mid nineteenth century.

The period of modern day allopathic medicine began to develop momentum during the earliest days of the twentieth century and reached a critical juncture around 1920 with the establishment of the first scientifically based medical school curriculum at the John's Hopkins School of Medicine. The scientific method's installation at the core of medical education gradually but pervasively changed the focus and meaning of the "healing profession's" self-perception. The focus on the organic, physical, and scientifically knowable aspects of humankind's suffering resulted in a total and cathartic transformation. It also insisted on a system of beliefs that may, to some degree, have contributed to the difficulties facing those who have espoused behavioral/developmental integration in pediatrics.

The demands of medical professionalization are marked not only by the personal sacrifice that is so commonly quoted. They also require surviving a process which Korsch (Werner, Adler, Robinson, & Korsch, 1979) has described as "the Medical Crucible"—which is significantly driven by the belief in the existence of a scientifically knowable "right answer" and "cure" for all ailments. This requires in turn a type of psychological equilibrium that must settle on the side of scientific absolutism at its extreme, and at the least an abhorrence of the ambiguous.

Greater specialization and categorization of human disorders as minutely analyzable mechanisms would naturally contribute to this view of medicine. The adoption of this professional life philosophy would leave little room for equivocation or relativistic thinking. Not surprisingly, the evolution of greater and greater medical scientific breakthroughs that has characterized the last 40 years of medicine has been paralleled by greater and greater subspecialization. This subspecialization has in turn, in many quarters of medicine, further amplified a de-emphasis on integrative thinking.

In contrast, child psychiatry, and psychiatry in general, owing to its focus on emotions, feelings, and models of interpersonal functioning, adopted during the same period of the 1920s and 1930s a more phenomenologic model. Psychoanalysis was less quantifiable than it was richly descriptive. Behaviorism, more popular with certain segments of experimental psychology and more quantitative and categorical, was not embraced by psychiatry on the whole. The schism that initially developed between the medical organic model of pediatrics and the phenomenology of child psychiatry has only deepened during more recent decades. Requiring psychiatrists to take less and less in the way of a traditional medical internship and residency prior to psychiatric training has been a recurring postgraduate educational theme. John Romano, renowned psychiatrist and medical educator from the University of Rochester, decried this trend throughout his distinguished academic and teaching career.

A distinct minority of proponents of integration have achieved some degree of prominence. From the arena of adult psychiatry were the classical psychosomaticists of the 1940s and 1950s, Franz Alexander being the most notable. In the field of internal medicine, George Engel, another Rochesterian, crossed over to conduct landmark research on the interplay of emotional and physical health. However, those who would integrate emotional and somatic considerations in health and illness swam against the main current of specialization in the academic world.

The decades from the 1950s to the present have seen the evolution of great structures of medical specialization and subspecialization. This is particularly true for the fields of pediatrics and internal medicine. Spectacular technologic and biochemical research advances have characterized medicine during the last 40 years. Infants born at 26 weeks gestation not only regularly survive, they have a high likelihood of developing normally. As little as 30 years ago, those infants would have been considered nonviable fetuses. Scientific advances in the subspecialty of neonatology have been responsible, and not surprisingly, that subspecialty has attained a prestigious place in most academic pediatric departments. Just as predictable has been the high proportion of revenue that neonatology presently brings into any hospital's department of pediatrics.

As has been the case for ambulatory general pediatrics, there has been significantly greater emphasis over the years on other inpatient-oriented subspecialties and on intensive care. During the 1978 Task Force on Pediatric Education's (American Academy of Pediatrics, 1978) deliberations, its chairman, Henry Kempe, noted that the relative underemphasis on areas such as general ambulatory practice and behavior and development in pediatric residency education ran contrary to real life pediatric practice and the needs of the nation's children. While no one would argue against the fact that the advances obtained by inpatient and intensive care oriented subspecialties have contributed to the health of children, there has clearly been a parallel shift in pediatric "subcultural emphasis" away from behavior and development.

Once again, there have been notable movements and pioneering contributions from pediatricians interested in behavior and development. Since the 1978 Task Force, there have been ever increasing demands on academic institutions to implement behavioral and developmental components in their pediatric undergraduate and residency curricula. Nevertheless, the amount of time, energy, and most importantly, resources, dedicated to behavior and development, have remained proportionately small. Moreover, and perhaps most telling, pediatric residents continue to face Korsch's "Medical Crucible" in medically intense settings and apparently identify strongly with role models in those arenas. Ironically, most residents surveyed immediately after entering into much more pedestrian settings, such as general ambulatory practice, will admit to being significantly more comfortable managing complex physical disease than common behavioral and developmental concerns of the family (Cheng, DeWitt, Savageau, & O'Connor, 1999).

History of Developmental and Behavioral Pediatrics—Swimming Against the Tide (Cohen, 1984)

Allusions to behavior exist even in the early medical writings of the Hellenistic period of medicine and certainly during ancient Roman times. Those and subsequent discourses over the centuries predating allopathic medicine often strayed from instructions on daily physical care involving feeding or changing of infants to how to respond behaviorally to an infant's disturbing cry (Kessen, 1965). However, paralleling physical medicine, attempts to consider children's behavior and their developmental "trajectory" in a formal manner, using even quasi-scientific methods, again waited until after the beginning of the twentieth century.

We first begin to see signs of individual pediatrician interest and involvement in the child development "movement" in this country around the 1930s and 1940s. Milton Senn, one of the founding fathers of developmental and behavioral pediatrics chronicled this in his section on "Pediatricians and Child Development" in his broader monograph on the child development movement in the United States (1975). Luminaries such as Arnold Gesell, Alfred Washburn, and C. Anderson Aldrich contributed to a rich and insightful early period, but not always within the mainstream of pediatrics or nascent pediatric academic departments. Senn himself, Sally Provence, Morris Wessell, Morris Green, Julius Richmond, T. Berry Brazelton, Arthur Hawley Parmelee, Barbara Korsch, Stanford Friedman, and others, continued to work to integrate their research findings into pediatric practice and training during the 1950s, 1960s and early 1970s.

Richmond, former U.S. Surgeon General, in 1967 made a strong case for behavior and development's inclusion into the practice of primary care pediatrics by calling it "the basic science of pediatrics" (1967). That period of time, as documented by the 1978 Task Force on Pediatric Education, was not, however, characterized by a significant inclusion of development and behavior in pediatric training. Nevertheless, there were, largely due to the perseverance of those pioneers, early fellowships in developmental and behavioral pediatrics. In 1959, the W. T. Grant Foundation first sponsored behavioral fellowships. By the following year, there were three such fellowships and an equal number in more traditional "developmental" pediatrics, emphasizing developmental disabilities. The disabilities arena, which would be destined to split away, contributed to the beginning of the "University Affiliated Facilities" in the 1960s for the training of professionals in developmental disabilities. In 1960, the American Academy of Pediatrics recognized the field by forming the Section on Developmental and Behavioral Pediatrics, one of its first formal sections.

By the late 1970s momentum had built within the pediatric educational, governmental, and philanthropic arenas to increase the amount of attention given to development and behavior in pediatric training. Starting in 1978, the W. T. Grant Foundation funded programs in 11 pediatric academic departments to provide fellowship training and also to foster residency training in developmental and behavioral pediatrics. This was further built upon in 1986 via additional funding for developmental and behavioral pediatric fellowships provided by the U.S. Maternal and Child Health Bureau.

In contrast to the building of a new subspecialty of developmental and behavioral pediatrics via the funding of fellowship programs, the Robert Wood Johnson Foundation began to fund general pediatric academic fellowship programs in six original university-based pediatric departments in the late 1970s. A major emphasis was to be placed on developmental and behavioral pediatrics. It is of interest that those original programs have produced an equal number of academic leaders in the subspecialty of developmental and behavioral pediatrics as the Grant Foundation fellowships. Another positive influence was massive federal support starting in 1977 to 48 departments of pediatrics throughout the country to heighten pediatric residency training in the areas of ambulatory care and continuity of care (Society for Developmental and Behavioral Pediatrics, 1999). Within those specific areas were strongly imbedded content and skills related directly to child development and behavior.

Advising and directing the governmental and private foundation funding of the training movement were many of the members of the original generation of pioneers in developmental and behavioral pediatrics. Visionaries such as Stanford Friedman and T. Berry Brazelton were advisors to foundations and the government and also directors of major fellowship training programs. These nationally funded programs and numbers of others to follow, collaborated with colleagues from the fields of child psychology, child psychiatry, and developmental disabilities to develop or expand already existing programs of research in various aspects of developmental and behavioral pediatrics. As of 1998, there were approximately 50 fellowship programs in developmental and behavioral pediatrics throughout the United States.

It should therefore not be surprising that a parallel movement developed to establish a professional society to organize the efforts of this pediatric subspecialty. The Society for Developmental and Behavioral Pediatrics (SDBP) was formed in 1982 and presently has a membership of approximately 640 members. The society is open to all professionals involved in clinical and/or academic pursuits in the field of developmental and behavioral pediatrics. While 80% of the membership is comprised of physicians, the decision to have open membership is a reflection of the collaborative nature of the discipline and its society (1999).

Professional colleagues from disciplines such as child psychology, child psychiatry, early education, and early intervention, have played active membership and leadership roles in the society. They have conducted research and described research models of collaborative practice in child development and behavior. They have directly reinforced the benefits of collaborative practice while helping to mold Society procedures and statements, affecting in turn regional and national public policy concerning collaboration.

The American Academy of Pediatrics (AAP) Section on Developmental and Behavioral Pediatrics, one of the academy's most active and largest sections, does not have the same emphasis on academic pursuit as SDBP. In theory, it also does not promote developmental and behavioral pediatrics as a subspecialty, and does not include the breadth of professional collaboration within its membership, as does SDBP. Nevertheless, the section has approximately 720 members, close in number to SDBP. In fact, there is significant overlap between the two groups, at least among pediatricians.

The original formation of SDBP was not without controversy. Perhaps the most significant debate was whether to split away from general ambulatory pediatrics to form a separate society in the first place. This would effectively define a separate subspecialty group, and might negatively affect long-standing efforts by the discipline to have development and behavior seen as essential to the mainstream of daily general pediatric practice.

When considering the relative success or lack of success in "winning over" trainees and general pediatric practitioners to an integrative approach to primary care, does defining oneself as a subspecialist do harm to the argument? From a practical standpoint, having a subspecialty of developmental and behavioral pediatrics could well lead to the typical general pediatrician ignoring development and behavior even more in deference to the "specialist" to whom he/she could always refer. The obvious flaw with that is, as defined by membership in either SDBP or the AAP section, there are far too few developmental and behavioral pediatricians to refer to.

The value of formal recognition as a pediatric subspecialty includes the status accorded subspecialties in academic and medical financial circles. The latter, for a cognitively oriented subspecialty such as developmental and behavioral pediatrics, is less strictly for monetary gain than for improved recognition of the discipline. As with other subspecialties, scientific endeavors by the workers in the field have increasingly been directed toward evidence-based research involving clinical interventions. In any event, much of the debate has been made moot by the recent granting of developmental and behavioral pediatrics subspecialty board certification status.

FACTORS AFFECTING DEVELOPMENTAL AND BEHAVIORAL INTEGRATION

As previously mentioned, evidence has existed for the relative lack of integration of developmental and behavioral pediatrics into the mainstream of pediatric practice. Major proposed impediments to progress—medical education and training, personality characteristics of pediatricians, lack of successful models of practice integration, and current patterns of pediatric office practice, will be reviewed. The broad issue of medical economics and managed care will not be directly addressed. We will conclude by considering implications for further program and research development.

Developmental and Behavioral Training and Its Use in Practice

Although, as noted, developmental and behavioral pediatric fellowships existed in the 1960s, the efforts of the Grant and Johnson Foundations and the federal government in the late 1970s and early 1980s were the main impetus to the training movement. The controversy of whether to approach integration via pediatric generalism and ambulatory care, or via the establishment of a defined subspecialty of developmental and behavioral pediatrics was lessened by the formal adoption by the Society for Developmental and Behavioral Pediatrics of integration via teaching as one of its major missions.

The relative lack of training and lack of attention to developmental and behavioral issues in primary care pediatric practice was both accepted and largely documented around the time of the 1978 Task Force on Pediatric Education (American Academy of Pediatrics, 1978). Shonkoff, Dworkin, Leviton, and Levine (1979), conducted an extensive pediatrician report survey covering the five New England states and revealed a significant lack of attention, lack of experience and training, and lack of informed approach to developmental and behavioral issues in general practice. Hickson, Altmeier, and O'Connor (1983), conducted a similar survey in Tennessee, including a parental report component. While not asking specifically about parental satisfaction, they did document confirmation by the parents of an apparent lack of interest in and expertise by pediatricians in parental developmental and behavioral concerns. Of note was that of the seven most common concerns parents had about their children, all but one were in developmental or behavioral domains. Costello (1986) performed an extensive review of the literature existent to the early 1980s and largely confirmed these findings.

In addition to the various educational efforts, the American Academy of Pediatrics, Committee on Psychosocial Aspects of Child and Family Health (1982) issued its report entitled "Pediatrics and the Psychosocial Aspects of Child and Family Health." It made reference to the term "The New Morbidity," a term used by Robert Haggerty and Julius Richmond describing the modern needs of families—needs involving children's development and behavior. A call to better prepare pediatricians to address development and behavior in daily practice was central to the report. With liberal grant and government funding and the apparent support of pediatrics as a profession, one could have reasonably expected major progress over the next 20 years. Several important caveats existed, and continue to exist, however.

First, the most effective training vehicle for developmental and behavioral integration in practice was only just being established in the early 1980s. The longitudinal, ideally weekly, attendance of residents in a "continuity clinic" practice was and is the ideal site for practical training on the integration of development and behavior in pediatrics. With the University of Rochester and a handful of other exceptions, most pediatric residency programs in that era, and for years to follow, either had no true continuity clinics or those clinics were indirectly undermined in various ways. The undermining of continuity clinic teaching continues to this day, largely due to the service demands of inpatient and intensive care rotations. Moreover, as the Ambulatory Pediatrics Association special interest group on continuity clinic education has noted, in the present era of Medicaid Managed Care, there are significant pressures to shorten visit lengths for residents and limit available formal faculty precepting. Moreover, not all continuity clinic programs have a formal developmental and behavioral integration curriculum, let alone developmental and behavioral faculty available to teach via the continuity model.

In addition, the relative amount of time and resources dedicated to development and behavior, while more than the 1970s, has been limited. Despite significant effort and lobbying, the most recent 1997 Pediatric Residency Review Committee (RRC) requirements for Developmental and Behavioral Pediatrics (Accreditation Council for Graduate Medical Education, 1997) are embodied by a one-month block rotation out of a potential 36 months of residency training. It should be noted that related rotations in adolescent medicine are required, and recent experiences in developmental disabilities "recommended." Faculty trained in development and behavior have, as a direct result of the fellowship movement, increased and many departments of pediatrics have sections or divisions of developmental and behavioral pediatrics (many others do not). However, these divisions are generally small and often underfunded, owing largely to the nature of cognitive versus procedural service reimbursement and recent federal cuts in academic program support. Frazier et al. (1999) recently surveyed 148 pediatric residency training programs concerning developmental and behavioral pediatric training. Fully 95% reported the required block rotation, with 87% noting a formal curriculum. However, consistently identified as barriers to success were lack of adequate faculty, time, money, and curricular resources.

Relatedly, an underinvestigated, but often discussed phenomenon is the relative lack of prestige in many academic departments that developmental and behavioral pediatrics holds. Some of this may be attributable to funding, the relative youth of the field, and the associated lack until recently of board certification. In addition, the ability to produce large numbers of scholarly works of substance in the field, especially given resource limitations and clinical productivity demands, is less than in more traditional organically oriented subspecialties. Moreover, in accordance with Korsch's "Medical Crucible" model of professionalization, it is not surprising that a significantly greater number of pediatricians, regardless of their eventual career paths, would tend to identify more with teachers of intensive care and technologically-based subspecialties.

Despite disadvantages faced by those pursuing academic career roles in developmental and behavioral pediatrics, efforts by that discipline to affect postgraduate pediatric education have continued. In 1997, a multidisciplinary committee of the Society for Developmental and Behavioral Pediatrics, partially funded by the Maternal and Child Health Bureau (MCHB) of the Department of Health and Human Services compiled and published extensive guidelines on pediatric residency training in developmental and behavioral pediatrics. Published in the *Journal of Developmental and Behavioral Pediatrics* as a supplement (Coury, Berger, Stancin, & Tanner, 1999), the guidelines spanned a number of important educational areas. Covered were core requirements for pediatric residency accreditation for developmental and behavioral pediatrics, an extensively crafted summary of essential elements of developmental and behavioral knowledge, methods for curricular implementation and evaluation, a nosology of childhood developmental and behavioral disorders and services, general resources, professional competencies, communication skills, and assessment methods.

Direct evidence of an effect of increased residency training in developmental and behavioral pediatrics over the last 20 years is sparse. Studies that document resident and new graduate practitioners' inclusion of developmental and behavioral considerations in typical practice contacts are essentially nonexistent. Descriptive follow-up surveys document mixed opinions by pediatricians about their developmental and behavioral pediatrics training experiences and their utility.

Nevertheless, there is evidence that some progress is being made at the level of primary care practice. Dobos, Dworkin, and Bernstein (1994), replicated Shonkoff et al., (1979) previously cited pediatrician report study 15 years later, using a more circumscribed population of New England pediatricians. They noted that pediatricians reported a significantly higher rate of both identification and referral of children with developmental problems than the sample 15 years previously. They also reported more appropriate approaches to further evaluation of children with suspected, but not yet confirmed problems.

Clearly, pediatrician self-report is not as accurate as a more formal assessment of clinician behavior. Horwitz, Leaf, Leventhal, Forsyth, & Speechley (1992) studied a cohort of 50 pediatricians and 20 pediatric nurse practitioners in the New Haven, Connecticut area. They documented the likelihood of behavioral problems and concerns in primary care patients prior to outpatient visits via administration of Achenbach's Child Behavior Checklist. They also provided pediatric practitioners a very simple 13-item developmental-behavioral screen to use with their patients. A much higher rate of identification of the problems was documented. Moreover, practitioners were much more involved with the problems and engaged in more appropriate referrals. Both positive findings were amplified in situations where the clinician had greater opportunities for a continuing care relationship with the family.

However, qualifications to this apparent success must be noted. In a recent broader study of pediatrician behavior during routine office visits, Cheng et al. (1999) note a much lower rate of physician involvement in both preventive and problem oriented counseling concerning behavioral issues versus biomedical issues. Reasons given by the pediatricians included inadequate time, lack of parental initiation of discussion about the behavioral concerns, and pessimism about being able to provide anything of help, including referral to competent behavioral health intervention.

A series of recent studies conducted by the American Academy of Pediatrics sponsored "PROS" Network (Pediatric Research in Office Settings) (Kelleher et al., 1997) have failed to show significant increases in the identification of developmental or behavioral problems by pediatricians. In fact, where increases were superficially apparent compared to past decades, those increases disappeared when the overall increase in prevalence or differences in patient population risk were controlled for. Insurance status, and hence socioeconomic status did not play a role in this lack of real improvement. One factor that did seem to result in greater pediatrician involvement in developmental and behavioral areas was, as in the Horwitz et al. (1992) study, if there was a more consistent continuing care relationship between the clinician and family.

This apparently conflicting body of research concerning pediatrician involvement after increased training efforts must be viewed cautiously. Studies quoted varied according to a number of different factors and dimensions. Critically important differences included whether data was from physician self-reporting versus parental report versus more objective measures, such as billing records and insurance referral information. Also important was whether the study was purely descriptive of otherwise unchanged patterns of office practice or whether quasi-interventions occurred, such as the use of the 13-item screen by physicians in the Horowitz et al. (1992) study.

From this review of the existing literature, reasonable conclusions about the effects of increased developmental and behavioral training over the last two decades include:

1. Practicing pediatricians appear more informed (or at least believe they are) about developmental and behavioral concepts and the potential approach to them.
2. Actual routine screening, intervention, and discussion of those areas with parents in standard office visits may be more variable, and may not have changed comparing the present managed care era versus 20 years ago. Factors affecting this may be perceived inadequate time and in given communities, perceived lack of effective behavioral health referral agencies.
3. Identification of problems, limited office interventions, and appropriate referral may be more likely if clinicians have at their disposal easily useable screening tools, or at least a practical means of actively eliciting parental concerns.
4. Involvement of pediatricians with developmental and behavioral concerns appears more likely, independent of screening aids, if the clinician has greater familiarity with and more of a continuing care relationship with the family.

Pediatrician Personality

The skills and types of patient interactions that are involved with developmental and behavioral issues and those required by more biomedically-oriented specialties could, in theory, attract different clinicians. Pediatricians who actively seek to incorporate developmental and behavioral issues could be different from others along intrinsic personality or cognitive style dimensions. This might also explain the findings of relative avoidance of development and behavior by some primary care pediatric practitioners in their daily family encounters.

Unfortunately there exists relatively little to support or refute that hypothesis in the medical literature. Sporadic studies of personality type have appeared over the decades involving other medical specialties. Work showing relatively distinct and homogeneous personality and temperament traits among surgeons (Schwartz et al., 1994) has been published recently. Other clusterings across specific specialties or subspecialties have not been discovered. Extensive personality trait research has been conducted by family medicine, particularly involving factors related to the choice of family medicine as a career track (Taylor, Clark, & Sinclair, 1990; Bland, Meurer, & Maldonado, 1995; and Carmel & Glick, 1996). Choice of an ambulatory general practice career in family medicine appears, from the literature, as much determined by external experiences, such as with role models, as by intrinsic personality factors. No such information exists concerning pediatricians or concerning pediatrician preference for or aversion to developmental and behavioral issues.

Screening Tools and "Practice Curricula" for Development and Behavior

While the issues of adequate reimbursement and the effects of managed care will not be directly discussed, economic and time limitations have been repeatedly cited as major disincentives to developmental and behavioral integration in pediatric practice. Given the high volume, brief contact nature of primary care pediatrics, there continues a constant tension between enough time and attention to important developmental and behavioral issues in the typical office encounter, and efficiency.

This has led over the years to proliferation of developmental and behavioral screening tools for use in primary care pediatric practices. Most of those tools are promoted for their ability to be rapidly self-administered by parents, or by non-M.D. office staff. On the other end of the spectrum have been extensive efforts to define specific "curricula" in development and behavior for practitioners to essentially add to already existing pediatric practice routines.

Developmental and Behavioral Screening

At a minimum, the pediatric practitioner who is involved with developmental and behavioral issues with her patients should be able to identify children and families at risk for potential problems in the developmental or behavioral domains. Several studies over the years have documented that informal pediatrician "impressions" of normality or risk for developmental and behavioral problems are largely inaccurate and will result in significant under identification. More reliable and systematic methods of identification of such children and families are therefore critical. One theoretical means of accomplishing this is via in office developmental and behavioral screening (Glascoe, 2000). Over the years, a number of developmental and behavioral screening tools have been developed and their promotion has become a central part of evolving national standards of primary care practice (Meisels, 1989).

Inherent to an objective consideration of the value of such screening is the basic question of accuracy versus facility and speed of use. Given survey feedback from pediatricians that they would be more likely to address development and behavior if they had at their disposal "quick" screening tools, the number of such instruments has increased steadily over the last several decades. The Denver Developmental Screening Test (DDST), the Child Behavior Checklist, the Pediatric Symptom Checklist, and the Parent's Evaluation of Developmental Status (Glascoe, 2000; Meisels, 1989; Achenbach & Ruffle, 2000; Jellinek et al., 1999), are better known examples of this growth. However, significant debate within professional circles continues concerning the accuracy and appropriateness of screening tools, whether their consistent use would lead to better outcomes, and whether even the shortest of screening tools are actually used with any regularity by most pediatricians (Stancin & Palmero, 1997).

Developmental Surveillance

As a counterpoint to the systematic use of screening tools, Dworkin (1989) has offered the alternative of "developmental surveillance," citing past difficulties in both integrating developmental and behavioral screening and limited intervention into primary care practice (Dworkin, Allen, Geertsma, Solkoskie, & Cullina, 1987), and limits on the accuracy of past tests, particularly the DDST. Developmental surveillance is a broadly-based "approach" during the longitudinal process of providing primary health maintenance visits ("Well-Child Care Visits"). It is a combination of observations made by knowledgeable clinicians during the multiple encounters that make up the standard schedule of well-child visits in addition to anticipatory guidance involving key, stage-specific developmental and behavioral issues. It includes the process of actively eliciting and responding to parental concerns, often, as the above noted studies reflect, concerning development and behavior.

As Dworkin points out, developmental surveillance does not preclude the concurrent use of well-chosen developmental screening tests. However, in many respects, developmental surveillance, in its fullest manifestations, requires a restructuring of typical office interchanges, imposing a type of developmental and behavioral "curriculum." Dworkin has successfully trained pediatricians in developmental surveillance as part of his ChildServ project (see below), although the vast majority of pediatric practices are not presently set up to accomplish such a shift.

Practice Curricula for Development and Behavior

Once having reliably discovered a potential or actual area of concern, the pediatric clinician is faced with how to proceed with that information. Should one immediately refer to a subspecialist? Should one begin to set up a plan for intervention? This raises the question of more extensive involvement with developmental and behavioral issues. In order to address this, several developmental and behavioral office-based practice "curricula" have been proposed. Unfortunately, as will be evident, this has added significantly to the dilemma of time limitation and modification of established daily practice routine.

Bright Futures

The National Center for Education in Maternal and Child Health (1994) via funding from the U.S. Maternal and Child Health Bureau, published in 1994 the 270-page "Guidelines for Health Supervision of Infants, Children, and Adolescents" titled "Bright Futures." It outlines in some detail recommendations at each of the American Academy of Pediatrics' preventive health care visits concerning physical assessment, laboratory screening, immunization, longitudinal and interval medical history taking, developmental and behavioral assessment, anticipatory guidance, nutrition and safety counseling, and advice about child rearing. It is without doubt the most comprehensive and detailed road map of children's health care supervision ever compiled. A major emphasis is on the areas of development and behavior. Ideas and examples of integration of the massive amount of material are part of the manual. Planned for release in early 2002, "Bright Futures in Practice: Mental Health" will develop consensus guidelines for mental health promotion and substance abuse prevention as integral parts of child health supervision. To date, there is no published information on systematic attempts at putting all or most of the Bright Futures curriculum into effect in primary care pediatric practices.

Advice Giving and Limited Preventive Intervention

In the area of advice giving and preventive intervention, Glascoe, Oberklaid, Dworkin, and Trimm (1998) have recently reviewed 114 studies of parent education and counseling that can be accomplished in office. The purpose was to determine what methods that were brief and realistic for pediatric offices could be considered for inclusion in an integrated approach. The methods included verbal suggestions, videotapes, information handouts, hand-held health records, role playing and modeling. They do note that such brief interventions and aids cannot be utilized with parents dealing with significant emotional/personal stress.

Touchpoints

The Touchpoints National Initiative is a program based on the lifelong work of T. Berry Brazelton and has been developed over the last several years. While not limited to pediatricians, it is being utilized to bring a more effective developmental and behavioral approach to pediatric practice. The Touchpoints model (Brazelton, 1999) focuses on prevention by establishing working and trusting relationships between parents and various professional providers. Basic principles taught to those trained in Touchpoints are:

1. Use of the overt behavior of the child as a language of communication with parents;
2. Focusing on and using as a basis of trust, the existing strengths of the given family;
3. Acknowledging and addressing strong underlying emotional themes of families; and
4. Valuing and using the evolving relationship between the provider and the family to effect change and acceptance of new approaches to child rearing.

An essential assumption of the model is its conviction that attracting families to a sound healthcare, educational, and family support system, and also ensuring their consistent participation, relies on a continuum of care that begins as early as pregnancy and continues seamlessly through early childhood. The implication is that a system of care provision and family support must be interlinked and provide consistent interventive input to parents. Therefore, in its ideal application, pediatric practitioners, their support staff, hospitals, social service support agencies, and entire communities would be trained on Touchpoints. There are no published reports or studies on the efficacy of Touchpoints applications to pediatric practice to date. Nevertheless, given the findings of Horowitz et al. (1992) and the PROS Network (Kelleher et al., 1997), improving the parent-pediatrician relationship via Touchpoints might further amplify the practitioner's involvement with development and behavior.

The "ChildServ" Project

Funded by the Hartford Foundation, the ChildServ Project (1999) is actually an extensive, practice-support service that provides expert triage of and case coordination for families requiring developmental or behavioral services for their children. ChildServ has, for the last several years, offered to pediatric practitioners of Hartford, Connecticut a telephone answering line for their families. Once referred to the telephone service, families have a coordinated assessment of need, formal evaluations where required, assignment of home-based services where necessary, and overall coordination of referral and follow-through for early interventive services.

A critical component of the service is the formal training of participating pediatricians in a highly effective model of developmental and behavioral surveillance. Supporting the telephone triage counselors is an extensive resource inventory for related services throughout the Hartford area. The case referral and triage system, whose entrée is the telephone answering line, is manned by expertly trained care coordinators. Those care coordinators are in turn supported by a child development and behavior consultation team.

In addition, a data collection and management system allows for the documentation of outcome and the identification of significant gaps in required services. This allows for both evaluation of the efficacy of the project and also objective data about necessary system improvement. While designed primarily to support primary care pediatricians' management of potential developmental problems for their Medicaid patients, ChildServ has documented a tremendous need for early behavioral intervention.

ChildServ, as a parallel service for fulfilling the developmental and behavioral needs of young children, requires significantly less modification of pediatric office practice daily routine. As such, it is less a "practice curriculum" than an extremely helpful practice resource.

Healthy Steps National Initiative

Perhaps the most ambitious of programs to incorporate development and behavior into pediatric primary care practice is the Healthy Steps National Initiative (Guyer, Hughart, Strobino, Jones, & Scharfstein, 2000; McLearn, Zuckerman, Parker, Yellowitz, & Kaplan-Sanoff, 1998). Originating in Boston, the Healthy Steps for Young Children Program is a comprehensive model of pediatric primary care practice that has fully integrated aspects of developmental and behavioral screening, preventive counseling, and intervention. It is a complete curriculum that is presently being studied for both its efficacy and its cost feasibility across a multisite clinical practice network. Written material, video and computerized teaching aids, and training vignettes are all included in a commercially available interactive multimedia training and resource kit.

It's major innovation is the incorporation of nonpediatrician, child development specialists and enhanced developmental and behavioral services directly into the standard pattern of health maintenance. The child development specialist may conduct well-child visits concurrent with the pediatric provider or in separate sessions in the same office. Many of the teaching methods, clinical skills, and educational materials span applications similar to Touchpoints and the multitude of parent education and counseling techniques summarized by Glascoe et al. (1998).

The formal evaluation of the Healthy Steps five-year project is still in process. However, its year four evaluation (Healthy Steps Phase Three, Year Four—Final Report, 2001), which summarizes findings for the first year of the 30-month actual clinical intervention, documents positive and impressive findings in terms of parental satisfaction, identification of early risk, and initiation of varying forms of early intervention. The actual cost of the total intervention versus efficacy will not be available for at least two more years. However, given the summary of hours provided by the "Healthy Steps Specialist" (child development specialist) in office and in home visits, and the other enhanced office services, the added cost will likely be substantial.

In summary, over the last two decades, a wide spectrum of practical screening devices, parent education interventions, and curricular approaches to modifying standard primary care pediatric practices have been developed, promoted, and made readily available. Nevertheless, despite the acknowledged need, as noted previously, evidence for daily primary care practice development and behavior integration is sparse. It is of note that in major national initiatives such as Bright Futures and Healthy Steps, curricular components must be added to already existing practice activities and routines. While brief, and at times self-administered by parents or by office staff, the same can be said for most screening tools. It is here that the recurring theme voiced by practicing pediatricians may be most relevant.

TIME AND THE TRADITIONAL STRUCTURE OF PRIMARY CARE OFFICE PRACTICE: THE EPSDT SAGA

Primary care pediatric office practice is typically characterized by an equal mix of visits involving self-limited illness and so-called health maintenance or "well-child care" office visits. Relatively small numbers of visits involve highly complicated patients with serious chronic disease. Since 1967, the American Academy of Pediatrics has issued eight revisions of its "Recommendations for Preventive Pediatric Health Care." Those recommendations include a periodicity schedule for visits, list of screening tests, immunizations, areas of medical history taking, and areas of physical assessment, including regular physical exams. The most recent revision (American Academy of Pediatrics, 2000) lists fully 11 visits in the first 24 months of life. This then continues at a rate of one visit a year to age 21.

The federal government's Early and Periodic Screening, Diagnostic, and Treatment (EPSDT) service is Medicaid's comprehensive preventive pediatric health program for eligible children under the age of 21. It was defined by law as part of the Omnibus Budget Reconciliation Act of 1989 and includes periodic well-child visits, screening, vision, dental, and hearing services (Health Care Finance Administration, 2000). The specific requirements, in essence, parallel and come from the same consensus process that establishes the AAP's Recommendations for Preventive Pediatric Health Care. Moreover, most private insurance carriers who provide comprehensive preventive health care coverage for children will also use EPSDT and/or AAP standards to determine what care is paid for and required of contracted physicians.

Tremendous pressure has been exerted over the years to make EPSDT and AAP periodicity standards the primary measures of preventive care quality. Moreover, what exactly is included in each set of standards has increased steadily since 1967 and 1989 respectively. In the early 90's, a collaboration of agencies undertook to write an all-inclusive set of ideal standards for preventive services to be provided via the vehicle of the pediatrician's well-child office visits. This was the previously described "Bright Futures" (National Center for Education in Maternal and Child Health, 1994). As a compendium of practice activities and topics, Bright Futures has been hailed publicly as a landmark in the establishment of quality markers for preventive care. It includes extensive screenings and limited intervention for risk for accidents, school function, sensory deficits, and development and behavior.

Over the last several years of escalating managed care "penetrance" and the associated increasing pressures to see more patients over less time, for less reimbursement, formal and expanded practice guidelines, such as EPSDT and Bright Futures, have been privately viewed by most pediatricians as totally impractical. As a tacit acknowledgement of this reality, neither the federal government nor the private insurance industry has sought to enforce any of the specific within visit recommendations save for the most basic of biomedically oriented, traditional services. Those have included the routine physical exam, immunizations, and a relatively limited number of strictly medical screening tests.

All of this must be viewed with the knowledge that the length of time that the average pediatrician is able to spend on each well-child visit now averages 17.8 minutes (Goldstein, Dworkin, & Bernstein, 1999). While this is woefully inadequate to even begin to address the addition of behavioral and developmental issues or for that matter the expansive expectations of Bright Futures, it is considerably more than the 10.3 minutes documented in 1980. Gavin, Adams, and Herz (1998) sampled EPSDT Medicaid performance and noted increasing pressure on providers to expand access to services and breadth of services provided. Little substantive improvement was noted. They concluded that inadequate base funding with increasing performance expectations is to blame. Perhaps even more of a hindrance has been the ever increasing demand by various public agencies for repetitive, time and office resource-consuming, paper-report generation.

In addition, several recent studies have documented that pediatricians and families do not themselves even comply with the periodicity schedules unless forced to (Byrd, Hoekelman, & Auinger, 1999; Richardson, Shelby-Harrington, Krowchuk, Cross, & Williams, 1994; Mustard, Mayer, Black, & Postl, 1996). In Monroe County, New York, pediatrician compliance with periodicity schedules for privately insured families was 68% and for publicly funded children 52%. The greatest degree of compliance was for the first two years of life when immunizations were most prevalent and at times when required for school entry. Many other factors, such as family no-shows for scheduled visits, also impacted the compliance rate.

Given the pressures that pediatricians state they face in terms of adequate time for behavioral and developmental integration, it would appear that the density of EPSDT and AAP requirements contribute significantly to the problem. Moreover, the typical busy pediatrician is often forced to approach each patient's well-child visit in a lock-step preconscribed manner, driven largely by the bare minimums of the biomedical EPSDT requirements with hardly enough time to complete them.

That would be bad enough, but it is not altogether clear what of the EPSDT and AAP well-child care visit requirements are of worth, aside from immunizations. Hoekelman, a strong advocate for preventive health care for children has for years argued that there is little evidence that the density of well-child visits, as presently constructed under EPSDT and AAP guidelines, provide valuable positive outcomes for children (Hoekelman, 1983, 1975). A review of the literature confirms this. There are no systematic studies showing that the present density of visits, or even much of the present preventive content, has any particular efficacy. In fact, the original backbone of visit periodicity was concretized by tradition, and to a lesser degree, the immunization schedule.

Hoekelman has argued that in an era of tight medical resources and financial remuneration we might do well to consider reallocating some precious health care dollars by cutting back the total number of well-child visits (1983). In fact, via an early study of the efficiency of pediatric nurse practitioners, he showed a number of years ago that similar health outcome could be obtained by both using nurse practitioners as well-child care visit providers and also cutting the total number of visits (Hoekelman, 1975).

Osborn (1994), has concurred with Hoekelman that "the value of office-based preventive interventions, such as child health supervision, is generally unproven." She has argued for a thorough and hard-nosed re-evaluation of the goals of well-child care visits and how to best attain them. Rosenbaum and Johnson (1986) have questioned whether we are clear about our goals for children's preventive health care, especially for children from lower socioeconomic conditions who are often on Medicaid and under EPSDT standards of care. They have emphasized the need for this given the long-standing tendency to fund Medicaid at a significantly lower level than employers for private insurance coverage. Stuart and Weinrich (1998) have suggested reconsideration of traditional assumptions about primary care preventive health visits given medical financing realities across socioeconomic strata.

Several others, including Haggerty (1987; Stickler, 1967; Yankauer, 1973) have questioned the actual value of the number repetitive nature of well-child visits over the last 25-30 years. The fact that no comprehensive studies documenting their value have been conducted would seem on the surface to raise a dilemma. However, Sardell and Johnson (1998), in recently reviewing the politics of EPSDT, have concluded that the major shift in funding that would be required by a more comprehensive consideration of all that is ostensibly required by EPSDT guidelines is unlikely to occur—primarily for political and economic reasons.

Margolis and colleagues at the University of North Carolina, in collaboration with the National Initiative for Child Healthcare Quality (NICHQ), have undertaken, with a network of other investigators throughout the country, an extensive project to redefine the nature of pediatric primary care practice. Funded by the Bureau of Primary Health Care and the Commonwealth Fund, that initiative has as its specific aim "to test and refine methods and tools to improve preventive and developmental care for children seen in community health centers." The ultimate goal of the collaborative is "to help practices and community agencies achieve improved preventive and developmental outcomes for families and children."

The collaborative intends to accomplish that goal by developing:

1. More efficient practice-based systems to organize prevention and developmental services,
2. Innovative approaches and tools for conducting preventive and developmental assessments,
3. Effective approaches for providing preventive intervention, and
4. Techniques for streamlining referral processes and making connections to community support agencies for the provision of developmental family-based services. (P. Margolis, personal communication).

A Practical Problem

As we have described, the history of developmental and behavioral pediatrics has been remarkably consistent in its repeated calls for greater involvement of practicing pediatricians with development and behavior in daily primary care practice. Despite the development of easily implemented screening tools, extensive practice guidelines, and major initiatives in postgraduate residency and subspecialty training, there appears to have been relatively little increase in the actual daily involvement of the practicing pediatrician with developmental and behavioral issues.

An equally consistent trend has been for governmental agencies and professional advisory bodies, primarily through the vehicle of EPSDT, to add increasing performance demands to the typical nonillness related pediatric "well-child" health maintenance visit. Highly desirable components such as advice on safety, safe sexual practices, and smoking cessation are only a few of the ever expanding recommended elements of the well-child visit. However, as Hoekelman and Osborne would agree, in some cases, the effectiveness of many such brief office interventions is simply not known.

In addition, liability concerns of schools, athletic programs for children, and child care centers have dramatically increased the repetitive and time consuming paper work load for primary care office staff and nurses. This is amplified even further in Medicaid predominated clinic practices where governmental report forms, insurance eligibility confirmation, child protection agency documents, and complex referral processes add dramatically to administrative workload. It should therefore not be surprising that many of the "quick" office screens for development and behavior that are meant to by-pass busy pediatricians and make use of their office staff and nurses may be valued, but not implemented.

A "Modest Proposal"

The dilemma of pediatric practice pattern inertia just described must be addressed by any serious effort to increase attention given to development and behavior by practicing pediatricians. As we promote the types of innovation and knowledge presented at this symposium, it will be critical to also consider how to aid pediatric practitioners in their attempts to reform their daily practice routines. This may well require future projects and research to focus not only on the content of developmental and behavioral integration, but also on the practical steps to actually bring implementation to fruition.

Above all else, it is critical to recognize the need to ally ourselves with practicing pediatricians in their struggles to be more efficient and effective. Simply adding more performance expectations on already saturated office sessions, as history has shown, will not likely bring about practice behavioral change among pediatric clinicians. Combined collaborative research by experts in developmental and behavioral practice content and in primary care practice efficiency will be essential.

Various limited studies, largely grant funded and based in academic centers, have documented how specific information system innovations can both save time, but also allow office staff and physicians to reallocate that time to more effective direct care activities (Shiffman, Brandt, & Freeman, 1997). Little if any research exists on both how to save time in offices and reallocate the savings to office-based efforts with development and behavior. Furthermore, in the present managed care era, we have very little data or objective evidence about whether capital and resources are available to either private or public Medicaid funded pediatric practices to install such systems.

Six years ago, an expansive article in the pediatric literature described the ideal pediatric primary care office of the twenty-first century (Zurhellen, 1995). That practice was characterized by efficiency, organization, but most of all modern time- and effort-saving information systems that would solve many typical office and nursing staff workload problems. We have little research data to convince us that even a small portion of primary care pediatric practices are presently equipped with such resources. We know even less about whether offices that are so equipped use those systems for anything other than more efficient billing. Linking studies of development and behavior integration in practice with improved practice time expenditure may lead the way to more practitioner acceptance of integration.

For example, studies displaying the effectiveness of parental report screening questionnaires that are administered by office staff may need to be linked to computer applications that save time for that same office staff. Implementation of developmental surveillance by groups of pediatric providers may need to be associated with concurrent reduction in repetitive EPSDT visit content that proves ineffective, superfluous, and time intensive. Evolving research efforts by organizations such as NICHQ should help us to identify what of ESPDT standards are worth retaining and what should be discarded in favor of other important elements, especially those related to development and behavior. A more direct collaboration between the Society for Developmental and Behavioral Pediatrics and the American Academy of Pediatrics' Section on Computers and Other Technologies ("SCOT") may be worthy of investigation.

Other "lower-tech" practice improvements that save time and effort for pediatric practice offices are also possible and need further investigation. As an example, a somewhat older practice innovation, the "group well-child care visit" has been described by Osborn as a means of providing more cost-efficient anticipatory guidance and preventive advice to families (Osborn, 1985). A more recent iteration of these pediatric practice parent-child group sessions investigated their efficacy with a socially high-risk parent group. Taylor and associates were able to show equal effectiveness of anticipatory guidance provided via high-risk parent-child groups with a single clinician as compared to high-risk parents and children who received traditional individualized sessions (Taylor, Roberts, & Kemper, 1997), implying greater cost benefit. Gaining time and efficiency while also developing another effective method of developmental and behavioral advice giving via group sessions would be a "win-win" situation. It would make development and behavior integration for many practitioners much more feasible.

It is important to take seriously the present generation of pediatricians who have at least received a modicum of training in development and behavior when they state they are overwhelmed by the volume and efficiency demands of managed care. Forging a research and clinical application alliance in this manner between those of us committed to development and behavior and the practicing pediatrician could eventually make possible a modern day "Modest Proposal" far more palatable than Jonathan Swift's—the restructuring of primary care pediatric practice toward greater integration of development and behavior.

REFRENCES

Accreditation Council for Graduate Medical Education, American Medical Association. (1997). *Pediatric residency review committee program requirements*. Chicago: American Medical Association.

Achenbach, T. M., & Ruffle, T. M. (2000). The Child Behavior Checklist and related forms for assessing behavior/emotional problems and competencies. *Pediatrics In Review, 21*(8), 265-271.

American Academy of Pediatrics. (1978). *Report of the task force on pediatric education: The future of pediatrics*, Evanston, IL.

American Academy of Pediatrics. (2000). *Recommendations for preventive pediatric health care* (RE9939). Evanston, IL: Author

American Academy of Pediatrics, Committee on Psychosocial Aspects of Child and Family Health. (1982). Pediatrics and the psychosocial aspects of child and family health. *Pediatrics, 70*,126-127.

Bland, C. J., Meurer, L. N., & Maldonado, G. (1995). Determinants of primary care specialty choice: Non-statistical meta-analysis of the literature. *Academic Medicine, 70*(7), 620-641.

Brazelton, T. B. (1999). How to help parents of young children: The Touchpoints model. *Journal Perinatol, 19*(6, pt. 2), S6-S7.

Byrd, R. S., Hoekelman, R. A., & Auinger, P. (1999). Adherence to AAP guidelines for well-child care under managed care. *Pediatrics, 104*(3), 536-540.

Carmel, S., & Glick, S. M. (1996). Compassionate-empathetic physicians: Personality traits and social-organizational factors that enhance or inhibit this behavior pattern. *Social Science and Medicine, 43*(8), 1253-1261.

Carnegie Task Force on Meeting the Needs of Young Children. (1994). *Starting points: Meeting the needs of our youngest children*. Waldorf, MD: Carnegie Corporation.

Cheng, T. L., DeWitt, T. G., Savageau, J. A., & O'Connor, K. G. (1999). Determinants of counseling in primary care pediatric practice. *Archives of Pediatric and Adolescent Medicine, 153*, 629-635.

Cohen, M. I. (1984). The Society for Behavioral Pediatrics: A new portal in a rapidly moving boundary. *Pediatrics, 73*(6), 791-798.

Committee on Integrating the Science of Early Childhood Development, Board on Children, Youth, and Families, National Academy of Sciences. (2000). In J. P. Shonkoff & D. A. Phillips (Eds.). *From neurons to neighborhoods: The science of early childhood development.* Washington, DC: National Academy Press.

Coury, D. L., Berger, S. P., Stancin, T., & Tanner, J. L. (1999). Curricular guidelines for residency training in developmental-behavioral pediatrics. *Journal of Developmental and Behavioral Pediatrics, 20*(2), S1-S38.

Costello, E. J. (1986). Primary care pediatrics and child psychopathology: A review of diagnostic, treatment and referral practices. *Pediatrics, 78*(6), 1044-1051.

Dobos, A. E., Dworkin, P. H., & Bernstein, B. A. (1994). Pediatricians' approaches to developmental problems: Has the gap been narrowed? *Journal of Developmental and Behavioral Pediatrics, 15*(1), 34-38.

Dworkin, P. H. (1989). British and American recommendations for developmental monitoring: The role of surveillance. *Pediatrics, 84*(6), 1000-1010.

Dworkin, P. H., Allen, D., Geertsma, M. A., Solkoskie, L., & Cullina, J. (1987). Does developmental content influence the effectiveness of anticipatory guidance? *Pediatrics, 80*(2), 196-202.

Eisenberg, L. (1988). The social context of behavioral pediatrics. *Journal of Developmental and Behavioral Pediatrics, 9*(6), 382-387.

Frazer, C., Emans, S. J., Goodman, E., Luoni, M., Bravender, T., & Knight, J. (1999). Teaching residents about development and behavior. *Archives of Pediatric and Adolescent Medicine, 153,*1190-1194.

Gavin, N. I., Adams, E. K., & Herz, E. J. (1998). The use of EPSDT and other health care services by children enrolled in Medicaid: the impact of OBRA '89. *Milbank Quarterly, 76*(2), 207-250.

Glascoe, F. P. (2000). Early detection of developmental and behavioral problems. *Pediatrics In Review, 21*(8), 272-280.

Glascoe, F. P., Oberklaid, F., Dworkin, P. H., & Trimm, F. (1998). Brief approaches to educating patients and parents in primary care. *Pediatrics, 101*(6), 10.

Goldstein, E. N., Dworkin, P. H., & Bernstein, B. (1999). Time devoted to anticipatory guidance during child health supervision visits: How are we doing? *Ambulatory Child Health, 5,* 113-120.

Green, M. (1993). Behavioral pediatrics: Its past and its future. *Journal of Developmental and Behavioral Pediatrics, 14,* 404-408.

Guyer, B., Hughart, N., Strobino, D., Jones, A., & Scharfstein, D. (2000). Assessing the impact of pediatric-based developmental services on infants, families, and clinicians: Challenges to evaluating the Healthy Steps Program. *Pediatrics, 105*(3), 33.

Haggerty, R. J. (1982). Behavioral pediatrics: Can it be taught, can it be practiced? *Pediatric Clinics of North America, 29*(2), 391-398.

Haggerty, R. J. (1987). Health supervision visits: should the immunization schedule drive the system? *Pediatrics, 79*(4), 581-582.

Hartford Foundation. (1999). *Child services annual report 1999.* Hartford, CT: Author.

Health Care Finance Administration, United States Department of Health and Human Services. (2000). *Medicaid and EPSDT.* Washington, DC: Author.

Healthy Steps Phase Three, Year Four—Final Report, The Healthy Steps for Young Children Program National Evaluation. (2001). The Johns Hopkins University School of Hygiene and Public Health, Baltimore, MD.

Hickson, G. B., Altmeier, W. A., & O'Connor, S. (1983). Concerns of mothers seeking care in private pediatric offices: Opportunities for expanding services. *Pediatrics, 72,* 619-624.

Hoekelman, R. A. (1975). What constitutes adequate well-baby care? *Pediatrics, 55*(3), 313-326.

Hoekelman, R. A. (1983). Well-child visits revisited. *American Journal of Diseases of Children, 137*(1), 12-20.

Horowitz, S. M., Leaf, P. J., Leventhal, J. M., Forsyth, B., & Speechley, K. N. (1992). Identification and management of psychosocial and developmental problems in community-based, primary care pediatric practices. *Pediatrics, 89*(3), 480-485.

Jellinek, M. S., Murphy, J. M., Little, M., Pagano, M. E., Comer, D. M., & Kelleher, K. J. (1999). Use of the Pediatric Symptom Checklist to screen for psychosocial problems in pediatric primary care: A national feasibility study. *Archives of Pediatric and Adolescent Medicine, 153*(3), 254-260.

Kelleher, K. J., Childs, G. E., Wasserman, R. C., McInerny, T. K., Nutting, P. A., & Gardner, W. P. (1997). Insurance status and recognition of psychosocial problems. A report from the Pediatric Research in Office Settings and the Ambulatory Sentinel Practice Networks. *Archives of Pediatric and Adolescent Medicine, 151*(11), 1109-1115.

Kessen, W. (1965). *The child.* New York: John Wiley.

Mahnke, C. B. (2000). The growth and development of a specialty: The history of pediatrics. *Clinical Pediatrics, 39,* 705-714.

McLearn, K. T., Zuckerman, B. S., Parker, S., Yellowitz, M., & Kaplan-Sanoff, M. (1998). Child development and pediatrics for the 21st century: The Healthy Steps approach. *Journal of Urban Health, 75*(4), 704-723.

Meisels, S. J. (1989). Can developmental screening tests identify children who are developmentally at risk? *Pediatrics, 83*(4), 578-585.

Mustard, C. A., Mayer, T., Black, C., & Postl, B. (1996). Continuity of pediatric ambulatory care in a universally insured population. *Pediatrics, 98*(6), 1028-1034.

National Center for Education in Maternal and Child Health. (1994). *Bright Futures: Guidelines for Health Supervision of Infants, Children, and Adolescents.* Arlington, VA: Author.

Osborn, L. M. (1985). Group well-child care. *Clinical Perinatology, 12*(2), 355-365.

Osborn, L. M. (1994). Effective well-child care. *Current Problems in Pediatrics, 24*(9), 306-326.

Richardson, L. A., Selby-Harrington, M. L., Krowchuk, H. V., Cross, A. W., & Williams, D. (1994). Comprehensiveness of well child checkups for children receiving Medicaid: A pilot study. *Journal of Pediatric Health Care, 8,* 212-220.

Richmond, J. B. (1967). Child development: A basic science for pediatrics. *Pediatrics, 39,* 649-658.

Rosenbaum, S., & Johnson, K. (1986). Providing health care for low-income children: Reconciling child health goals and child health financing realities. *Milbank Quarterly, 64*(3), 442-478.

Sardell, A., & Johnson, K. (1998). The politics of EPSDT policy in the 1990's: Policy entrepreneurs, political streams, and children's health benefits. *Milbank Quarterly, 76*(2), 175-203.

Schuster, M. A., Duan, N., Regalado, M., & Klein, D. J. (2000). Anticipatory guidance. What information do parents receive? What information do they want? *Archives of Pediatric and Adolescent Medicine, 154,* 1191-1198.

Schwartz, R. W., Barclay, J. R., Harrell, P. L., Murphy, A. E., Jarecky, R. K., & Donnelly, M. B. (1994). Defining the surgical personality: A preliminary study. *Surgery, 115*(1), 62-68.

Senn, M. J. E. (1975). Insights on the child development movement in the United States. *Monographs of the Society for Research in Child Development, 40*(3-4, Serial # 161).

Senn, M. J. E. (1977). Quality of services to children. *Pediatrics, 60*(5), 768.

Shiffman, R. N., Brandt, C. A., & Freeman, B. G. (1997). Transition to a computer-based record using scannable, structured encounter forms. *Archives of Pediatric and Adolescent Medicine, 151,* 1247-1253.

Shonkoff, J. P., Dworkin, P. H., Leviton, A., & Levine, M. D. (1979). Primary care approaches to developmental disabilities. *Pediatrics, 64,* 506-514.

Society for Developmental and Behavioral Pediatrics. (1999). *Petition for subspecialty boards in developmental-behavioral pediatrics.* Submitted to the American Board of Medical Specialties.

Stancin, T., & Palmero, T. M. (1997). A review of behavioral screening practices in pediatric settings: Do they pass the test? *Journal of Developmental and Behavioral Pediatrics, 18*(3),183-194.

Stickler, G. B. (1967). How necessary is the "routine check-up?" *Clinical Pediatrics, 6*(8), 454.

Stuart, M. E., & Weinrich, M. (1998). Beyond managing Medicaid costs: Restructuring care. *Milbank Quarterly, 76*(2), 251-279.

Taylor, A. D., Clark, C., & Sinclair, A. E. (1990). Personality types of family practice residents in the 1980's. *Academic Medicine, 65*(3), 216-218.

Taylor, J. A., Roberts, L. D., & Kemper, K. J. (1997). Health care utilization and health status in high-risk children randomized to receive group or individual well child care. *Pediatrics, 100*(3), 1.

U.S. Public Health Service Report of the Surgeon General's Conference on Children's Mental Health. (2000). *A national action agenda.* Washington, DC: Department of Health and Human Services.

Werner, E. R., Adler, R., Robinson, R., & Korsch, B. M. (1979). Attitudes and interpersonal skills during pediatric internship. *Pediatrics,63*(3), 491-499.

Yankauer, A. (1973). Child health supervision - is it worth it? *Pediatrics, 52*(2), 272-277.

Young, K. T., Davis, K., Schoen, C., & Parker, S. (1998). Listening to parents. A national survey of parents with young children. *Archives of Pediatric and Adolescent Medicine, 3,* 255-262.

Zurhellen, W. M. (1995). The computerization of ambulatory pediatric practice. *Pediatrics, 96*(4), 835-842.

DISCUSSION SUMMARY
written by Thomas M. Yerkey

Dr. Geertsma's presentation at the Kent State Psychology Forum began with a discussion of his concerns that in spite of a long history of acknowledgment of the need for physicians to identify children who have psychosocial problems and of the need for physicians to collaborate with mental healthcare professionals, identification and collaboration occur too rarely. The discussion finished with a few comments from other forum attendees.

Dr. Geertsma stated that very little progress has been made in identification of child psychosocial problems or on physician collaboration with mental healthcare professionals. Training and practice guidelines have been written to encourage physicians to focus more of their efforts on identification of children with psychosocial problems. Still, Dr. Geertsma asserted that physicians tend to focus on "quick and dirty treatment" of these children. The presentation included discussion of several factors that Dr. Geertsma believed might influence physician behavior when dealing with child psychosocial problems. Dr. Geertsma asserted that physicians' training, such as the type of residency or whether or not a physician had attended a pediatric residency, their knowledge of psychosocial problems, their skills in addressing psychosocial problems, and their personality could impact physician behavior. Additionally, a physician's role models, both during and after, training might impact how he or she addresses psychosocial issues. Identifying with a role model who does not believe it is a physician's role to address child psychosocial problems could reduce the chances that a physician would choose to identify and treat these problems. Further, the availability of tools that physicians can use in office settings could impact their behavior when dealing with a patient with a psychosocial problem.

Dr. Geertsma stated that collaborative work between physicians and mental healthcare professionals has been happening since the 1970s and has worked in some settings and failed in others. He asserted that the primary factor determining the success or failure of collaboration was support. In settings where the political and financial supports were there, collaboration was successful. However, Dr. Geertsma claimed that this support has been rare. Even in training settings, support for collaboration to address psychosocial problems is frequently resisted. Dr. Geertsma reported that while pediatricians have tended, in some studies, to identify more children with psychosocial problems than physicians from other disciplines, changes in pediatric residency training programs to include more focus on psychosocial issues is frequently and strongly resisted. He concluded that those working to increase physician focus on child psychosocial issues are "swimming against the tide."

Discussion following Dr. Geertsma's presentation was brief but enthusiastic. Dr. Deborah Plate, a family practitioner pointed out that the training of family practitioners is different from the training of pediatricians. She stated that the focus of the entire first month of residency for family practitioners was primarily on psychosocial issues. She emphasized that family practitioners frequently have long standing professional relationships with their patients long before they have children. Dr. Geertsma responded that family medicine is often more receptive to working with psychosocial issues than is pediatrics.

Dr. Geertsma was also asked where he would suggest putting research funds. He replied that he felt that research on collaborative programs such as that described by Carolyn Schroeder would be among the most important.

Dr. Geertsma's presentation and the discussion which followed the presentation underscored the complexity of the issues that affect the identification of children with psychosocial problems. The general feeling following his presentation was that there was still a great deal of research to be performed in this area. Additionally, Dr. Geertsma's chapter and presentation illuminated the need to understand the history of the relationship between medicine and psychology when performing research on identifying children with psychosocial problems in primary care medical practice. Much has already been tried and has not been as effective as we would like. In creating the solutions of the future, we need to avoid the pitfalls of our past.

CHAPTER 4

NEW DIRECTIONS FOR RESEARCH AND TREATMENT OF PEDIATRIC PSYCHOSOCIAL PROBLEMS IN PRIMARY CARE

Joseph Hagan, Jr.
University of Vermont College of Medicine

Mental Health needs of Children and Adolescents are increasing while access to behavioral health, mental health, and substance abuse service is decreasing.

—American Academy of Pediatrics (2000a).

INTRODUCTION

The rate of psychosocial problems identified by primary care physicians in the children they care for has increased from 7% to 18% in the past 20 years (Kelleher et al., 1997). Information accumulated by the Pediatric Research in Office Settings (PROS) Network confirmed what practicing pediatricians already know: the children we see for earaches bring with them the symptoms of their behavioral health. These children may have attentional difficulties, conduct issues or significant problems of mood. They may suffer acute adjustment difficulties or evidence posttraumatic

Treating Children's Psychosocial Problems in Primary Care, 93–115

stress from physical, emotional, or sexual abuse, family poverty, family divorce or a host of other intrinsic or situational problems that impact on their health and the ability of their family and caregivers to provide for their health.

Why this near tripling of psychosocial problems? Is this simply a phenomenon of better identification? Given better training of professionals and greater sophistication of patients and families, perhaps psychosocial problems that previously went undetected and unattended are now noted. However, Kelleher, McInerny, Gardner, Childs, and Wasserman (2000), in a further discussion of the previously cited PROS data found no association between advances in training (described below) and increased identification.

Has the experience of the child sufficiently changed in the past 20 years to bring about such an increase? Changes in perceived family structure and function have occurred. Are these changes detrimental and problem causing, or are we falsely accusing these changes simply because they are change? In comparing studies of similar populations in Rochester, New York in 1979 to 1996 (Kelleher et al., 2000), found increases in psychosocial problems, excluding mental retardation, and especially Attention-deficit Hyperactivity Disorder (ADHD). Parallel demographic changes are identified, notably poverty and single-parent families. In its soon to be published report, the American Academy of Pediatric's' Task Force on the Family (AAP, 2003) describes the contemporary American family and its many compilations and functional styles. Potential strengths and weaknesses are described, but conclusive statements regarding sources of psychological problems cannot yet be made.

Are the psychosocial issues that now surface in pediatrician's offices problems which were previously cared for in other professional settings? In the past when sadness or school failure were observed, reactive depression may have been suspected. Referral was initiated as few primary care physicians were sufficiently facile with this diagnosis or its treatment. ADHD was referred to school psychologists or psychiatric colleagues. Today's pediatrician must be prepared to deal with depression and ADHD in the primary care setting, for that is where most children receive their care. Certainly changes in health care insurance have driven changes in access to mental health services.

Most communities have greater numbers of mental health providers currently than historically, so access overall may not be diminished. But few mental health providers will see children, leading most pediatricians to complain anecdotally of little or no access. This will be discussed further later in this chapter; Dr. Rappo also considers this problem in Chapter 6.

Today's pediatrician wears many hats. The traditional morbidities related to infectious disease, congenital malformations, nutrition and others are complicated by the "new morbidities" of psychosocial problems (American Academy of Pediatrics' Committee on Psychosocial Aspects of Child and Family Health, 1993). The average office day of 25 to 30 patient visits is a mix of sick calls, well-child and problem visits, with an occasional parent conference added in. While the day might start with URI's and gastroenteritis, traditional health problems, the schedule also includes well-child visits which are preventive in focus, including social issues and growth and development, nutrition, family issues and behavior in addition to the physical exam. Problem visits and parent conferences deal with diverse issues such as headaches and sports injuries or sleep problems, or anticipatory guidance for family divorce or school failure.

Case One—Alex

Alex is new to our practice. He was fist seen for a sick call Visit soon after he and his single mom moved to the community. She works at a local bank and notes that she has had difficulties with childcare for Alex. He has been "expelled" from two childcare centers; the third has recommended referral to the state's Child Development Clinic. His first office visit if brief as his sick Problem is readily addressed. The pediatrician notes that the Child Development Clinic referral is appropriate and notes that the child was fairly active and difficult for his mother to manage, in spite of illness.

The office's next contact with Alex is in the form of a phone call from the developmentalist who saw Alex at the clinic. He notes Alex's immaturity and struggles in the social mileau. He has initiated several referrals for community-based services, especially in speech and language. He discusses that at age four "you really can't diagnose ADHD." When asked about impairment, the developmentalist agreed that there were many social impairments but was unwilling to recommend pharmacotherapy or even behavioral therapy outside of the community supports that would be provided by his local Early Essential Education program.

Soon Alex was seen for a four-year old check-up by a pediatric resident on rotation in our primary care office. This thorough evaluation included not just his physical exam and review of his medical history but also evaluation of his social needs. This is a single-parent family with few social supports in this community. Extended family are elsewhere and Alex's father has never been involved. Alex's mother has a low-level managerial job at a local financial institution and Alex is now on his sixth day care placement and again at risk for expulsion.

Continued ...

Case Two—Clancy

Clancy is a 14-year-old high school freshman. His mother called and spoke with an office nurse, expressing her concern that Clancy was depressed. She noted sad mood, flattened affect and waning interest in his schoolwork, which has been accompanied by falling grades. When the nurse astutely inquired about suicidality, Mother noted that she did not feel that he was at risk but agreed to discuss this with her husband and son.

The nurse inquired if there were firearms in their home and instructed that they be removed immediately. The nurse agreed to discuss the case with the pediatrician and would call her back within the hour. This was a family well-known to the practice, and the nurse and the pediatrician were concerned about this mother's observations. Resources to address this were not available at Clancy's school. As urgent evaluation did not appear to be warranted, a mental health referral was initiated through standard processes.

In this chapter, we will discuss the American Academy of Pediatrics' (AAP) "renewed commitment" to these new morbidities and how pediatricians do and could assist children and families who struggle with psychosocial stressors (American Academy of Pediatrics, 2001).

PRIMARY CARE AND MENTAL HEALTH SERVICES

Practitioners

Many healthcare professionals come into contact with children and families and contribute to their behavioral healthcare. In this chapter, I will discuss primary care pediatricians specifically. The distinction between family practitioners providing primary care for children and pediatricians is noted, as the training in pediatrics is distinct between these two primary care specialties. Both pediatrics and family medicine have three-year postgraduate residencies, including continuity care training. Pediatric care specializes in infants, children, and adolescents; family practice residents must also be trained in adult and geriatric care, limiting the training time available to focus on younger patients. In addition to primary care pediatricians and family physicians, other providers caring for children include pediatric nurse practitioners and family nurse practitioners. Nurse practitioners receive postgraduate nursing training in diagnosis and treatment in primary care settings. Like their pediatric and family practice colleagues, the pediatric nurse practitioner's training is focused on children and adolescents while the family nurse practitioner's training is broadened to include training of adults. Nurse practitioner training programs are similar in duration.

Residency Training in Pediatrics

Pediatrics is a science of human development. Now increased training is required in the field of child development, both normal and abnormal. Likewise, as behavioral problems have become more intrinsic to primary care pediatrics, one in five encounters reported in the PROS study, practice demands have led to research, research to expertise, expertise to focused training requirements. The Residency Review Committee of the American College of Graduate Medical Education now publishes specific requirements that a residency program must meet to graduate pediatric trainees (http://www.acgme.org/rrc/peds/PedReq_Comp.htm). In addition to training in hospital based pediatrics, neonatal intensive care and pediatric intensive care, residency programs provide a continuity primary care practice experience. Residents learn to appreciate the long-term commitment and relationship of general pediatric care "including aspects of physical and emotional growth and development, health promotion/ disease prevention, management of chronic and acute medical conditions, family and environmental impacts, and practice management" (http://www.acgme.org/rrc/peds/PedReq_Comp.htm). In this continuity experience, residents in effect create small practices under supervision. "They must devote at least one-half day per week to their continuity experience" (http://www.acgme.org/rrc/peds/PedReq_Comp.htm, p. 12) over three full years, allowing exposure to sufficient patient numbers and variety to meet educational objectives, including specific objectives in developmental and behavioral pediatrics. Residents are trained in the generalist approach to common outpatient pediatric issues, in contradistinction to the subspecialist approach of their inpatient training experience.

Residency programs must provide specific training in normal and abnormal behavior and child development from infancy through young adulthood. "The program must educate their residents in the intrinsic and extrinsic factors that influence behavior to enable them to differentiate behavior that can and should be managed by general pediatrician from behavior that warrants referral to other specialists" (http:// www.acgme.org/rrc/peds/PedReq_Comp.htm, p. 14). Components of this required training can be found at the ACGME website. (http:// www.acgme.org/rrc/peds/PedReq_Comp.htm).

On the other hand, the time available for focused study of developmental and behavioral pediatrics in the 36-month residency program is typically one month, or occasionally two. Training programs certainly vary in content and quality. It is no wonder that pediatricians entering practice feel ill prepared to deal with the large proportion of psychosocial problems their patients bring.

Pediatric Grandmothers and Grandfathers

What of the many pediatricians in primary care who completed their training in the era before the current guidelines were developed? There are few truly new diagnoses among children's psychosocial problems, but substantial advances in screening, diagnosis and, most significantly, in management techniques. Consequently, it is likely that many development or behavioral problems in children go unidentified, untreated or are under treated. Skill among board certified pediatricians in the areas of developmental pediatrics varies.

While experience is an important teacher, quality measures in behavioral health care in primary care practices are lacking. Clinical guidelines are a recent development and they are not widely known, consulted or utilized. For example, the AAP Guidelines of Diagnosis of ADHD (American Academy of Pediatrics, 2000b) were published in Spring of 2000 and the companion Treatment Guideline in Fall 2001 (American Academy of Pediatrics , 2001b). Diagnosing clinicians are reminded to apply dsm-iv criteria for diagnosis, to rule out entities that mimic ADHD but require different treatments, and to search for comorbidities. ADHD is identified as a chronic condition, indicating that treatment and follow up must be long term.

Alex, Concluded

By history and observation, Alex meets *DSM-IV* criteria for ADHD, combined type, in spite of his age. The development clinic report has just become available and its data supports this diagnosis.

Stimulants are indicated in an attempt to rescue Alex socially so that he might not lose yet another child care placement. Goals of therapy are discussed and side effects are reviewed. He is begun on a low-dose stimulant.

Phone follow-up the next week reveals remarkable response to a morning dose of a short-acting stimulant with return of his typical problem behaviors in the afternoon. Stimulant therapy is adjusted by phone and over the next four weeks a follow-up visit is scheduled. In the follow-up conversations it is noted the great difficulty that Alex's mother has in providing historic information in a clear and concise manner. A 10-item checklist is recommended for mother and school so that Alex's response can be more properly evaluated.

Continued.....

Will the guidelines be followed? An AAP Project Advisory Committee has been convened to encourage adoption of, and adherence to the new guidelines, seeking to impose a higher community standard of care. Substantial energies are being directed to AAP members to inform and to enable them to use these guidelines. Those caring for children who are not Fellows of the AAP might not benefit from this outreach.

Clinical guidelines have not yet been developed for other behavioral health disorders which could be useful to pediatricians, such as depression in childhood and adolescence, obsessive compulsive disorder and the disorders of oppositionality and conduct.

Continuing Medical Education

Consistent with its "renewed commitment" to behavioral and developmental morbidities, training in this area is a key and essential part of the American Academy of Pediatrics' continuing education efforts. This commitment reflects the AAP's core values, but also responds to practicing pediatricians, who know they need these skills and desire to provide treatments that are sensitive to child and family needs and that have good outcome.

Developmental and behavioral topics are a substantial component of the AAP's six year cycle of continuing education. At the annual National Convention and Exhibition of the AAP, a specific tract of developmental and behavioral pediatric topics is woven through a week-long, broad-based curriculum. Psychosocial teaching opportunities are well attended and (Kelleher et al., 2000) suggests a positive effect in this continuing training for pediatricians in practice.

The AAP convenes a Section on Developmental and Behavioral Pediatrics for AAP Fellows with interest or special education in this area. Through committees, the AAP derives practice guidelines, position statements, and continuing education goals. AAP was a contributor to the *Diagnostic and Statistical Manual for Primary Care* (*DSM-PC*) (American Academy of Pediatrics, 1996). This manual, with its companion, *Bright Futures for Mental Health* (National Center for Education in Maternal & Child Health, 2002), will become valuable tools for practitioners.

In 2002, the American Board of Pediatrics bestowed subspecialty board status in developmental and behavioral pediatrics to those pediatricians who complete a two-year postresidency fellowship and demonstrate certain competencies. While some of these colleagues will provide primary care, most will teach or staff referral clinics. The positive impact on residency training is obvious. The impact on practices may be more subtle and less timely. It is unclear how these colleagues will be able to combine primary care practice with subspecialty practice. Dr. Geertsma, a developmental and behavioral pediatrician discusses this further in Chapter 3.

Consultations and Referrals

Just as generalists may need to call on subspecialists for assistance with their patient's medical problems, generalists must have access to mental health professionals for assistance in management of behavioral and psychosocial problems. While it is important that general pediatricians take a more active role in these frequently occurring morbidities, they cannot be expected to provide this type of service with out appropriate backup. All pediatricians know *when* to call the pediatric cardiologist for help, and *who* to call. Do they know *when* to call mental health colleagues? Actually, *when* varies—based on experience and professional comfort level. The *who* they can call depends on the availability of the mental health specialist.

Will consultants be available? In recent years, primary care physicians have taken on an ever-increasing role in prescribing psychotropic medications. This is a complex and ever expanding pharmacology, often with only subtle differences between agents but perhaps remarkable differences in appropriate use and outcomes. Noting our expanding understanding of brain function on the cellular and molecular levels, one managed care company medical director (name withheld, personal communication) noted, "In ten years all mental health will be pharmacology." While few would agree with his assessment, the source and impact of this attitude are clear. Psychopharmacology will be the treatment of choice and primary care physicians will be expected to expand their treatments with these agents.

Primary care doctors will need help. They will need to stay current with a new literature. They will need to assure themselves and their patients that they are providing up to date treatments of the highest quality, so that primary care pediatrics does not become the second balcony of children's psychopharmacology.

Select cases will need to be referred, and *referral sources must be available*. The American Academy of Child and Adolescent Psychiatry notes that 30,000 child psychiatrists are needed but only 6,300 are available. There is a maldistribution in child psychiatric and children's mental health services, and rural areas as well as areas of low SES have the least access. The "carve out" of mental health coverage (discussed below) has resulted in limitations on services that are provided by a family's health insurance and often a reduction in provider availability.

Managed care health insurance complicates this process. Is the needed consultant in the same network as the primary care physician? If in a different network, can the patient be referred to that consultant? Is the referral process uniform, and does it insure ready access, or is it cumbersome with delays and restrictions?

Clancy, Continued

Mother was encouraged to call the mental health number on the family's insurance card, inquire about therapists experienced with young adolescents and to begin the process of calling to find a therapist. Recognizing the difficulty of finding therapists in the community, specific referrals were not given. Rather, the family was encouraged to take the first available appointment with whatever therapist was on their insurance company's plan.

The family was reminded that they could call back at any time in the event of an emergency. In addition, the phone number for the community mental health service emergency call service was also provided.

Several days later, the office confirmed that the family had found a therapist for Clancy in the near future. After a few weeks Clancy's mother called again seeking further advice. Clancy's doctorate psychologist had recommended antidepressants and the family was seeking Clancy's pediatrician's opinion about the appropriateness of this course of therapy as well as guidance in obtaining psychopharmacologic agents. The pediatrician agreed to see Clancy the following day and requested that the therapist be in contact prior to the visit. Clancy's therapist confirmed a diagnosis of major depressive episode, not otherwise specified, code 311.

Clancy was scheduled in the next day's sick call session at the practice. The pediatrician's impression confirmed the diagnosis of depression and it was noted in the chart that *DSM-IV* criteria were met. Antidepressant therapy was deemed appropriate.

However, in taking a family history it was noted that Clancy's father carries a diagnosis of bipolar disorder and has been successfully managed on a mood stabilizer for many years.

The father related that he had substantial problems with mania as well as deep depression prior to this therapy, but thankfully his disease had been well-controlled all during his later adult life as a parent.

Could Clancy's depression be a manifestation of bipolar disorder?

Difficult cases need be discussed with other pediatricians or with specific mental health consultants. Consultation might include discussion of the pediatrician's own management, with specific recommendations and direction in the use of psychopharmacological agents.

Clancy, Concluded

The primary care pediatrician recognized the risk of initiating antidepressant therapies in someone who might indeed have bipolar disorder. This dilemma was shared with the family and discussed at length with Clancy. A prescription was not given at this visit, but the primary care pediatrician agreed to consult with a psychiatric colleague and communicate with the family by phone to further discuss therapeutic options.

This primary care pediatrician had enjoyed a long collegial relationship with several child psychiatric colleagues in his community; one of these colleagues had encouraged "curbside" and telephone consults. In the ensuing consultive discussion, the child psychiatrist suggested that there were two options. Certainly an antidepressant selective seratonin reuptake inhibitor could be initiated if the clear instruction to the family that should hyperactivity or mania be observed, that the medication should be stopped immediately. Alternatively, a mood stabilizer could be initiated and antidepressant added as needed.

The primary care clinician elected to begin an SSRI, providing careful caveats to the family. Follow-up was arranged by phone for dosage adjustment and in the office for reevaluation.

Clancy has done well.

The Collaborative Care Model described by Dr. Carolyn Schroeder in the monograph (Chapter 1) offers promise as a new approach in the primary care setting. Drawing from the community health clinic model or the hospital inpatient model where interdisciplinary colleagues have been traditionally available, this new system places primary care pediatric providers and mental health providers in the same clinical practice and overcomes many existing barriers. Will it be available beyond larger centers and in more rural areas? Some states have ear-marked Medicaid funds for case management of mental health in primary care offices, to help offset cost barriers (Moseley, personal communication).

Reimbursement

The pediatric office today should provide behavioral health screening and anticipatory guidance in the context of every well-child and sick visit. The pediatrician must be prepared to uncover and effectively address psychosocial issues at every encounter: some earaches are complicated by parental divorce. While a sick call visit does not include the necessary time to address the child's and family's adjustment to this or other significant psychosocial stressors, there is time for identification, perhaps brief patient education and anticipatory guidance, and certainly an opportunity to make arrangements for a later meeting.

To provide this care, pediatricians need training, collaboration, and reimbursement. Training will enhance primary care skills and new collaborations may overcome barriers to consultation. But, fee schedules for well-child care or sick care are not adequate to compensate time spent in training for, consulting on, or providing care for the behavioral and psychosocial problems uncovered in those visits. Primary care pediatricians can assume responsibility for mental health services of variety and depth, but will they be paid for it? If primary care providers are not reimbursed for their services, behavioral health care will not find a home in primary care.

CURRENT REIMBURSEMENT SYSTEMS

Medicaid

A significant minority of children's mental health services are accessed only through state Medicaid systems. Nationally, 20% of children are insured by Medicaid (American Academy of Pediatrics, unpublished), but the rate of coverage varies widely by state.

Primary care providers struggle with reimbursement for mental health in the Medicaid system. State Medicaid programs vary in the services or codes they will allow primary care physicians to bill, limiting the provision of mental health services which will be reimbursable. Billing for primary care services including mental health requires both a diagnosis and a procedure code. State Medicaid offices often limit providers both in the diagnoses they might be allowed to care for and in the procedures that they will be allowed to provide.

For example, a pediatrician may always bill under CPT (Current Procedural Terminology, American Medical Association, 2000a) codes 99211 to 99215, which designate evaluation and management of a problem, whether it be a physical or behavioral problem. However, might be restricted in using codes 90804 and 90806, typically used by mental health providers for counseling. Some payors incorrectly insist that counseling, and these counseling codes, are only the purview of mental health providers.

Curiously, some diagnoses are accepted by third party payors, while others are refused. A diagnosis code of 311.x indicating clinical depression might be allowed while services provided under the diagnosis of mood problem, v40.3 will be rejected. Specific diagnosis is essential to patient care, and an improperly applied diagnosis could be considered fraudulent. But, the problem to child and family is significant to the family regardless of the diagnosis, and the services provided are of value.

Traditional Medicaid programs, that is programs not enhanced by specific waiver, limit mental health providers to psychiatrists, psychologists and other mental health providers *only* when supervised *on site* by a psychiatrist. Thus, access to clinical social workers or other masters of level professionals, key providers for children, is limited. In this era of Medicaid expansion and the State Child Health Insurance Program (SCHIP), many states have included new provisions for mental health care access in their Medicaid expansion programs, increasing the availability of services. The Caring for Every Child's Mental Health: Communities Together Campaign of the U. S. Department of Health and Human Services Substance Abuse and Mental Health Administration has been recently initiated with the stated goal "to increase the likelihood that children and adolescents with emotional disturbances and their families are appropriately and effectively served and treated" (CMHS National Mental Health Knowledge Exchange Network).

Access to providers in the Medicaid system continues to be limited by reduced reimbursements, often a fraction of already low Medicare rates. It is common for mental health providers to limit the number of Medicaid referrals they will accept to preserve a mix of practice reimbursements. The extra, out of session, and unreimbursed time spent talking with parents, teachers and others in the child patient's life is a further disincentive to these providers for children, in both the Medicaid and private systems (see Geertsma, Chapter 3, this volume).

Managed care Medicaid is found in some states. While these programs are designed to improve access to medical services, mental health services may be handled differently, similar to the private insurance programs described below.

Private Third Party Systems

Private pay systems are not necessarily more family or pediatric friendly than the public system. Third party coverage for health care and mental health care may take many forms, ranging from traditional fee for service to varied levels of care management. Managed care contracts vary in their restrictions, from the lenient preferred provider contracts to the stringent capitated systems. The system of reimbursement is essential to the consideration of providing mental health services in a primary care office.

With fee for service, services billed are paid at published rates. Limitations might exist on fees allowed or on allowable diagnoses based on provider credentials. For example, some insurers may refuse to pay primary care physicians for services rendered for certain psychiatric diagnoses and procedure codes might also be limited by provider type, as described previously. But fee for service provides reimbursement for specific work done on the individual patient.

Managed care contracts may use a modified fee for service reimbursement mechanism or rely on capitated reimbursement, where a practice receives a small monthly capitation to provide all primary care services for a patient over the length of the insurance contract. Practitioners receive the same amount per month for high service utilization as for nonutilizers; that is, the same payment is received for patients seen infrequently as for those seen excessively. Consequently, there is *no financial incentive* to take the extra time to deliver mental health services; indeed there is a disincentive. Capitation inadvertently rewards the practitioner who ignores psychosocial issues.

Mental Health "Carve Out"

Most health insurers, private and Medicaid, now "carve out" the mental health portion of the benefit packages. Carve outs allow a separate system for claims for mental health. Often the mental health portion of coverage is subcontracted out to a separate care management organization or third party provider. While carve outs may serve to reduce cost, they will have an impact on access.

Consultants might be in another network and therefore unavailable. There may be decreased opportunities for coordination of care and services.

More importantly, if mental health diagnoses are carved out of the insurance contract they are also carved out of primary care. Pediatricians cannot bill for services provided for these diagnoses. Cost can be contained by effectively limiting access to both primary care and specialty mental health services.

NEW SCHEMA FOR REIMBURSEMENT IN PRIMARY CARE

Recognizing the importance of behavioral health services in primary care, the American Psychiatric Association in collaboration with the American Academy of Pediatrics and the Society for Developmental and Behavioral Pediatrics, the American Psychology Association and the Society for Pediatric Psychology, the American Academy of Child and Adolescent Psychology, the National Institute for Mental Health and the Maternal and Child Health Bureau of the U.S. Department of Health and Human Services developed the *DSM-PC* (Kelleher et al., 2000), *DSM-PC* utilizes diagnoses consistent with *DSM-IV* (American Psychiatric Association, 1994) and *ICD-9* (American Medical Association, 2000b) and includes diagnostic descriptors. Each diagnostic category is considered from normal variant, through problem behaviors, to full diagnosis. In addition to diagnostic criteria, each category is described, exemplified, and differential diagnoses and comorbidities are noted. *DSM-PC* is useful not just for coding, but also as a reference source. We are fortunate that one of the *DSM-PC* authors, Dr. Dennis Drotar, participated in this symposium. Dr. Drotar's chapter (this volume) provides additional depth to this discussion.

DSM-PC now provides primary care pediatricians with the diagnostic codes necessary to bill for these psychosocial problems they address in their practices. While barriers remain, there are opportunities to utilize specific diagnoses to bill for services provided. While insurers may continue to reject claims from primary care physicians for certain diagnoses, types of services or supplementary situational morbidities, a schema for demonstrating the breadth of psychosocial service problems cared for and time spent in the provision of services is an important first step. Proper diagnostic coding allows the assessment of outcome and justification that effective services were provided. It allows the primary care physician to more fully describe their interventions than could be accomplished with simply medical diagnoses. A new standard of care can be established and documented. Now the insurance companies may argue "pediatricians don't do that." If primary care pediatricians would simply tell insurance companies what they do, the groundwork for reimbursement is established. If it is billed, a new standard is defined and reimbursement must follow.

An important contribution of *DSM-PC* to primary care pediatrics is its inclusion of both normal variant and problem level diagnostic criteria and codes. In addition, a series of situational codes are included, allowing consideration of environmental factors which impact on the child and family's mental health, for example marital discord and family divorce or homelessness. These ICD codes are "v codes," characterized as "supplementary classification of factors influencing health status and contact with health services: a problem is present which influences a person's health." Unfortunately, many pediatricians are convinced that the "v" stands for "v̲ery unlikely to be reimbursed." But adding a second "v" code diagnosis to the primary medical diagnostic code of the patient encounter can justify "up coding" to a higher procedure code for reimbursement for the office visit. For example, when a child is seen for abdominal pain, a common procedure or billing code might be 99213 (office visit expanded focus). If it was determined that the child's parents had recently separated, a savvy pediatrician might find no medical cause to the tummy aches and correctly identify the child's pain a reaction to his family's marital disruption. But this is time consuming—more so than the typical abdominal pain office visit. Using a diagnostic code of 789.00 for abdominal pain will only justify the 99213 level of billing. Including the additional diagnostic code of v61.1, marital discord, justifies an up coding of 99214 (office visit, detailed history and evaluation) or even 99215 (office visit, highly complex). All codes in the 99211 to 99215 group can be based on time spent, appropriately allowing for higher reimbursement. It is important that primary care physicians understand the subtleties of billing for behavioral health services so they can reflect the nuance of their practice and be appropriately reimbursed for services provided.

Additional coding opportunities exist. In the fee for service system a number of special codes, which are poorly utilized, are allowed to primary care physicians (see Table 4.1). These specific codes reimburse for some of the medical minutia, but they are often forgotten.

In the managed care environment, primary care pediatricians who provide developmental and behavioral services should be encouraged to

Table 4.1. Behavioral, Attention-Deficit/Hyperactivity Disorder/ Special Needs Codes

DESCRIPTION	*TIME SPENT*	*CODE*
Care Conference	30 min	99361
(with or without patient present)	60 min	99362
E&M Codes (existing patient codes)	OV Minimal	99211
	OV Problem Focused	99212
	OV Expanded Focus	99213
	OV Detailed	99214
	OV Highly Complex	99215
Family Psychotherapy		
Without Patient (child) present	Not Time-related	90846
With Patient (child) present	Not Time-related	90847
OV with Physical (link to another diagnosis)	Problem-Focused	99212-99225
	Expanded Focus	99213-99225
	Detailed	99214-99225
Phone Case Management	Brief Call	99371
	Intermediate Call	99372
	Complex Call	99373
Physician Supervision		
(Covers 30-d period)	15-29 min	99374
	30+ min	99375
Preventative Counseling	15 min	99401
	30 min	99402
	45 min	99403
	60 min	99404
Prolonged Physician Services		
(face-to-face)	First 60 min	99354
	Each additional 30 min	99355
Prolonged Physician services		
(without face-to-face)	First 60 minutes	99358
Review Testing		
Psychological/School	Not Time-related	90887

negotiate special contracts for these services. Two options are proposed. The argument can be made that pediatricians with expertise in psychosocial problem management could be seen as both primary care physicians and subspecialists. This is a familiar model that has been utilized by gynecologists who provide primary care general medical services for women as well as specialty obstetric and gynecologic care. While insurance companies will not welcome this proposal, properly credentialed and experienced pediatricians should draw attention to their special skills that make them different from all other primary care providers who receive the same capitation or negotiated reimbursement, but do not provide the developmental and behavioral pediatric services.

An alternative (although not mutually exclusive) argument has to do with the cost of consultants. Experienced pediatricians might argue that it is less costly to the insurer for the experienced pediatrician to care for children with ADHD, family adjustment problems or uncomplicated depression than it would be to refer that child to a specialist. One argues that the long-term relationship with the child and family provides a more cost effective opportunity for intervention.

In addition to contracting, pediatricians providing special services must be prepared to defend and challenge denied claims. An example of such a defense is found in Table 4.2.

SUMMARY

The Surgeon General's Report of Children's Mental Health (U.S. Public Health Service, 2000) notes, "mental health is a critical component of children's learning and general health." Eight goals for addressing all of America's children are proposed. While all eight goals are in the purview primary care pediatrics, goal number seven deserves special mention: "train frontline providers to recognize and manage mental health issues."

The medical model of our training can and will work for us as we provide these broader services addressing our patients behavioral health needs. We must take thorough histories and, to do so, enhance our interviewing skills. Pediatricians must become familiar with tested screening tools and checklists, to assist in developing appropriate differential diagnoses and to assess the presence of co-morbidities. Additional effective primary care interventions are needed and primary care pediatricians will learn to use them. Each generalist must develop his or her own network for case discussion, consultation and referral. New models for the collaborative practice of primary care and mental health practitioners working side by side must be developed which are community based and not lim-

Table 4.2. Challenge to Denied Third-Party Payments

Any Pediatrician
Anytown, USA
December 27, 2001

ATTN: Case Manager

RE: ___________
DOB: ___________
INSURANCE #: ___________

To Whom It May Concern:

I saw ______________________________ on ____________________
for ____.

This letter documents the components of the services billed under diagnosis code ______________.

The following services were provided:

_______ Parent Conference, regarding the diagnosis, etiology, management and medical treatments of ________________. This conference lasted approximately ________________ minutes.

_______ Face-to-face visit with _______________ for additional discussion and initiation of therapy; ____________ minutes.

_______ Correspondence with the school ____________________ attends.

_______ Review of School Records.

_______ Phone Consultation(s): ____________ minutes.

_______ Other:

____

Should you have any additional questions or wish these services to be coded in a different way, please contact ______________________________ in my office.

Thank you for your consideration.

Sincerely,

ited only to universities or training centers. Dr. Carolyn Schroeder's chapter describes one collaborative care model, and other models are in development (Morseley, personal communication).

The treatment of pediatric psychosocial problems will begin in primary care and the systemic changes necessary to allow this standard of care are within our reach.

REFERENCES

American Academy of Pediatrics. (1996). *The classification of child and adolescent mental diagnoses in primary care. Diagnostic and Statistical Manual for Primary Care (DSM-PC) Child and Adolescent Version.* In M. L. Wolraich, M. E. Felice, & D. Drotar (Eds.). Elk Grove Village, IL: Author.

American Academy of Pediatrics. (2000a). Insurance coverage of mental health and substance abuse service of children & adolescents: A consensus statement. *Pediatrics, 106*, 860-862.

American Academy of Pediatrics. (2000b). Clinical practice guideline: Diagnosis and evaluation of the child with attention-deficit/hyperactivity disorder. *Pediatrics, 105*, 22-36.

American Academy of Pediatrics. (2001). Clinical practice guideline: Treatment of the school-aged child with attention-deficit/hyperactivity disorder. *Pediatrics,108*, 1033-1044.

American Academy of Pediatrics, Task Force on the Family. (2003). Family pediatircs. *Pediatrics, 111*, 1539-1569.

American Academy of Pediatrics' Committee on Psychosocial Aspects of Child and Family Health. (1993). The pediatrician and the "new morbidity." *Pediatrics, 92*, 731-733.

American Academy of Pediatrics' Committee on Psychosocial Aspects of Child and Family Health. (2001). The new morbidities revisited: A renewed commitment to the psychosocial aspects of pediatric care. *Pediatrics, 108*, 1227-1230.

American Academy of Pediatrics. Unpublished data.

American Medical Association. (2000). *Current procedural terminology CPT 2001.* Chicago: Author.

American Medical Association. (2000). *International classification of diseases ICD-9-CM 2001.* Chicago: Author.

American Psychiatric Association. (1994). *Diagnostic criteria from DSM-IV,* First MB, ed. Washington, DC: Author.

CMHS National Mental Health Knowledge Exchange Network, PO Box 42490, Washington, DC, 20015. www.mentalhealth.org

http://www.acgme.org/rrc/peds/PedReq_Comp.htm

Kelleher, K. J., Childs, G. E., Wasserman, R. C., McInerny, T. K., Nutting, P. A., & Gardner, W. P. (1997). Insurance status and recognition of psychosocial problems: A report from PROS and ASPN. *Archives of Pediatric Adolescent Medicine, 151*, 1109-1115.

Kelleher, K. J., McInerny, T. K., Gardner, W. P., Childs, G. E., & Wasserman, R. C. (2000). Increasing identification of psychosocial problems: 1979-1996. *Pediatrics, 105*, 1313-1321.

Jellinek, M., Patel, B. P., & Froehle, M. C. (Eds.). (2002). *Bright Futures in practice: Mental health practice guide*. Arlington, VA: National Center for Education in Maternal and Child Health.

U.S. Public Health Service. (2000). *Report of the Surgeon General's conference on children's mental health: A national agenda*. Washington, DC: Department of Health and Human Services.

DISCUSSION SUMMARY
written by Courtney Fleisher

Dr. Joseph Hagan practices as a pediatrician in a rural setting. As such, he was able to address the ways in which primary care physicians attend to the psychosocial issues of children when financial, temporal, and professional expertise resources are not readily available. Dr. Hagan's comments generated discussion about ways to improve mental health treatment of children in three arenas: deficits in knowledge requiring research evaluation, necessary changes in clinical practice, and political issues about which professionals need to be knowledgeable. The following summarizes the ideas discussed and conclusions drawn in the three areas noted above.

Research

The dearth of professionals available to treat the psychosocial problems of children has resulted in management of behavioral and emotional problems largely with psychotropic medication. Participants discussed concerns about this method of treatment due to the fact that most research evaluating the efficacy of psychotropic medications has been conducted on adults. It has been assumed that the same medications, modifying dosage for the height and weight of the child, would work therapeutically in a similar fashion to that of adults. Forum participants expressed concern that studies to date have not considered the impact of developmental issues on the efficacy of pharmacological therapies, nor have they investigated the effect of the medications on children's development. Participants acknowledged the need for methodologically sound studies on the efficacy of psychopharmacological treatments for children that consider their physical and psychological development in their design and conclusions.

Clinical

In addition to the research implications of psychopharmacological treatment, the clinical use of medications was discussed following Dr. Hagan's presentation. Participants voiced concerns that psychiatrists prescribe psychotropic medications for children when psychological treatments should be considered. Some participants argued that psychiatrists are not solely to blame for this problem. It was noted that sometimes referrals are made to psychiatrists when a mental health specialist's training is insufficient to design and administer effective psychological treatment. Children with acting out behaviors consistent with Oppositional Defiant Disorder diagnoses are being referred for pharmacological treatment, but these behaviors are unlikely to remit with medication. A well-planned and administered course of behavioral treatment, on the other hand, can be effective in improving the situation. The number of children treated pharmacologically for ADHD has caused public concern over the past decade. These symptoms, however, often respond better when pharmacological treatment is paired with behavioral interventions and manipulations to the child's environment. Collaborative care models, where physicians and mental health therapists work together, are ideal in these situations because they allow titration of medication to be accomplished in the context of the behavioral work being conducted with the family. One individual pointed out that when mental health therapists and psychiatrists consult on cases, treatments other than pharmacotherapy are often agreed upon as the indicated method of intervention.

Participants agreed that when professionals reach an impasse in the treatment of a patient, consultation, rather than referral, might be the most efficient first step. Although consultation can be a challenge when limited resources are available, some effective models for collaborative care exist. For example, mental health specialists practicing out of the same office as physicians, as has been done in Chapel Hill, North Carolina, allows professionals to have convenient access to each other, as well as having the benefits of sharing overhead costs. Weekly or bi-monthly meetings held in a rotating fashion at local offices for mental health specialists and physicians to discuss challenging cases are another opportunity for network building and cost-effective consultation.

When referrals are indicated and made, participants noted the importance of communication between the referring and treating professionals. Collaboration across disciplines on a professional level is essential in achieving treatment of psychosocial problems, or the "new morbidities," in primary care pediatricians' offices. Participants representing referring primary care pediatricians and treating mental health specialists complained that treating specialists rarely report back to the referring physician following the therapist's assessment. In addition, concerns were raised that when mental health specialists intervene, referring physicians seldom report observations about the effectiveness of the intervention following future contact with the family. Although the traditional medical model of referrals allows the referring professional to shift responsibility to a specialist believed to be better qualified to address the identified issue, this model may not serve the patient most effectively when addressing psychosocial problems in children. Feedback by primary care physicians and mental health providers can independently verify the need for and effectiveness of the treatment. Furthermore, communication between professionals consistently conveys the importance of the intervention to the family, which, in turn, may improve family involvement in addressing the issue and ultimately, the effectiveness of the intervention. In practice, collaborative care models have been well-utilized and well-received by physicians, patients, and mental health specialists when they have been available (Schroeder, Chapter 1).

The need for improved communication between psychiatrists and primary care pediatricians was also raised. While psychiatrists and pediatricians "round" together during residency, professionals representing both fields pointed out the lack of communication between the professions following training. Because primary care pediatricians are increasingly managing children's psychotropic medication, forum participants argued the shortage of child psychiatric services could be partially ameliorated by psychiatrists educating primary care pediatricians about the process of monitoring psychotropic medication in children and adolescents. Primary care physicians could then consult with psychiatrists when concerns arise that pose a problem for the primary care physician.

Political

Discussion surrounding the need for improved communication across the varied professions yielded ideas about future directions in clinical work. Participants were also anxious to understand how primary care pediatricians are currently coping with the increased demands of handling children and adolescents' mental health issues. Lack of available services and funds appeared to be themes with which practitioners are constantly struggling. In particular, with the dearth of child mental health professionals, if there is a child specialist in the area, it can take several months for the family to be seen. Additionally, poor reimbursement to primary care physicians for treatment of mental health issues makes the idea of taking the time to intervene with these complex problems less appealing. Discussion, in turn, focused on creative ways in which physicians have been culling local resources to assist with the treatment of children's psychosocial issues. One professional noted having requested monies from the county mental health and recovery board to fund a collaborative-care model entailing placement of mental health professionals in well-child care clinics. Dr. Hagan indicated that he compensates for the under-reimbursement for time he spends addressing psychosocial problems with the over-reimbursement vis-à-vis the time he spends with simple medical problems like ear infections. Dr. Hagan also reported that he has made it his priority to develop strong relationships with local mental health practitioners with whom he regularly consults and to whom he regularly refers patients. Practicing professionals emphasized that solutions are locally focused in that practitioners need to develop local networks of trusted professionals and that accessing funds may best be accomplished at the local governmental level. Participants noted, however, that local politics regarding funding largely impact the attempts communities can make to address the new morbidities in primary pediatric health care.

While participants discussed the importance of actively creating and fostering local networks and being aware of and involved in local politics regarding medical spending, the solution forum participants appeared to support as being most successful was modeled after that presented by Dr. Carolyn Schroeder. Many participants agreed that improved communication occurs when professionals are housed in the same building, and results from Dr. Schroeder's research were cited confirming that referral rates were higher when professionals occupied the same facility. Dr. Schroeder recalled that when the mental health professionals were moved into an adjoining building, there was concern that communication would falter. She noted that while forms were created and used to facilitation communication between professionals, communication was still not as facile as when all were housed in the same office.

An additional issue with political implications sparked by Dr. Hagan's presentation surrounded the issue of the American Academy of Pediatrics' (AAP) Guidelines of Diagnosis and Treatment of ADHD. Professionals representing the psychological sciences were interested in physicians' thoughts about the published guidelines. Dr. Hagan initially summarized the guidelines indicating that they suggested physicians talk with the teacher and the parents in addition to assessing the problem using screening tools. Next the guidelines encourage the physician to go over the *DSM-IV* checklist to identify presence of the disorder. Finally the AAP Guidelines recommend evaluating the child to rule out other disorders accounting for the symptoms. Representing a primary care pediatrician's point of view, Dr. Hagan indicated that he already knew the information included in the guidelines, and that he had also sought out information from the Health and Education guidelines, although he was not certain to what extent other pediatricians might have done the same. Some physicians suggested that the guidelines were not particularly user-friendly for physicians less familiar with assessing and treating ADHD, as would particularly be the case for physician's trained before the inception of the "new morbidities." Dr. Hagan indicated that the AAP was committed to implementing the guidelines, and that hopefully the commitment would extend to education to bridge the gap in knowledge for those less familiar with the disorder. Forum participants acknowledged the importance of these types of guidelines while noting the ADHD guidelines only covered one psychiatric disorder commonly treated by primary care pediatricians. The political implication is that professionals within organizations may be able to affect change by encouraging attention to be paid to mental health issues.

In conclusion, Forum participants discussed new directions in the areas of research, clinical work, and political involvement. Participants called for research examining the efficacy of medication used to treat psychiatric illnesses in children on an age-appropriate sample and taking developmental issues into consideration. With respect to clinical work, participants concluded that improved communication and more collaborative models of intervention would improve the treatment of mental health issues in pediatric primary care settings. Finally, from a political perspective, physicians ought to become increasingly engaged in their communities to develop a network of mental health professionals with whom they can collaborate. Additionally, physicians in professional organizations must lobby for further action in recognizing and prioritizing mental health issues, as was done by the AAP with the ADHD guidelines.

CHAPTER 5

ISSUE OF MENTAL HEALTH IN AMERICAN POLITICS

Courtney Fleisher
From a Presentation by Congressman Ted Strickland

Politics and health care service delivery are inextricably entwined in America's health care system. Ohio congressman Ted Strickland (D-OH), a psychologist by training, represented the political atmosphere surrounding the issue of pediatric psychosocial problems in primary care in a presentation at this forum. He highlighted political efforts he has made to impact the mental health of Americans, as well as providing insight on ways professionals might influence legislators' attention to important issues. This chapter will provide an historical view of the recent attention to the general issue of mental health in American politics. In addition, the role Congressman Strickland has played in prioritizing these issues will be highlighted. Finally, Congressman Strickland's remarks about ways to encourage prioritization of the specific issue of pediatric psychosocial problems in primary care will be shared.

During well-child visits, in addition to assuring the child's general physical health, physicians are mandated to conduct screenings for problems such as lead poisoning and ensuring immunization of all children. Such guidelines impact the way physicians spend their time during fifteen-minute office visits. Issues not prioritized by legislators are likely to be neglected in favor of those that are mandated to be evaluated during

Treating Children's Psychosocial Problems in Primary Care, 117–127

office visits. Furthermore, research funding generally stems from government-funded agencies. Monies are more abundant for studies investigating illnesses receiving public attention due to the role of important spokespeople whose lives have been directly affected by the illness. If health professionals are interested in prioritizing the mental health of children, practitioners must be aware of the political workings necessary to receive research funding and government monies for screening and intervention. The following pages will highlight information valuable to practitioners about the history of the political view of mental health in the United States, as well as methods to gain the attention of those responsible for funding in this country.

Beginning with the Clinton-Gore administration, and Mrs. Gore's public disclosure of her personal struggle with clinical depression, there has been a shift in the priority of the issue of the mental health of Americans. Over the past several years political conferences have been held, legislation has been proposed and passed into law, and preparation of the first Surgeon General's Report on mental health has brought the issue of mental illness into the homes of average American citizens. National attention paid to the mental health of Americans impacts identification and treatment of pediatric psychosocial problems in primary care in several ways: (1) it increases the economic priority of psychosocial problems in health-care delivery, (2) it helps determine whether treatment of psychosocial issues in the primary care setting is covered and reimbursed by insurance, (3) it drives funding of research in the area of identification and treatment of pediatric psychosocial problems, and (4) it impacts funding for training professionals.

HISTORICAL CONTEXT OF MENTAL HEALTH LEGISLATION AND GOVERNMENT-SUPPORTED PROGRAMMING

During the mid to late 1990s, the Clinton-Gore administration addressed the issue of mental illness on many levels. In order to equalize insured individuals' benefits for mental and physical health, the Clinton-Gore administration advocated for and passed into law the Mental Health Parity Act. This legislation required the same annual and lifetime spending caps be in place for mental health as for medical and surgical benefits. Regulations were also issued toward ending discrimination against the mentally ill in the issuing of health insurance. These measures are being enforced by the Departments of Labor, Treasury, and Health and Human Services who are working toward preventing unjustly denied benefits under the Mental Health Parity Act. Organizations serving Medicaid populations were also encouraged to recognize mental health needs in serving their patients. On a financial level, the Clinton-Gore administration increased Mental Health Services Block Grants from 289 to 359 million dollars for the 2000 fiscal year, an unprecedented increase of 24 % in one year. These grants provide resources for state governments to offer comprehensive community-based care for the seriously mentally ill and their families. Finally, the Department of Defense piloted a program at Tinker Air Force Base which provided specialty behavioral healthcare in primary care clinics. The goals of this program were to decrease stigma associated with mental illness, enhance access to mental health care, and to enhance efforts to prevent mental illness (The Clinton-Gore Administration: Improving Mental Health Website, 2001).

Several Clinton-Gore initiatives have been more directly related to children's mental health. As a part of the 1997 Balanced Budget Act, President Clinton ensured that 24 billion dollars was set aside to provide full range benefit health care coverage for millions of uninsured children through the Children's Health Insurance Program (CHIP). A wide range of programs designed to protect or improve the mental health of children were funded by the Clinton-Gore administration. Some programs were geared toward preventive interventions promoting resilience, while others pointed severely emotionally disturbed children toward healthy, productive adult lives. In the schools, over 180 million dollars per year have been awarded through the Safe Schools/Healthy Students Program to school districts in conjunction with law enforcement and mental health agencies to promote healthy childhood development and prevent violence. Within the juvenile justice system, a 1999 competitive grant was offered to fund research on programs designed to substantially increase the quality of mental health services provided to detained and committed youth (The Clinton-Gore Administration: Improving Mental Health, 2001).

In December of 1999, the first-ever Surgeon General's Report on Mental Health was released. This report provided an up-to-date review of scientific advances in the study of mental health and of mental illnesses. The Surgeon General's Report approached understanding of mental illness and mental health from a developmental perspective, emphasizing the period during childhood because it serves as the foundation for the individual's psychological adjustment. The report highlighted that symptoms and behaviors present at one point in a person's life may be indicative of illness while being considered within normal limits at another point. In addition, the Surgeon General's Report identified the roots of stigma of mental illness and how it has changed over the years. Furthermore, the impact of stigma on help seeking for mental health and paying for treatment was discussed. The report concluded that many efficacious treatments exist to address the array of mental and behavioral disorders that occur throughout one's life. As such, the Surgeon General concluded that all individuals should be encouraged to seek help when questions arise about mental health. Finally, this document pointed out the fragmentation of mental health services in the United States and how many individuals in need of help fall through the cracks, especially the disenfranchised often in the most need of assistance (U.S. Public Health Service [USPHS], 2000).

Two major political conferences were held in the late 1990s to demonstrate the priority status of mental health issues during the Clinton-Gore administration. In June of 1999, President Clinton and Vice President Gore convened the first-ever White House Conference on Mental Health. The major goals of this conference were to debunk myths about mental illness, reduce stigma surrounding these diseases, showcase innovative treatments, and to push full parity for treatment of mental illness. President Clinton took the opportunity of the conference to announce a campaign to inform Americans about their rights under the Mental Health Parity Act as well as an advertising campaign to dispel myths surrounding mental illness and encourage individuals to seek help. He also unveiled an outreach program to educate consumers and health-care professionals about the risk of depression in the elderly, and a five-year National Institute of Mental Health (NIMH) study to examine prevalence of mental illness in a representative sample of adolescents and adults in America (Rabasca, 1999).

A meeting at the White House regarding the mental health of children followed in March of 2000. This meeting, involving political leaders and governance representatives from 14 major mental health, health care, educational, and consumer organizations, was called following the well-publicized results of a study revealing the extensive use of medications to treat psychosocial problems in preschool children published in the *Journal of the American Medical Association* (Zito et al., 2000). The purpose of the meeting was to launch collaboration between the public and private sectors to ensure appropriate diagnosis, treatment, monitoring and management of children with emotional and behavioral conditions by qualified health care professionals, parents and educators. Four initiatives were derived from this meeting: (1) the development and release of a fact sheet on treating children with psychosocial problems geared at parents, (2) five million dollars of funding by the NIMH to study the effects of psychotropic medication on children under the age of seven, (3) improvement of pediatric labeling information for young children by the FDA, and (4) the development of a national conference sponsored by the Surgeon General's office on the treatment of children with behavioral and mental disorders (Levant, 2001).

In September of 2000, the Surgeon General held a conference on children's mental health whose purpose was to develop a national action agenda. This conference yielded eight major goals ranging from reducing impediments to mental health services for children to improving available treatment, and to coordinating and monitoring delivery of services. A few of these goals and their associated action steps are particularly relevant to identification and treatment of pediatric psychosocial problems in primary care settings. One goal strove to improve the assessment and recognition of mental health needs in children. Several steps were recommended for practitioners serving in the many services in which children have regular contact. In order to achieve better assessment and recognition of mental health needs in children, tangible tools must be created to assist professionals in assessing social and emotional needs, in discussing mental health issues with parents, children, and caregivers, and in making appropriate referrals for additional assessment or intervention. Furthermore, primary healthcare providers and educational personnel should be trained in ways to enhance mental health and recognize early signs of mental health problems in at risk children. An additional step in improving assessment and recognition of mental health needs in children involves educating practitioners, policymakers, and the public about the role of untreated mental health problems in placing youth at risk for entry into the juvenile justice system. It was also considered necessary for healthcare providers to make appropriate referrals when additional assessment and/or intervention was necessary as untreated mental health problems play a major role in placing mentally ill youths at risk for entering the juvenile justice system (USPHS, 2000).

Another goal relevant to treating children with mental health problems in the primary care setting was improvement of the infrastructure for children's mental health services across professions. Action steps recommended in accomplishing this goal included reviewing incentives and disincentives for healthcare providers to assess children's mental health needs. Furthermore, providing infrastructure for cost-effective, cross-system collaboration and integrated care was encouraged. The third pivotal goal relevant to primary care treatment of mental health problems in children focused on training frontline providers to recognize and manage mental healthcare issues and educating mental health providers about scientifically-supported prevention and treatment services. This goal could be attained by engaging professional organizations in educating new frontline providers in various systems in child development, equipping these providers with skills to address and enhance children's mental health, and training them to recognize early symptoms of emotional or behavioral problems. This education was suggested to be included in existing curricula of professional programs as well as offering training support to encourage on-going training opportunities across disciplines to develop effective partnerships and keep abreast of the newest developments in the field of children's mental health. Finally, it was suggested that monitoring mechanisms be established to examine the effectiveness of newly instigated training efforts (USPHS, 2000).

CONGRESSMAN STRICKLAND'S INVOLVEMENT

While conferences held and legislation passed remains imperfect, the political environment is ripe for addressing the issue of mental health care provided in primary care settings. To allow a more first hand account of how the political agenda is impacted by the concerns of patients and providers, Congressman Strickland spoke at the forum about his involvement in various legislative efforts as well as the circumstances that influenced his activity on these issues. The following paragraphs summarize his work.

As the first psychologist elected to congress since 1992, Ted Strickland has prioritized children, mental health issues, and patient's rights in his political agenda. His efforts have ranged from identifying the importance of mental health issues in social problems to supporting improvements in training for mental and physical health professionals. Congressman Strickland's motivation for addressing these concerns stems from his own training as a psychologist as well as his continued exposure to these issues through stories shared by his wife, who continues to work in the education field, and interactions with his constituents.

In 1997, as part of the Balanced Budget Act, Congressman Strickland attached an amendment to the bill that prohibited states from mandating children with special needs (behavioral, emotional, intellectual, or physical) to be serviced by managed care plans. According to Congressman Strickland, managing serious and chronic ailments of children with short-term, cure-based treatments is an inappropriate approach to health care for these children. Congressman Strickland indicated that a faction of representatives in the Congress actively sought to override the amendment arguing that these types of decisions are better left to states where representatives are closer to and more able to accurately reflect the will of their constituents. However, Congressman Strickland argued that state representatives often forgo the needs of their weakest constituents, including children, for the goals of special interest lobbyists, and thus he believed addressing these issues at a federal level is more effective. Since the passing of the Balanced Budget Act and Congressman Strickland's amendment, the struggle has been in enforcing the language of the amendment in health-care facilities. Congressman Strickland noted that

Children's Hospital in Columbus, Ohio, as well as other Children's Hospitals across the country have been particularly active in working with him to ensure the legislation is followed when it comes to administering health care to individual children with special needs.

Also born out of the Balanced Budget Act, hospitals and other health-care facilities are about to experience increased funding for psychology internship training programs. Recently, the U.S. Department of Health and Human Services (HHS) agreed to subsidize training of psychologists under Medicare's Graduate Medical Education program. This agreement allows for services rendered by psychology interns to Medicare patients to be billable by the facilities at which the treatment was provided. This change represents increased parity for mental health treatment as services rendered by medical residents have been covered by Medicare payments for many years. The new rule has been under development since 1997 when Congressman Strickland and other representatives urged the HHS to reimburse for psychological training. Up to two hundred million dollars over the first five years could be allocated to hospitals and other health-care facilities for psychology internships; thus helping to ensure quality training and more comprehensive care of Medicare beneficiaries.

Congressman Strickland has focused attention on laws specific to the needs of the mentally ill. Over the past several years, Congressman Strickland has joined forces with Congressman Roukema (R-NJ) to seek parity for mental health with physical health insurance coverage. The Roukema Bill was subsumed under the 1996 Mental Health Parity Act which mandates insurance companies to cover treatment for certain mental health conditions at the same level as treatment for physical health conditions, as mentioned prior.

Congressman Strickland has initiated other legislation to establish mental health courts for hearings on criminal offenses perpetrated by adult individuals with mental health problems that may mediate their crimes. Such courts have been piloted in Florida, Washington, California, Indiana, Ohio, and Alaska with promising results. In a University of Washington study, the program was praised for its success at breaking the cycle of arrest-jail, arrest-jail experienced by many mentally ill people. It has reportedly resulted in faster case processing time, improved access to public mental health treatment services, improved well-being, and reduced recidivism (Trupin, Richards, Lucenko, & Wood, 2001). In 2000, with the help of Senator DeWine (R-OH), the federal bill to establish mental health courts was passed. Currently Congressman Strickland's efforts are aimed at funding this bill and proposing a similar measure to address the criminal justice system's handling of child and adolescent offenders whose crimes may also be mediated by mental illness. As many children and adolescents with mental health problems eventually become involved with the juvenile justice system, Congressman Strickland's involvement in this area is aimed at bolstering tertiary care for these youth.

In an attempt to address the quality of mental and physical health care of individuals insured by managed care companies, the House and Senate have both introduced a Patient's Bill of Rights. Provisions of this bill include: (1) the right for women to choose an OB/GYN as their primary care physician; (2) the right for a parent to see that his or her child who needs pediatric specialty care receives it, and (3) the right to reimbursement for emergency room treatment if a patient used prudent judgement in choosing to go to an emergency room even if the problem could have been addressed in a primary care physician's office. According to Congressman Strickland, one of the most important provisions of the bill is patient's and their family's right to pursue justice in a court of law if a patient is harmed or loses his or her life due to an insurance company's denial to pay for a necessary service.

Congressman Strickland indicated he believed that managed care companies currently have no incentive to put patient need above profit because if a poor decision was made, the patient can only litigate for the cost of the denied procedure, not damages that have resulted because of the denied treatment. As an illustration of this belief, Congressman Strickland shared a story about a 31-year-old, female, leukemia patient living in Ohio who is in need of a bone-marrow transplant. The congressman was contacted by the patient's husband who indicated that even though the patient has a brother who is a perfect match and a doctor who indicated this surgery was necessary to improve her chance of survival, the patient was being denied coverage of the procedure due to the fact that the insurance company deemed the surgery experimental. Currently the family is in the process of holding fund-raiser events to pay for the needed surgery as the insurance company will not pay for this likely life-saving procedure.

Polls show that the American public wants a Patient's Bill of Rights passed, and Congressman Strickland believes it may pass this congress due, in large part, to the involvement of Senators McCain (R-AZ) and Kennedy (D-MA) who have introduced a strong bill in the Senate. Those who oppose the law argue that matters of treatment should not be handled in the courts, but in doctors' offices. Congressman Strickland indicated that Texas' Patient's Bill of Rights, which passed without then Governor Bush's signature, resulted in very few trials to resolve such medical issues. However, Congressman Strickland argued that the mere threat of legal action appears to be incentive enough for managed care companies to operate in a more patient-friendly manner. Recently, members of the Senate have invested much energy into negotiating a Patient's Bill of

Rights that President Bush will not veto, but according to Congressman Strickland, whether or not the bill passes will depend largely on whether the public demands it.

ROLE OF PROFESSIONALS IN EFFECTING LEGISLATIVE ACTION

Professionals, including physicians, can have significant impact on whether this and other health-related legislation is passed. The most effective way professionals can accomplish this feat is by being organized and vocal about their views on the issues. Congressman Strickland emphasized that the American public respects the opinion of their physicians, and thus legislators are particularly receptive to the viewpoints of physicians. Congressman Strickland offered suggestions about how physicians and other health and mental health professionals can effectively get their message across. Congressman Strickland urged all professionals to take advantage of opportunities to serve on advisory boards. He emphasized the importance of this type of involvement when the inviting representative holds a differing stance on the issue from that which the invited professional believes is good for his or her patients. In addition, Congressman Strickland advocated professionals putting themselves in positions to talk to and be heard by legislators. For example, Congressman Strickland encouraged professional organizations to host opportunities for its members to converse with representatives and to share their viewpoints on the legislative issues that impact their patients.

According to Congressman Strickland, health-care professionals can take effective action to impact passage of legislation that is pertinent to their patients by developing strong relationships with their state senators and congressional representatives. He offered that meetings with knowledgeable individuals who discuss, in depth, their concerns and problems regarding particular issues are very influential. Congressman Strickland urged professionals to contact their representatives to request an hour of their time in their state or district office. He offered that it is most effective to bring a small group of like-minded professionals to a face-to-face meeting where the professionals can share stories about how their patients are affected by the issue at hand. While writing letters and e-mails and making phone calls to your representatives can communicate where constituents stand on certain issues, Congressman Strickland argued that face-to-face meetings are the most persuasive method of lobbying on health-related issues. For comparison, big businesses hire lobbyists to further their interests. They do not expend efforts on having their employees contact their representatives.

Congressman Strickland bemoaned the predominant approach in our society that people who are good and moral thrive and those who are disenfranchised are entirely responsible for their lot in life. He called this the "survival of the fittest mentality", and he believes it is ever present in our society. This approach blames the victim if he or she should fall sick or come upon misfortune. Congressman Strickland voiced his belief that greater numbers of people in our society embrace the concept of helping those in need by investing in prevention, but that they are less organized and effective at conveying their message. As a result, he suggested the better-organized voices of those with financial interests overpower, thus prevention issues fall to the background. Congressman Strickland advocated lobbying representatives to take on such initiatives as the American Association of Pediatrics' (AAPs) Kids First proposal. He further noted that the CHIP has made some progress.

With the changeover of administration, mental health care is unlikely to receive as much support as it did during the Clinton-Gore years. The 1996 Mental Health Parity Act is expected to sunset in the fall of 2001, resulting in elimination of the requirements on health insurance policies to cover annual and lifetime caps for mental health problems at the same level as those for medical and surgical issues. Congressman Strickland urged mental and physical health care professionals to take an active stance in encouraging their representatives to focus on issues of mental health care. As long as improving primary care treatment of children's psychosocial issues is dependent upon financial support for research and treatment, it will be important for health care providers to lobby representatives about the importance of the issue so that it will be brought to the political forefront. If we are not the spokespeople for our children, who will be?

REFERENCES

The Clinton-Gore Administration: Improving Mental Health. (2001, November 24). [On-line] Available: http://www.nimh.nih.gov/whitehouse/accomplish.asp

Levant, R. F. (2001, November 24). [On-line] Available: http://www.fenichel.com/WHmeeting.shtml

Rabasca, R. (1999). White House conference on mental health. *APA Monitor Online, 30*(7).

Trupin, E., Richards, H. J., Lucenko, B., & Wood, P. (2001, November 24). *The Washington institute for mental illness research and training* [On-line]. Available: King County District Court, Mental Health Court Phase site: http://www.metrokc.gov/kcdc/execsum.htm

U. S. Public Health Service. (2000). *Report of the surgeon general's conference on children's mental health: A national action agenda*. Washington, DC: Department of Health and Human Services.

Zito, J. M., Safer, D. J., dosReis, S., Gardner, J. F., Boles, M. & Lynch, F. (2000). Trends in the prescribing of psychotropic medications to preschoolers. *Journal of the American Medical Association, 283*, 1025-1030.

CHAPTER 6

NEW DIRECTIONS FOR DIAGNOSIS, TREATMENT, AND RESEARCH OF PEDIATRIC PSYCHOSOCIAL PROBLEMS IN THE PRIMARY CARE OFFICE

Perspectives from the Pediatric Community

Peter D. Rappo
North Easton, MA

Primary care pediatrics, as a medical specialty, is a uniquely American institution with no international counterpart. Although pediatricians are represented worldwide as individuals specially qualified to care for infants, children, adolescents, and young adults, in most medical environments they function as specialty consultants who practice referral or problem-based pediatrics. With America having 55,000 pediatricians who are board-certified (with a two-thirds/one-third split between generalists and specialists) it is clear that the marketplace has shaped the practice environment to allow this largesse of physicians to function. Primary care pediatrics focuses primarily on treatment of acute illness (usually respira-

Treating Children's Psychosocial Problems in Primary Care, 129–143

tory) and so-called well-childcare that involves periodic assessment of growth, development, nutritional status, and anticipatory guidance around health and safety issues. Any intervention which can be made at the time of a well-child encounter could be included as part of the content for that visit. However, empiric data is demanded to support the insertion of such an intervention. Over the years, a variety of special interest groups have lobbied pediatric organizations to include screening questionnaires, mental health assessments, domestic violence evaluations, searches for sexual abuse, and specific reviews for information related to a host of safety and environmental issues. If the intervention cannot be readily accomplished in the context of a well-child encounter, or if the activity does not result in the opportunity for risk modification, it will not be included as part of the anticipated action around well-child care. The average consumer has little idea as to how much thought and effort is expended by primary care pediatricians to "fit" all of the items deemed to be necessary for a complete, comprehensive, and coordinated visit. However, with the increasing number of immunizations that must be received by children in the first two years of life (21 immunizations, at a minimum), the visits in the minds of some parents and pediatric staffs have become "the time when the kids get their shots." Recent data from the National Ambulatory Medical Care Survey (NAMCS) suggests that the average length of a pediatric office visit has increased to 20 minutes per patient, with 54% of pediatric office encounters ranging from 11 to 30 minutes (U.S. Department of Health and Human Services, 1999). When one considers the range of subjects and topics that might be covered at an office visit, it is clear that some information or necessary counseling might be given short shrift. Although the average pediatric encounter lasts for 14 minutes, the average well-child encounter is minimally expected to last for 20 to 25 minutes. Since a discussion of the list of anticipated topics—nutrition, health, well-being, growth, development, safety, sensory concerns, immunization counseling, and so forth would require 45 to 60 minutes per visit, it is obvious that some of the transmission of information is accomplished by ancillary staff, and other data is digested by patients and family members through the use of handouts and Internet resources subsequent to the office visit. The reader is referred to Sherry Glied's chapter in this volume regarding changes in the length of the medical encounter.

The Academy of Pediatrics' periodicity schedule outlines the range of interventions that need to be accomplished at a well-child exam, if the appropriate level of insurance coding is to be satisfied, so that the pediatrician can receive "appropriate" levels of reimbursement. From an administrative point of view, the encounter is reported to an insurer through the use of two numeric or alpha-numeric coding systems: the Current Procedural Terminology System (*CPT-IV*) which reports the procedure performed on behalf of a patient at the time a service was rendered (what was done) and the *International Classification of Disease System (ICD-9cm)* which reports the diagnosis linked to the procedure (why it was done). Since the insurer does not receive a copy of the medical record documentation at the time that the service is reported, it is implicit that the documentation is capable of supporting the level of service provided and reported. Although it is intuitive that each CPT code could and should be honored by an insurer, it is well documented that health plans pick and choose those services which they choose to cover (uncovered services) and those which are not covered under an individual patient's plan (not allowed services). Since the interventions are outlined, items not covered in the schedule are not accorded appropriate levels of attention and, by inference, payment. When pediatricians are queried what they are most frequently asked by parents, the most common answer is "ear infections." However, when parents are asked what are their most urgent concerns, the list includes discipline (19%), sleep problems (17%), eating problems (15%), toilet training (14%), speech development (9%), colic and disorders of temperament (9%), and for adolescents, issues around substance use and abuse (19%) (*Contemporary Pediatrics 2001 Factbook*, 2002). Clearly, none of these topics lend themselves well to interventions such as an injection or an antibiotic. What is common to all of these clinical concerns is their fundamental psychosocial basis, the need to do both general and focused inquiry, the need to have an appropriate training background to respond to information received, and the need to have the appropriate time to respond to these concerns.

An efficient pediatric office operates with a marginal overhead of 50% or less; some offices with favorable-rent allowances can approach 40% overhead. Sadly, some offices have levels of expense that approach 70% of net revenue. With these sorts of numbers, the breakeven point on a daily basis is 25-30 patients per provider per day. The average pediatrician will see 35-40 patients a day, with some seeing significantly more. The present reimbursement system for pediatrics has been keyed to pay for and, in fact, reward treatment of acute illness and well childcare. Although primary care pediatricians suggest that the care of children with developmental, behavioral, mental health, and chronic illness concerns is outside their area of expertise, in point of fact, most training programs have included these areas of study as part of a core curriculum. What drives pediatricians away from the evaluation and treatment of these patients is concern about lack of time for adequate assessment coupled with a historical realization that even when the time and assessment are appropriate, such efforts are poorly or nonrecompensed.

In an effort to break through this impasse regarding concerns related to screening, diagnosis, treatment, and reimbursement for behavioral and mental health issues in the primary care office, the National Institute of Mental Health (NIMH) convened a meeting in Washington, D.C. in 1991 to review the use of the psychiatric coding manual, *DSM-III-R* (*Diagnostic and Statistical Manual* [3rd ed., rev.]), to see what its applicability could be for the primary care arena. In addition to government experts, there was representation from the American Psychiatric Association, the American Academy of Pediatrics, the American College of Obstetricians and Gynecologists, the American Society of Internal Medicine, the American Academy of Family Practice, and the American Medical Association, among others. After an energized and, at times, contentious series of discussions, it was concluded that *DSM-III-R* and the soon-to-be released, *DSM-IV*, would not meet the mental health diagnostic needs for primary care physicians. It was determined that a new volume to be labeled *DSM-PC* would need to be adapted for user friendliness for the primary care community. This process was undertaken by the shareholder groups of the original Washington, D.C. meeting and a simplified version was created. A number of anecdotal vignettes from the conference participants described the difficulties encountered when coding for mental health diagnoses, challenges around payment for these diagnoses, and the insensitivity of *DSM-III-R* in describing subsyndromal problems which did not fully satisfy that system's diagnostic criteria. The pediatric representatives at these subsequent meetings felt that even this "new volume" did not meet their needs since most of the developmental, behavioral, and mental health issues presenting to the office-based pediatrician or family physician caring for children would not approach the level of diagnostic rigor as specified in the existing *DSM* manuals. With an acknowledgement that 30% of children have psychosocial problems, a more sensitive tool was felt to be necessary for use by the pediatric community. Thus, the Academy of Pediatrics was simultaneously involved in two parallel working task forces: creation of the broad-based *DSM-PC* and creation of the unique child and adolescent version of *DSM-PC*, entitled *The Classification of Child and Adolescent Mental Diagnoses in Primary Care* (Wolraich, Felice, & Drotar, 1996). The reader is referred to Dr. Dennis Drotar's discussion in this text of the development of the *DSM-PC* for pediatrics.

In addition to the American Academy of Pediatrics, other shareholder organizations for the pediatric *DSM-PC* included the American Psychiatric Association, the American Psychological Association (Society for Pediatric Psychology & Section on Clinical Child Psychology), the Society for Developmental and Behavioral Pediatrics, the American Academy of Child and Adolescent Psychiatry, and the National Institute of Mental Health. The task force was divided into a number of working groups that created the content, and all proceeded from the rationale that psychosocial issues were of critical importance in primary care, that the system had to describe what clinicians did in primary care settings around mental health issues and that such activities, whether preventative or treatment-focused, needed to be fairly reimbursed. Basic rules assumed as integral to this endeavor were that *DSM-PC* would be compatible with *DSM-IV* and *ICD-10*, would cover the spectrum of clinical findings from normal to disorder, that the disorder diagnoses would be the same as those found in *DSM-IV*, that the volume would be user friendly and intuitive with indices and symptom-based algorithms, that the volume would have an overall developmental perspective, would include environmental risk and modifying factors, and finally, would be empirically-based as much as possible.

The pediatric *DSM-PC* includes diagnostic lists, a severity rating system, a situation section, a symptom or manifestation section, common chief complaints, diagnostic vignettes to assist clinicians in their coding, and a listing of relevant criteria from *DSM-IV*. The situations section lists children's responses to environmental problems and possible stressful events (e.g. marital discord, divorce, child or parental illness, birth of a new sibling, etc.). The symptom or manifestation section includes broad categories including problems of eating, sleeping, elimination, negative and antisocial behaviors, impulsivity and inattention, amongst others. The volume is particularly useful at creating distinctions between the ways issues are addressed in the primary care office-the spectrum of developmental presentation from variation to problem to disorder. A **variation** is a concern that brings a parent or child to a pediatrician's office and upon evaluation, the issue is found to be a variation of normal, a misperception or the euphemism "worried well." A **problem** is a constellation of signs and symptoms that require medical intervention, but does not approach the number of criteria to qualify for the appropriate *DSM-IV* diagnosis; in other words, the problem is "subsyndromal." Finally, for patients with a complex set of symptoms, **disorder**, as used in *DSM-PC*, will meet the same diagnostic criteria as *DSM-IV*. With this remarkable tool at the disposal of primary care pediatricians, the ideal outcome should have been that our reimbursement and medical necessity problems should have disappeared. The outcome is an unqualified "maybe." Since the pediatric *DSM-PC* needed to be compatible with *DSM-IV*, and since there was no opportunity to create new codes to characterize subsyndromal diagnoses, existing "V codes" were pressed into service. V codes are a section of the *ICD-9cm* text that describe symptoms, undiagnosed problems, risk factors in terms of family history or environmental characteristics, and anticipated problems not found. Health insurers prefer documentation of diagnoses rather than anticipated or potential diagnoses. Insurers' computers are frequently programmed to refuse V codes as a primary diagnosis. Thus, the traditional statement among cynics is that the "V" in V code means, "very unlikely to be paid."

As managed care has emerged as a dominant model for the American health care market, it is clear that what is being managed is cost rather than care. Fortunately for pediatricians, prevention is a dominant mantra for health maintenance organizations (HMOs). Under a system which prizes anticipatory guidance, pediatricians have been well rewarded for doing what they thought was important. However, some health futurists believe that managed care is increasingly perceived as a failed model, and the failure of health maintenance organizations to demonstrate consistent cost savings through prevention has led to the dual catastrophe of significantly reduced payments to providers coupled with spiraling, double-digit rate increases. It is even less clear that managed care understands how best to deal with mental health benefit structure and parity. After some well publicized failures of managed health to provide open access to patients for behavioral services, many plans have acknowledged that "they don't get it" and have moved to a behavioral or mental health carve out. A carve out refers to a group of services (vision, durable medical equipment, mental health, etc.) that has been removed from an employer's health benefit plan and then is contracted out to a separate health care provider to provide those services. Pediatricians are desirous of treating the whole child, and believe that the concept of mind-body duality is not a separable construct. Insurers, however, have separated these spheres and have created barriers-separate credentialling and non-payment of *ICD-9* diagnoses based on internally generated lists, on a plan-by-plan basis. Although the illogic of this concept will be addressed in a subsequent section, it is mentioned here since it overshadows issues that impact on the appropriate provision of care for the primary care physician to his patients with mental health issues.

If we assume that pediatricians will use the *DSM-PC* system to initiate appropriate case finding for their patients with behavioral, developmental, and mental health issues, where this system fits in the overall coding and data aggregation model, must be clearly understood. *DSM-PC* is a diagnosis-based system compatible with *ICD-9* and, ultimately, *ICD-10*. Insurers require this type of diagnosis, coupled with a procedural code, usually from the *CPT-4* system, as copyrighted and developed by the American Medical Association. *CPT-4* is updated yearly, and by inference, codes are deleted, added or altered on a daily basis. It is necessary for the volume to be purchased each year, not only to assure coding accuracy, but also to avoid charges of fraud or abuse due to inappropriate coding, even if such errors were inadvertent. Provisions of the Kennedy-Kassebaum (HIPAA) legislation and the False Claims Act of 1860 impose severe potential civil and criminal prosecution for providers who deal with data inappropriately or submit inappropriate claims.

Primary care physicians should familiarize themselves with the section of the *CPT Manual* entitled "Evaluation and Management Service Guidelines." These brief introductory pages review the seven components and determinants of levels of evaluation and management service. These components include history, examination, medical decision making, counseling, coordination of care, nature of the presenting problem, and time. Four of these components, specifically, medical decision making and its complexity, counseling, coordination of care, and time, have enormous potential implications for the use of the *DSM-PC* codes, because most evaluation and management codes can be paired with the *DSM-PC* diagnosis codes. Table 1 in Rappo (1997) illustrates a number of evaluation and management codes that primary care physicians might consider using as part of the *DSM-PC* process. If the common documentation criteria for the CPT codes are not used, and time is used as the determinant as the level of service, "time spent" should be entered into the medical record. "Time spent" is considered the determining factor for a counseling visit when time spent counselling is equal to greater than 50% of the visit.

A major question is whether primary care providers will be reimbursed for the time and effort spent in assessment and coding of diagnoses and procedures. If we assume that health insurers are neither evil nor Machiavellian, why would they not be willing to pay for mental health services provided by primary care pediatricians? The overly simplistic answer relates to systems issues associated with behavioral health carve outs. Most HMOs acknowledge that their previous efforts at controlling mental health costs, and managing care for patients in the behavioral arena, have failed and it is easier to contract with outside vendors for required services. The allotment of capital to a mental health entity requires that the entity perform credentialling and quality initiatives involving their service providers. It is to that entity's advantage (although not necessarily to the advantage of patients or outside providers) to limit the number of plan providers since access is determined on a referral basis. The health plan has already directed resources to the carve out provider. Payment to physicians for a service that, in a sense, they have already contracted for with the behavioral health entity, would be viewed as duplicative waste. The only obvious solution is dual credentialling that allows pediatricians with special training and/or experience in handling patients with behavioral, developmental, or mental health needs to provide such services. Organized medicine must play a role in educating third-party payers and other carriers concerning the importance of mental health and behavioral screening. For example, each state chapter of the American Academy of Pediatrics should suggest to insurance carriers that there could be significant behavioral cost offsets from appropriate mental health screening and care. A study by Hellman, Budd, Borysenko, McClellamd, and Benson (1990) suggested that a group of "over-utilizing" primary care patients, who presented with frequent physical and psychosocial symptoms, could benefit from an intensive mental health intervention. After six months, patients in this program reported less physical and psychological discomfort and began averaging two fewer visits per year to their health plan than did patients with similar symptoms that did not participate in the program. Net savings after costs of the program to the health maintenance organization was approximately $85 per participant during the subsequent six-month follow-up. Current research suggests that a variety of such interventions can reduce overall health care costs. These interventions can include brief mental health consultations, support groups, and psychosocial counseling. The reader is referred to Dr. Douglas Tynan's chapter in this text to see additional discussion of such interventions. Obviously, for these interventions to have an impact on health care costs, case identification as facilitated by the *DSM-PC* must occur.

At the present time, insurance companies give lip service to the mantra of quality as it relates to patient care. Most of the assumptions concerning healthcare have been based on concerns of cost, rather than quality of care. Introduction of the National Committee for Quality Assurance Measures Health Plan Employer Data and Information Set (1997) is critically important to the future of managed care because mental health screening and assessment are included as performance standards. The National Committee for Quality Assurance (NCQA) is a nonprofit, independent organization that reviews and assesses the quality of managed care plans. Its mission is to examine health plan capability, managed care services, to report on the quality of the marketplace, and to promote quality improvement. In a competitive marketplace, the lack of NCQA accreditation is a barrier that most health plans find insurmountable when marketing to potential employer clients. As an acknowledgement of the importance of mental health services, HEDIS 3.0 (NCQA, 1997), listed a large number of quality measures related to mental health issues. They included follow-up after hospitalization for mental illness, availability of mental health providers, mental health utilization data, chemical dependency services, readmission to a hospital for mental health disorders, and pediatric mental health services. The HEDIS testing measure set included office screening for chemical dependency, continuation of treatment for depression, appropriate use of psychotherapeutic medications, and family visits for children undergoing mental health treatment.

It is ironic that the cost-offset argument for savings related to effective mental health services must be advanced to justify continued existence of behavioral health services because such biomedical care as chemotherapy, hospice care, and surgery for severely disabled or chronically ill infants is not based on some offset measure, but rather on individual patient need and the ethics of quality medical care. It must be remembered that the primary purpose of health care is not to save money, but to improve health outcomes. Behavioral and mental health services should be judged by the same criteria as biomedical services. The American Academy of Pediatrics issued a policy statement in October, 2000, entitled, "Insurance Coverage of Mental Health and Substance Abuse Issues for Children and Adolescents." The statement acknowledged that the mental health needs of children and adolescents are increasing while access to needed services is decreasing. A review by Kelleher, McInerney, Gardner, Childs, and Wasserman (2000, pp. 313-1321) demonstrated that in the past 20 years, the rate of psychosocial problems has increased from 7-18% of the pediatric population. The consensus statement of the AAP calls for mental health parity. Although most professional organizations support parity for mental health services, opposition has come from two disparate groups—politicians and the Church of Scientology (both of whom apparently believe that the provision of mental health services will weaken the nation through the provision of psychiatric and psychopharmaceutical interventions). Although there is an increasing movement towards attempts at guaranteeing parity for behavioral services, such attempts seem to be circumscribed by carve-out methodologies.

A carve out is a separately capitated or financed pool of monies dedicated to paying for a specific healthcare benefit within the structure of a health plan or risk arrangement. From an insurer's perspective, the benefit of such a model is obvious: the plan can precisely budget all of its costs for a group of services and avoid administrative entanglements for a benefit structure that has been traditionally difficult to monitor and direct. Additionally, the carve-outs administration would be responsible for analysis of and reporting of such quality parameters as the NCQA's HEDIS Performance Measures. The benefit to patients and the individual primary care physician is somewhat less clear. In an ideal world, a behavioral carve out should increase access, should improve service quality, should facilitate benefits management, and should facilitate and centralize operational efficiencies. Potential problems emerge quite quickly, however. Regulatory mandates by state agencies may restrict or prevent operational streamlining. Parity legislation may differ significantly from the benefit structure of the carve out entity and may make the carve out less profitable from an administrative perspective. Limitation of numbers of mental health providers may discriminate against providers who care for traditionally high-cost patients, such as children with multiple simultaneous comorbid diagnoses, such as attention-deficit hyperactivity disorder (ADHD), obsessive cumpulsive disorder, oppositional defiant disorder, and Tourette's syndrome. Although health plans should be interested in promoting the health of all patients, it is clear that "cherry-picking" of patients without chronic medical or mental health needs is rampant. Any managed-care entity which holds itself out as the "best provider" for patients with chronic needs, would quickly be overwhelmed with a largesse of patients whose diagnoses would create an adverse risk situation to the insurer. Insurance is ultimately about spreading risk, not accepting risk. The issue of adverse risk and selection can only be dealt with on a retrospective basis, that is, any plan that assumes the care of more involved patients should be rewarded by an external risk pool quaranteed by state, federal, or insurance oversight entities. Additionally, a pass-through mechanism would allow enhanced payment for pediatricians who willingly and expertly care for complicated patients.

Technically, the carve out entity would be responsible for the administration of and payment for all mental health, behavioral, and substance abuse issues for a plan with which it has contracted. The infrastructure would need to include divisions of member services, network development, utilization review, credentialing, and claims management. Performance measurements would include member satisfaction, provider satisfaction, claims adjudication, case management, appropriate prescriptive practices, and demand management strategies to facilitate prompt patient referral to appropriate levels of care.

Where does the primary care physician, who is interested in evaluating and treating patients from a mental health perspective, fit within a carve out paradigm? Frequently the answer is "nowhere." Such a primary care physician is not credentialed by this outside entity and even if the program has provisions for payments to "nonplan" providers, they are usually based on geographic isolation criteria or special competency or need rather than specialty or interest. In fact, there have been numerous anecdotal reports at a national level, that the use of diagnoses contained in *DSM-IV* will preclude payment to a nonpsychiatric primary care pediatrician (PCP). Since the mental health coding manuals include diagnoses such as attention deficit disorder, enuresis, encopresis, anorexia nervosa, and so forth, physicians have, at times, used catch-all diagnostic codes such as "adjustment disorder" to facilitate payment. Adjustment disorder is accepted as a diagnosis, not because it is particularly descriptive, but because it has been entered into diagnostic coding databases. This shortcut sacrifices diagnostic rigor and makes obtaining data about the true frequency of behavioral disorders in pediatrics difficult, if not, impossible.

The inappropriate coding/lack of reimbursement for behavioral and mental health issues is certainly an annoyance for primary care pediatricians, but it is a disastrous problem for a subsegment of the pediatric community—developmental and behavioral pediatrics. Such individuals have devoted their academic and practice careers to the issues covered in *DSM-*

PC. Additionally, they have taken on oversight for children with severe chronic illness, another group of patients whose care has been traditionally under appreciated, at times, avoided by the primary care community, and frequently, poorly reimbursed. Although board certification for this subgroup of pediatricians will help to clarify their roles and should improve opportunities for enhancement of professional self-esteem, it will not solve the problem of how to distinguish care that they provide so that it is differentiated from that provided by primary care colleagues. The developmental and behavioral community is uniformly the most dissatisfied group of pediatric professionals when asked about perception regarding appropriateness of reimbursement. Insurers, however, tend to ask discomforting questions: If a primary care pediatrician requires a one-hour assessment to diagnose ADHD, and the developmental and behavioral specialist requires six hours for the same diagnosis, and the interventions in both cases include behavioral, educational, adjustment, medical, and medication manipulations which are identical, how does one justify the traditional value equation, Value = Quality outcome/Cost. If the quality outcome is the same, dramatic increase in costs clearly decrease the value proposition for the insurer. Analysis of this simple proposition will either assure or doom the specialty of developmental and behavioral pediatrics. This is indeed a conundrum. If I evaluate a patient with ADHD for 1.5 hours and recommend behavioral and pharmacologic interventions, and my developmental/behavioral brother spends 6 hours and recommends the same interventions, the value equation does not work. It is difficult to demonstrate differential outcomes.

Although some health plans are moving to point of service options that allow patients to seek consultation with a specialist without a referral from their primary care physician, most managed care organizations still employ the gatekeeper system that hopefully facilitates referral of patients to appropriate levels of care. Ironically, such gatekeeper methodologies almost never exist around mental health referrals, irrespective of a plan's use of carve in versus carve out models. This disconnect, and its obvious consequent tendency to limit or prohibit communication, under the guise of confidentiality, between the PCP and the mental health professional, has created a situation that would normally be intolerable to a patient, family, and provider-lack of information exchange around an ongoing clinical problem. The notion that the mind/body duality can some how be segmented into separate components where little opportunity for interchange exists, has potentially disastrous implications for the continued well being of our mutual patients.

The literal explosion of new medications to treat a variety of mental health conditions has enormous implications for putting back together, that which may be best not to divide: the biomedical/psychosocial interface. Since psychologists are unable to prescribe psychopharmacologic agents, in most venues, and pediatricians are unfamiliar with the treatment options presently available, such prescriptive practices would seem to fall to psychiatrists who are particularly adept at evaluating the appropriate selection and need for such medications. However, such individuals are in short supply. Interestingly, the law of supply and demand, in the medical marketplace, has allowed psychopharmacologists to opt out of traditional managed care arrangements, and has allowed them to utilize the concept only dimly recalled by most physicians: fee for service. Although such a model is good for psychiatrists, it clearly limits access to care for children and families with limited resources. Since it is the obligation of health plans to provide access to psychopharmacologic services, new models will need to be carefully considered and implemented. For example, after a psychologist determines that a trial of medication might be appropriate for a child's condition, consultation would need to occur with the child's primary care clinician, and an evaluation would include not only an assessment of the child by the PCP, but also a telephonic or virtual consultation with a designated plan psychopharamacologist or pediatric developmentalist adept at medication selection, manipulation, and monitoring. The reader is referred to Dr. Carolyn Schroeder's chapter for further examples. Generally accepted guidelines for dosage alteration, expected side effects, and necessary laboratory assessment could be provided by electronic communication and, due to the nature of virtual algorithms, could be updated in real time, as opposed to the inevitable lags with paper publications. When all of the involved disciplines realize that our intent is to improve access and outcomes for children around increasingly complex mental health concerns, the mandate for cooperative change becomes more compelling. To quote Antoine de Saint-Exupery, "As for the future, your task is not to foresee, but to enable it."

In the year 2000, the American Academy of Pediatrics and other members of the pediatric community completed and published the Future of Pediatric Education II Report. This document, a follow-up to the original report published in 1978, laid out the expected necessary course and requirements as to how the next generation of pediatricians would need to be educated. The ever improving health status of America's children with continued expected decreases in the acquisition of acute infectious illness due to improved hygiene, new immunizations, and improved overall immunity is overshadowed by the increasing prominence described in the 1970s as the "New Morbidity of Pediatrics"—abuse, neglect, and biopsychosocial problems. Although the healthcare system has rewarded pediatric practice in the past for illnesses which should have decreasing future relevance, it is incumbent on the pediatric community to anticipate the inevitability of change and to address the crushing burden of unmet mental health and developmental needs for America's children.

If the 8,000 pediatric trainees, who are presently passing through the postgraduate educational system, are not enlightened about the real needs that they will be asked to address in practice, then pediatrics could find itself in an environmental niche which would be an evolutionary dead end. A robust future would require the ability to view pediatric care as an opportunity for enhanced cooperative, compassionate, collaborative, coordinated care as a team approach linking services to a variety of interested participants in the medical and mental health communities.

REFERENCES

American Medical Association. (2000). *Physicians' current procedural terminology: CPT 01*. Chicago, IL: Author.

Contemporary Pediatrics 2001 Factbook. (2002). Medical Economics Publications.

Hellman, C. J. C., Budd, M., Borysenko, J., McClellamd, D. C., & Benson H. (1990). A study of the effectiveness of two groups behavioral medicine interventions for patients with psychosomatic complaints. *Behavioral Medicine, 16*, 165-173.

Kelleher, K. J., McInerney, T. K., Gardner, W. P., Childs, G. E., & Wasserman, R. C. (2000). Increasing identification of psychosocial problems: 1979-1996. *Pediatrics, 105*, 1313-1321.

National Committee for Quality Assurance. (1997). *The health plan employer data and information set, 3.0.* Washington, DC: Author.

Rappo, P. D. (1997). The care of children with chronic illness in primary care practice: Implications for the pediatric generalist. *Pediatric Annals, 26*.

U. S. Department of Health and Human Services. (1999). *National ambulatory medical care survey.* Washington, DC: Author.

Wolraich, M. L., Felice, M. E., & Drotar, D. (Eds.). (1996). *The classification of child and adolescent mental diagnoses in primary care; diagnostic and statistical manual for primary care (DSM-PC) child and adolescent version.* Elk Grove Village, IL: American Academy of Pediatrics.

DISCUSSION SUMMARY
written by Christine Golden

Dr. Rappo offered a realistic glimpse into the challenges that pediatricians face in attempting to address psychosocial problems in primary care. His extensive personal experience and work with various national agencies allowed him to provide Forum participants with a comprehensive view of these challenges set within the national milieu.

Dr. Rappo began his presentation by discussing the uniquely American framework that has been developed for the practice of primary care pediatrics. Dr. Rappo noted that on an international basis, pediatricians are primarily used as "specialty consultants," whereas in the United States, the primary care pediatrician is working within a practice-based context. Within this context, the primary care pediatrician focuses primarily on treatment of acute illness, and well-childcare that includes assessment of growth, development, nutrition, and anticipatory guidance regarding health and safety issues. The challenge of incorporating assessment of psychosocial issues was raised at this point. Dr. Rappo and Forum participants pointed out that in order for this to occur successfully there is a need for brief, empirically supported interventions as well as screening tools for primary care pediatricians to use as part of the content of a visit. Clearly, being able to implement all of these various goals within the context of a primary care pediatric visit is difficult. Dr. Rappo highlighted the fact that it would require "45 to 60 minutes per visit" to include all of the areas required and recommended the primary care pediatrician cover. He aptly pointed out that ancillary staff, handouts, internet resources, and subsequent office visits are necessary to accomplish transmission of all this information.

An ongoing discussion throughout the Forum of the impact of insurance plans, managed care, and general financial constraints placed on the primary care pediatrician followed. Dr. Rappo emphasized the fact that there are serious repercussions of inappropriately or incorrectly using the required CPT codes that insurance companies demand. He pointed out that inaccurate coding could lead to charges of fraud or abuse, as there is potential civil and criminal prosecution for providers who deal with data inappropriately or submit inappropriate claims. For example, if a pediatrician submits a diagnosis of Adjustment Disorder it may get reimbursed by the insurer but could also be considered fraudulent if the patient is actually "subsyndromal" and does not meet the full criteria for this diagnosis, as specified by the *DSM-IV.* Dr. Rappo reminded Forum participants that this need for precision in diagnosis places the primary care pediatrician in a difficult position as they desire to attend to psychosocial issues, many of which are subsyndromal, but also need to receive financial reimbursement for their time. Dr. Rappo stated that, "what drives pediatricians away from evaluation and treatment of these patients (those with psychosocial problems) is concern about lack of time for adequate assessment coupled with a historical realization that even when the time and assessment are appropriate, such efforts are poorly or nonrecompensed."

Dr. Rappo discussed the fact that our health care system currently deals with the need to address psychosocial issues by establishing mental health "carve outs." He explained that a carve out is a "separately capitated or financed pool of monies dedicated to paying for a specific healthcare benefit within the structure of a health plan or risk arrangement." While the benefit of carve outs for mental health services is clear for the insurers, the benefit to patients and the primary care physician are not as clear. Dr. Rappo discussed that having mental health carveouts leaves the primary care physician who is interested in evaluating and treating patients from a mental health perspective in an awkward position. He stated that the answer is frequently "nowhere," since the primary care physician is not credentialed by the mental health carve out to provide such services. Dr. Rappo indicated that "there have been numerous anecdotal reports at a national level that the use of diagnoses contained in the *DSM-IV* will preclude payment to a nonpsychiatric primary care provider." This would remove the possibility that a primary care pediatrician could even hope to attain reimbursement for assessment and treatment of psychosocial issues.

With this vast array of challenges set before the primary care pediatrician, it is not surprising that many experience "rust out" as Dr. Rappo discussed. He indicated that many people refer to "burn out" in the medical field, but that he felt primary care pediatricians "rust out" from prolonged, repeated attempts to manage these challenges. Dr. Rappo suggested, and Forum participants agreed, for example that the mundane work of treating repeated ear infections in order to ensure reimbursement and cover costs rather than being able to freely work with more special needs children leaves the primary care pediatrician unchallenged, and over time they grow weary of their work; they "rust out."

Dr. Rappo concluded his realistic presentation of what the primary care pediatrician faces with an injection of hope and motivation. He challenged those present at the Forum to rise to the occasion and advocate for change in the current system. He indicated that although the healthcare system has rewarded pediatric practice in the past for a focus on illness, this focus should have decreasing relevance in the future as the health status of American children improves. Recognizing this important reality, Dr. Rappo encouraged those present to realize that it is critically important for the pediatric community to advocate for children so that unmet mental health and developmental needs are met for them.

CHAPTER 7

THE ECONOMIC AND HEALTH SYSTEM CORRELATES OF DIAGNOSIS IN PRIMARY CARE

Sherry Glied and Adam Neufeld
Columbia University

Epidemiologists estimate that as many as 20% of school-age children seen in a pediatric ambulatory setting have a diagnosable behavioral disorder (Costello, 1986; Costello et al., 1988). Yet only about half of American children with a diagnosable psychiatric disorder receive treatment in a given year. And of the approximately 21% of children receiving mental health services in a year (not all of whom have a diagnosable disorder), only about 15%—just 3% of all children—receive such care from primary care physicians (U.S Department of Health and Human Services, 1999).

Unfortunately, most studies find that primary care physicians often fail to identify and properly treat psychosocial disorders in their patients (e.g., Kessler, Cleary, & Burke 1985; Klinkman, Coyne, Gallo, & Schwenk, 1997, 1998; Williams et al., 1999). The RAND medical outcomes study, for instance, found that primary care practitioners recognized only about half of all cases of depression (Wells et al., 1989). Even when primary care providers do recognize psychiatric problems, they often provide inappropriate or no treatment or referral to specialists (Mechanic, 1990; Rogers, Wells, Meredith, Sturm, & Burnam, 1993). These patterns also hold for

Treating Children's Psychosocial Problems in Primary Care, 145–170

pediatricians in particular (e.g., Costello, 1986; Costello et al., 1988; Lavigne et al., 1993; Horwitz, Leaf, Leventhal, Forsyth, & Speechley, 1992).

Yet this picture of poor diagnosis and treatment may be excessively gloomy. Many children who are not identified for treatment by their primary care practitioner do receive treatment. While the focus of this volume is on primary care, it is important to remember that an extensive network of mental health services for children is provided outside the health system. While according to the 1992 Methods for the Epidemiology of Child and Adolescent Mental Disorders (MECA) Study, only 3% of children with a diagnosable mental health condition received care for it in the general health sector, over 36% of children with a diagnosable condition did receive care. Most children with a diagnosable condition, 27%, received care in school (Leaf et al., 1996). This extensive complementary service system helps mitigate the effect on child health of the poor diagnosis rates in primary care.

Moreover, the diagnosis of psychosocial problems in children by pediatricians and family practitioners appears to have improved substantially over the last 20 years. Kelleher, McInerny, Gardner, Childs, & Wasserman (2000) compared diagnosis rates in 1979 and 1996 among children ages 4 to 15 years presenting for nonemergent services in private practice offices of primary care pediatricians and family practitioners. Clinician-identified psychiatric problems increased from 6.8% of all pediatric visits in 1979 to 18.7% in 1996.

Nonetheless, further improvement is certainly needed. Since pediatricians have regular contact with their patients and, in some contexts, also serve as gatekeepers to specialty mental health services, they often have the best opportunity to recognize psychosocial problems in children. Their diagnostic ability can have substantial effects on access to care through their diagnosis, and treatment of psychiatric disorders in children.

This chapter uses an economic model of diagnosis in primary care to evaluate the potential for policy to yield further improvements in these rates of diagnosis and treatment. This model, based loosely on the fundamental economic theory of the production of health (Grossman, 1972), suggests that a physician's diagnosis of depression depends on inputs, including patient characteristics, provider characteristics, and resources available, and on the production technology available to the physician—that is the methods available to diagnose and treat depression. Improvements in the diagnosis of depression in primary care, according to this model, are likely to stem from changes in these inputs or technologies.

From a policy perspective, key input and technology characteristics to evaluate are those that both affect the likelihood of diagnosis (such as those that affect the underlying prevalence of depression in practices) and are amenable to policy change. Policy has its most direct effects on the resources available at a visit. Policy affects resource availability by influencing the organization and funding of the health care system. Thus, the central focus of this chapter will be on system organization and funding. We begin, however, by examining policy relevant aspects of patient and physician characteristics and in the technologies of treatment available to providers.

PATIENT CHARACTERISTICS, PROVIDER TRAINING, AND TECHNOLOGY

The rate of diagnosis of psychosocial problems in primary care depends, in part, on the epidemiology of depression in the population seeking care. Since the prevalence of psychosocial problems varies with age, sex, and socioeconomic status, the prevalence of psychosocial problems in primary care is affected by the sociodemographic characteristics of the population that seeks care. Although policy has little impact on these characteristics of all children, it can certainly alter the profile of children who actually seek care. The main factor that affects the characteristics of children who appear in primary care is the availability of health insurance.

There have been significant recent changes in access to health insurance for low income children. During the late 1980s and early 1990s, Medicaid eligibility expanded so that in 2002 all children under age 19 throughout the United States from families with incomes below 100% of the federal poverty line are eligible for Medicaid, and eligibility is broader in many states. In 1997, the Federal Government passed the State Children's Health Insurance Program (SCHIP), which further expanded coverage to children. In most states, children from families with incomes below 200% of the federal poverty line are eligible for SCHIP (Rosenbach et al., 2001). Both these programs provide coverage for mental health services provided in primary care.

Children on Medicaid and CHIP have lower incomes than privately insured children and are more likely to come from families with only one parent. Both these sociodemographic characteristics increase the underlying prevalence of mental health problems (Glied et al., 1998). Having health insurance coverage increases the propensity of children to make primary care visits (Glied, Hoven, Moore, Garrett, & Regier, 1997). Thus, expansions of these programs may have led to increases in the prevalence of mental health problems in the population seen by primary care physicians. Indeed, Kelleher et al. (2000) associates the increased primary care diagnosis rate in children over the past 20 years in part with an increase in Medicaid enrollment.

A second way that expanded Medicaid enrollment may affect the prevalence of disorder in primary care is through the interaction of Medicaid eligibility and child eligibility for Supplemental Security Income (SSI) benefits. When a child becomes eligible for SSI because of a disability, the child is also automatically made eligible for Medicaid. In response to the Supreme Court's 1990 ruling in *Sullivan v. Zebley* (1990) the standards for determining SSI-qualifying disability in children were made more flexible. Additionally, in 1990, new mental health functional criteria were implemented for children and certain child mental health problems, such as attention deficit hyperactivity disorder (ADHD) and eating disorders, were added to the list of disabilities qualifying for SSI. Between 1989 and 1992, the share of SSI children receiving payments due to a psychiatric disorder increased from 6.4% to 16.6% (Kennedy, 1993). Although new regulations have limited child eligibility for SSI, almost 30% of children receiving federal SSI payments in 2000 had a psychiatric diagnosis. Overall, 850,000 children received a federal or state SSI payment in 2000, up from 227,000 in 1985 (Social Security Administration, 2000). Children who become eligible for Medicaid through an SSI-qualifying mental health disability are, by definition, more likely to have a mental health problem than other, nonqualifying children.

A second policy-relevant input into the rate of diagnosis and treatment is provider training. The ability of providers to diagnose psychosocial problems in primary care is a function of their training. Physicians receive general and specialty training. Both the content of general training and the mix of specialties in the primary care physician population may affect the propensity of physicians to make a diagnosis. Furthermore, physicians also obtain training after finishing medical school, and this training, too, may affect diagnosis rates. Policy can affect the content of training, the specialty mix, and the availability of continuing educational efforts.

Some researchers have asserted that many primary care physicians do not feel adequately prepared to diagnosis and treat psychosocial problems (Badger et al., 1994; Main, Lutz, Barrett, Matthew, & Miller, 1993; Sharp, Pantell, Murphy, & Lewis, 1992). In a survey of pediatricians and family practitioners who see children, only 8% reported adequate training in the treatment of childhood depression and 16% agreed with the statement "I am comfortable with treatment of childhood depression."

Some studies find that specialty training is important. Pediatricians appear more likely to refer patients with depression and somewhat less likely to treat with selective serotonin reuptake inhibitors (SSRIs) than family practitioners (Rushton, Clark, & Freed, 2000a, 2000b). On the other hand, Gardner et al. (2000) found that a primary care clinicians' training, practice type, and beliefs about mental health issues had no effect on treatment choices for children who had an identified psychosocial problem but were not already receiving specialty mental health services. Similarly, Kelleher et al. (2000) concluded that the increase in primary care diagnosis of children over the past 20 years was not associated with a change in clinician characteristics.

Considerable attention has been focused on ways of improving the ability of primary care physicians to diagnose and treat mental illness, even after they complete their medical education. The U.S. Department of Health and Human Services sponsored the creation of clinical practice guidelines for the detection of mental illness in primary care (e.g., Depression Guideline Panel, 1993). Research agendas also reflect the growing importance of the primary care physician in the recognition and treatment of mental illness. By 1997, the Services Research and Clinical Epidemiology branch was allocating $8.8 million to study provision of services for psychiatric disorders in primary care (National Institutes of Health, 1999). For instance, there have been efforts focused on training primary care practitioners to effectively locate depressed patients within their practices.

A third component of diagnosis and treatment is the availability of technology. The menu of diagnostic tools and therapies available to practitioners has significantly expanded over the past 15 years. There have been stiking innovations in psychopharmaceuticals and more information is now available on previously existing modalities.

There has also been considerable innovation in the methods available for diagnosis of psychosocial disorders within the context of an office visit (e.g., Brody et al., 1999; Jellinek et al., 1999; Leon, Olfson, Weissman, Portera, & Sheehan, 1996; Mulrow et al., 1995; Spitzer, Kroenke, & Williams, 1999; Weissman et al., 1998). Standardized behavioral screening instruments, such as questionnaires for parents, behavior-rating scales, and checklists (e.g., Child Behavior Checklist, Pediatric Symptom Checklist), have been suggested as ways to improve physicians' ability to make a diagnosis. Despite this innovation in the design phase, however, it is not clear that use of these instruments actually improves diagnosis in practice (Stancin & Palermo, 1997). Furthermore, there is little evidence that these screening instruments are widely used in primary care.

By contrast, innovations in psychopharmeceuticals have disseminated widely. Most significant of these innovations are the new selective serotonin reuptake inhibitors (SSRIs) which were introduced in 1988. Because they had fewer side effects than the traditional tricylic antidepressant (TCA) medications, Prozac and other SSRIs were widely adopted for treatment of depression beginning in 1989. The introduction of SSRIs has contributed to a large increase in the share of visits to primary care physicians associated with psychotropic drugs (in terms of prescription, supply, administration, and continuation). Indeed, if SSRIs are excluded, the number of psychotropic drugs visits remained basically unchanged (Pincus et al., 1998). New antipsychotics, such as Clozapine and Risperdal, were also approved in the late 1980s and the 1990s (Coffey et al., 2000).

Psychotropic prescriptions, counseling, and referrals in primary care for children in particular have increased over the last 20 years (Kelleher et al., 2000). Ambulatory care prescriptions for psychotropics even for the youngest children, those ages 2 to 4, increased from 1991 to 1995 (Zito et al., 2000).

For children, psychopharmaceuticals used are primarily stimulants for attention deficit hyperactivity disorder (ADHD) and SSRIs for depression and anxiety. ADHD is the most commonly diagnosed childhood psychosocial problem and is generally effectively treated with stimulants such as Ritalin. Although stimulants have been used for childhood behavioral problems since the 1930s, stimulant prescriptions of ADHD have increased greatly since 1989 (Goldman, Genel, Bezman, & Slanetz, 1998; U.S. Department of Health and Human Services, 1999). In 1996, SSRIs began to be used for treating major depression in children, after the previous standard, tricyclic antidepressants, showed higher toxicity and lower efficacy in children (U.S. Department of Health and Human Services, 1999).

The influence of innovations in psychopharmaceuticals on diagnosis and treatment would not be expected to be as great among children as among adults, because research on the use of these medications in children has lagged. Except for stimulants prescribed for ADHD, most psychotropic drugs used in children have only undergone extensive safety and efficacy testing in adults, and are either inadequately labeled or not labeled for pediatric use (Vitiello & Jensen, 1997). Extrapolation of adult drug data to children has been the typical route. Children are thus exposed to greater risk of over- or underdosing. Many physicians may decide the drugs have not been sufficiently researched to prescribe, thus denying children potentially effective therapies. Physician choice is further limited because many drugs are not produced in forms, such as chewable tablets, young children can use (U.S. Food and Drug Administration, 2001).

The outlook for pediatric psychotropics has improved recently. The Food and Drug Administration (FDA) Modernization Act of 1997 included a pediatric exclusivity provision, which granted six months exclusivity to manufacturers for conducting pediatric studies of drugs. The marketing incentive has been fairly effective in encouraging more pediatric research and in providing new information for product labeling. The FDA has also recently begun requiring pediatric studies in certain circumstances, although the effect this regulation will have is unclear (U.S. Food and Drug Administration, 2001).

SYSTEM AND VISIT CHARACTERISTICS

Health care system organization and financing are the inputs into diagnosis and treatment that are most amenable to policy change. The organization and financing of care for mental health problems is quite distinctive within health care. Health insurers have controlled mental health care service use much more tightly than general health use.

Mental health care has traditionally been associated with higher copayments and deductibles and more stringent lifetime limits than other forms of health spending. The reason for this is that mental health service use is much more sensitive to the provision of insurance than are other forms of health service use (Frank & McGuire, 2000). A person who can obtain mental health services at no cost uses about four times as many services as would an identical person who had to pay full cost for these services. By contrast, a person who can obtain general health services at no cost uses only about two times as many services as would an identical person who had to pay full cost (Newhouse, 1993).

Unfortunately, these higher copayments and deductibles, while reducing excessive service use, have also kept some children in need from seeking care altogether. They have also meant that families of children with mental health problems have had to bear significant financial burdens for care. These problems have led to the recent policy interest in parity for mental health coverage. Parity legislation would require that plans impose identical limits for both general and mental health services.

Although full parity has not yet passed at the federal level, more than 20 states have adopted parity legislation (Frank, Goldman, & McGuire, 2001). One reason for the growing acceptability of parity legislation is that managed care offers insurers new ways of controlling service utilization without imposing high out-of-pocket costs on service users. These new techniques, including provider capitation and utilization review, allow insurers to monitor service use and restrict services to those most in need. These new restrictions may not bring equity between mental and general health coverage, because access to mental health care can still be more tightly controlled than access to general health services (Burnam & Escarce, 1999). By reducing copayments, however, these new forms of controlling access may reduce financial burdens on severely affected families. They also substantially reduce the impediments to seeking out care for an initial visit and, thus, several studies suggest, increase the proportion of the population receiving some care (Burns, Teagle, Schwartz, Angold, & Holtzman, 1999; Stroul, Pires, Armstrong, & Meyers, 1998).

Managed care has spread rapidly in mental health and among children. Almost 80% of privately insured Americans are covered for mental health services through a specialized managed behavioral health carve out (Findlay, 1999). Children are disproportionately enrolled in managed care. Youths under the age of 20 made up around 33% of HMO enrollment in 1994. Twenty-two percent of that age group, or 16.7 million, were enrolled in managed care plans (Hughes & Luft, 1998). Of particular importance to children, Medicaid plans are increasingly turning from fee-for-service insurance to managed care. By 1999, 42 states operated some form of managed mental health care (Substance Abuse and Mental Health Services Administration, 2000). Some of these arrangements include children with serious emotional disorders in all plans; others carve out such children to special plans. In both these cases, private plans are paid a capitated fee to care for children with these disorders.

In principle, the organization and financing of the mental health care system, including the ways in which it differs from the general health system, may affect diagnosis and treatment in several ways. One important way is by affecting the time and resources that physicians are willing to commit to a patient. Several analysts have argued that the time constraints of primary care practice inhibit diagnosis and treatment of psychosocial problems (Eisenberg, 1992; Kroenke, 1997). Others, though, have suggested that identification of mental health disorders is mainly a function of the first few minutes of treatment and longer visit lengths do not lead to a higher rate of diagnosis (Goldberg, Jenkins, Millar, & Faragher, 1993; Marks, Goldberg, & Hillier, 1979).

Although there has been great concern about the effects of managed care on the time constraints of practice, the evidence suggests that primary care visits have been growing longer, not shorter. Mechanic, McAlpine, and Rosenthal (2001) found that the mean length of prepaid visits to primary care physicians by individuals of all ages increased by 2.0 minutes from 1989 to 1998. The mean duration of nonprepaid visits increased by 2.6 minutes. The visit duration for patients with common and serious primary diagnoses increased or stayed the same over the period from 1989 to 1998.

Managed care may restrict the resources available to primary care physicians in other ways. For example, physicians who are capitated for specialty referrals may try to avoid incurring the cost of specialty care and treat patients who might be better served in specialty care.

Evidence on how diagnosis and treatment of mental health problems varies by physician payment type is limited to adults, studies are dated, and results are mixed. One large study found that outcomes for adults with depression were worse for those enrolled in managed care plans than in those enrolled in fee-for-service plans. The principal reason for this difference was the greater use of primary care physicians in diagnosing and treating depression under managed care (Keeler, Manning, & Wells, 1988). Similarly, the RAND health insurance study, which compared primary care providers in fee-for-service settings and in-group practice HMOs found that primary care providers in the HMO had lower rates of diagnosis and treatment for mental health problems (Wells et al., 1989). In contrast, two other studies found no differences in recognition, treatment, or outcomes among adult respondents with mental health problems who had HMO or fee-for-service coverage (Leaf et al., 1988; Wells, Manning, & Valdez, 1990).

The organization of the system may affect the frequency with which patients seek care, and hence, the number of problems presented at a single visit. Patients often present a host of health problems and complaints to a primary care provider in a single visit (Kroenke, 1997; Lemelin, Hotz, Swensen, & Elmslie, 1994). If patients make fewer visits annually, mental health needs are more likely to compete for physician attention with other important health problems. Again, there has been no significant change in the annual number of visits per child to outpatient health care providers (Kirby, Machlin, &Thorpe, 2001).

Similarly, the organization of the system may affect the complexity and nature of problems seen in primary care. In particular, under managed care gatekeeping systems or capitated payment arrangements, the severity of problems seen by primary care providers may increase. Thirty percent of primary care practitioners in a recent survey reported that the scope of care for which they are responsible has expanded (St. Peter, Reed, Kemper, & Blumenthal, 1999).

Characteristics of the health care system changes may affect the rate at which patients switch providers and thus, the continuity of care. Kelleher et al. (1997) suggest that continuity of care is the best predictor of clinician recognition of psychosocial problems in children who screened positive on the Parental Symptom Checklist. The growth of managed care arrangements in which patients have limited choice of physicians has raised concerns about continuity of care. People with HMO coverage are much more likely to report that they changed providers because of a change in health plan than are those with other coverage. Nonetheless, the difference in the overall rate of provider switching is not great. About 14% of people with HMO coverage changed providers in 1998-1999, compared to just over 11% in non-HMO plans (Reed, 2000).

Finally, the nature of the health care system may affect the ability and willingness of physicians to make referrals to other specialties. If physicians find it difficult to make appropriate referrals for psychosocial problems, it is plausible that they would not make special efforts to identify such problems. The expansion of managed care, and particularly of behavioral health carve-outs, has raised concerns about further deterioration in the coordination between physical and mental health services. Carve-out plans do not generally require a primary care referral for access to mental health specialty care. Instead, mental health specialty care is carved out to a dedicated behavioral health provider (Feldman, 1998). Often in carve-out arrangements, the referring physician and the mental health professional have no direct contact.

Although further studies are needed to assess this threat fully, separating the financing of mental health from that of physical health appears to maintain, and may even improve, access and quality of mental health services (Burns et al., 1999; Stroul, Pires, Armstrong, & Meyers, 1998; Sturm & Klap, 1999). The likely reason for these optimistic results is that carve-out plans are compared not to an ideal system, but to the system in place before the carve outs entered the market. Behavioral carve outs typically replace plans that have very high copayment rates for mental health service use. Under carve outs, people who would have been shut out of care by these financial limits are able to receive treatment. At the same time, the poor prior record of primary care physicians in diagnosing and treating mental health problems before carve outs makes it more difficult to detect any deterioration due to diminished coordination.

In sum, the institutional and financial context in which pediatric visits take place has profoundly changed and there is reason to believe that organizational and financial context are important in the rate of diagnosis and treatment. But the magnitude and importance of these effects is less clear.

THE MAGNITUDE AND IMPORTANCE OF SYSTEM AND VISIT CHARACTERISTICS IN CHILD MENTAL HEALTH DIAGNOSIS AND TREATMENT

Research on primary care diagnosis in adults provides some evidence of the relative importance of these various inputs. Glied (1998) used the National Ambulatory Care Survey (NAMCS), a large nationally representative annual survey of office-based physicians to study how system and provider characteristics affect diagnosis. She found that physicians who usually spent more time with patients were no more likely to diagnose mental health problems than were those whose typical visits were shorter. Similarly, physicians who saw more patients with HMO coverage were no less likely to diagnose than those who tended to see patients with fee-for-service coverage (Glied, 1998). In this study, physicians specializing in family practice were more likely to make a mental health diagnosis than were internists and general practitioners. Physicians who more frequently reported that they had counseled a patient to stop smoking were also more likely to diagnose mental health problems, suggesting that practice style may be an important determinant of diagnosis (Glied, 1998).

The results of this study suggest that system changes have not been important drivers of diagnosis in adults. But similar analyses have not yet been conducted about diagnosis rates in children. We repeated our analyses of the NAMCS to explore changing patterns in the treatment and diagnosis of psychosocial disorders in children by primary care physicians over the past 15 years.[1] We restricted our analysis to general practitioners, family practitioners, and pediatricians. As in the prior study, we examined both patient and practice level measures. For example, we examined how insurance status affects diagnosis and treatment by comparing rates among children with different types of coverage. Physician's practice characteristics, including features such as visit length and content, however, may not vary according to a specific patient's insurance coverage. Instead, physicians may organize their practices according to the characteristics of their average patient (Glied & Graff Zivin, 2002). To test this, we also examined whether diagnosis was affected by the percentage of a provider's patients who hold managed care or Medicaid coverage.

As prior research has suggested, our analyses show that the rate of mental health diagnosis in children in visits to primary care providers has increased over the past 15 years. In 1998, 2.57% of children seen in primary care visits had a mental health diagnosis, up from 0.82% in 1985 (Figure 7.1). This trend is strong and significant (Table 7.1, Column 1).

Patients whose reasons for visiting included mental health symptoms were much more likely to receive a psychiatric diagnosis. Over time, the share of visits at which patients report mental health symptoms has increased significantly. Again, however, changes in the rate of mental health symptom presentation alone do not explain the increasing diagnosis trend. Indeed, the psychiatric diagnosis rate for children whose reasons for the visit do *not* include mental health symptoms shows a strong and significant increasing time trend over the past 15 years. This suggests that primary care providers are getting better at identifying mental health problems that are not directly flagged.

How might changes in patient, physician, and system characteristics, and in technologies have affected diagnosis?

In our data, as elsewhere, children who are male, older, or white are more likely to be diagnosed with a psychiatric disorder (Table 7.1, Column 2). However, the increasing trend in diagnosis rates is not related to changes in patient demographics. The share of children visiting primary care physicians who were covered by Medicaid increased from 10% of the

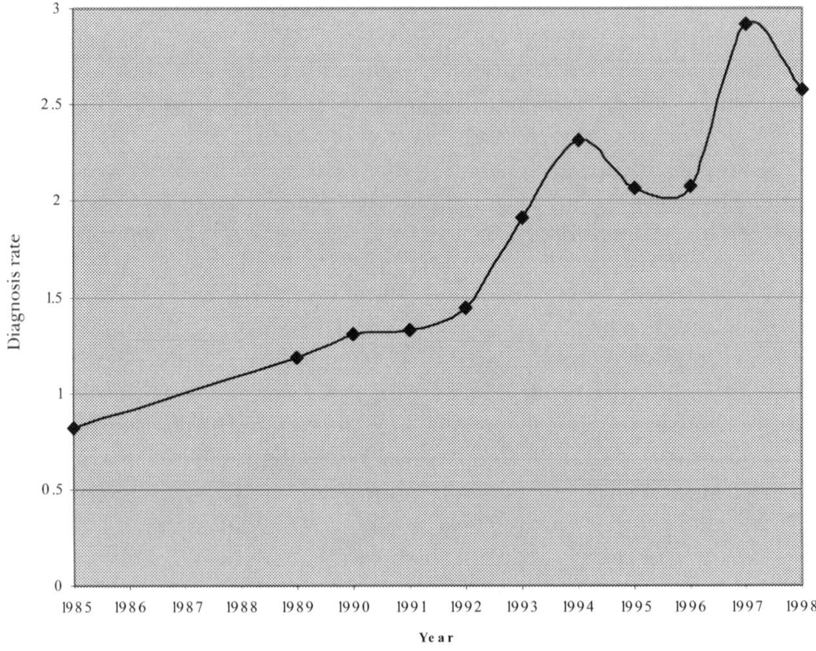

Figure 7.1. Diagnosis rate for children in visits to primary care providers.

caseload in 1985 to 18% in 1998. Psychiatric diagnosis was significantly more likely for patients who had Medicaid coverage. The Medicaid effect is not just a product of greater mental health symptom presentation among the Medicaid population as would be expected if SSI incentives were driving this result. Controlling for mental health symptoms does not affect Medicaid's significance, suggesting an independent effect on diagnosis. Although we find that children with Medicaid were more likely to be diagnosed with a mental health problem, Medicaid expansions explain only a part of the overall time trend. Kelleher et al. (2000), comparing two points in time (1979 and 1996) finds that increased Medicaid coverage explains part of the observed increase in diagnosis.

Pediatricians were significantly more likely to make a psychiatric diagnosis than were (self-described) general practitioners, while family practitioners were somewhat, but not significantly, more likely to make a psychiatric diagnosis than general practitioners. Like Kelleher et al. (2000), we find that changes in the specialty composition of physicians do not appear to be responsible for the increase in primary care diagnosis rates over the past 15 years.

Our main focus is on changes in visit and system characteristics, and these changes have been large. The percentage of children seen in pri-

Table 7.1. Psychiatric Diagnosis, Patient Characteristics (1985-1998)

	Year only *N = 46,838*	*Year, Demographics, Insurance, Symptoms, Visit* *N = 44,106*
Time trend	1.102** (0.028)	1.078** (0.029)
Male		2.050** (0.296)
Age		1.849** (0.121)
Age^2		0.975** (0.0033)
Black		0.542** (0.145)
Asian/Native American/Other		0.513 (0.237)
Hispanic		0.546* (0.177)
Medicaid		1.645* (0.453)
HMO		0.787 (0.170)
Mental health symptoms		65.64** (13.66)
2+ symptoms		0.744 (0.139)
Patient seen before		0.900 (0.219)
Pediatrician		1.876* (0.618)
Family practitioner		1.667 (0.564)
Mean visit duration in practice		1.009 (0.014)
Medicaid composition in practice		1.329 (0.643)
HMO composition in practice		1.480 (0.640)
R^2	0.011	0.251

Notes: *Odds Ratios with $p < 0.10$; **Odds Ratios with $p < 0.05$; *SE* accounts for clustering and stratification (40% inflation)

mary care who held HMO coverage has increased in the past 15 years, from 12.3% in 1985 to 37.7% in 1998.

Although more children belong to HMOs, we found no evidence to suggest that the growth in HMOs had affected diagnosis. Belonging to an HMO did not have a direct significant effect on psychiatric diagnosis. While a growth of managed care may have increased the complexity of problems seen in primary care, we found that children with multiple symptoms were not significantly less likely to be diagnosed with a mental health problem than were those who reported only a single problem. Similarly, while HMOs may lead patients to switch providers more often, diagnosis rates were not associated with whether the patient had seen the provider before.

The average duration of primary care visits by children has increased over the past 15 years, from 12.6 minutes in 1985 to 15.2 minutes in 1998. Physicians spent about 50% more time during visits with children with a psychiatric diagnosis than for other children. A provider's average visit length had a small and insignificant effect on diagnosis.

We also looked at whether the insurance composition of the practice affected the likelihood of psychiatric diagnosis. The Medicaid share of a practice was not a significant predictor of diagnosis, suggesting that physicians serving low-income populations are not more (or less) likely to make a psychiatric diagnosis. The share of a provider's patients who belonged to an HMO also did not affect the likelihood of diagnosis.

In sum, patient and provider characteristics have substantial effects on diagnosis rates. Together with symptom presentation, these characteristics explain about one fourth of the variation in diagnosis. Changes in these characteristics over the past 15 years, however, have not been large enough to alter population-level diagnosis rates. Changes in system characteristics, by contrast, have been very large. These characteristics, however, appear to have very little effect on diagnosis rates and contribute little to either the diagnosis rate at a point in time or to changes in that rate over time.

What Explains Improvements in Diagnosis and Treatment?

If patient, provider, and system characteristics do not explain improvements in treatment, what does? Most health economics studies identify changes in medical technology as the most important reason for increases in health care costs and, in the recent past, improvements in health care outcomes (Newhouse, 1993; Cutler & McClellan, 2001). Evidence on adult mental health suggests that technological changes also explain changes in adult diagnosis rates.

In adults, the rate of diagnosis of mental illness in primary care has increased over the past 10 years. From 1987-1997, the rate of outpatient treatment for depression increased from 0.73 per 100 to 2.33 per 100. This change appears to be largely a consequence of the introduction of new therapies (Olfson et al., 2002). New therapies tend to be easier to prescribe and are more frequently prescribed by primary care doctors.

The pattern for children may differ in important ways because, as discussed above, developments in psychopharmacology have been less significant for children. To assess this, we compared diagnosis rates with and without an accompanying psychotropic prescription. If developments or marketing in drugs were responsible for changes in diagnosis, we would expect the rate of diagnoses with accompanying prescriptions to increase relative to the rate of diagnoses without drugs (Figure 7.2).

Diagnoses with an accompanying mental health prescription rose dramatically in 1993 and 1994, while diagnoses without psychotropics jumped in 1997. Over the past 15 years, the likelihood of having psycho-

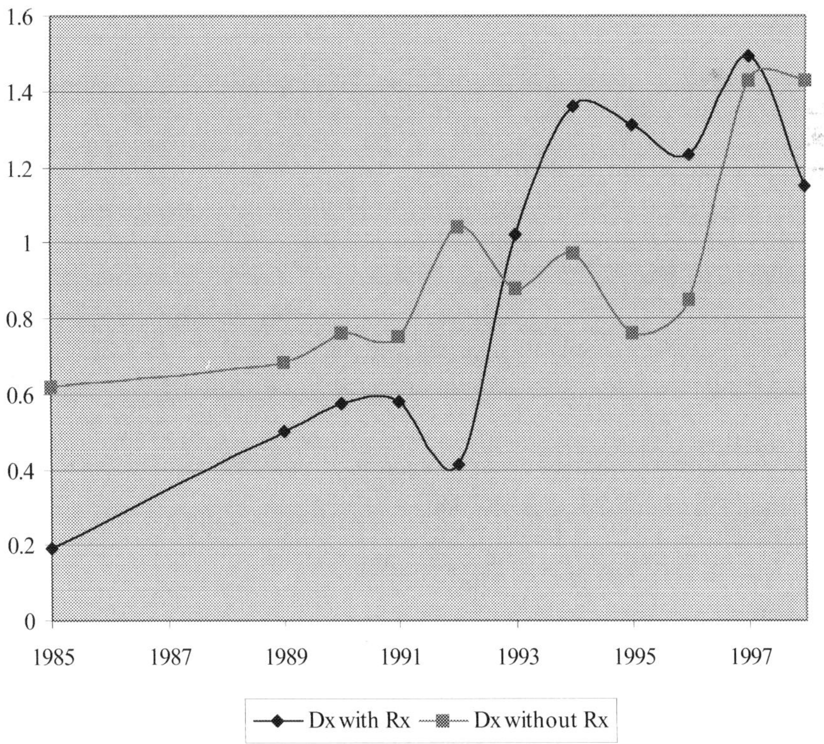

Figure 7.2. Diagnosis rates with and without psychotropic drugs

tropic medication accompany a diagnosis increased substantially, yet unlike the situation for adults, the diagnosis rate increased both with and without an accompanying psychotropic prescription. In a regression framework controlling for all individual characteristic variables including mental health symptom presentation and Medicaid, however, the time trend was substantially greater for diagnosis with accompanying psychotropic medication than diagnosis without psychotropics. For children, as for adults, dissemination of treatment technologies that make treatment fit more easily into standard office practice appears to be correlated with increases in diagnosis rates.

Increased diagnosis of ADHD accounts for most of the trend in psychiatric diagnosis over the past 15 years. In 1985, ADHD accounted for 31% of mental health diagnoses. By 1998, ADHD accounted for fully half of all mental health diagnoses. The rate of diagnosis of ADHD grew most among children who did not report mental health symptoms as a reason for their visit. In fact, the time trend in diagnosis for all psychiatric disorders other than ADHD was not significant.

Changes in technology also affected treatment patterns. The psychotropic prescription rate has increased significantly over the past 15 years, but it has increased less than has the diagnosis rates. In 1985, only 23% of children with a mental health diagnosis received a prescription for psychotropic medication. By 1998, the figure had increased to 45%. Insurance did affect the rate of psychotropic medication. Physicians whose practices had a higher share of patients covered by Medicaid were much more likely to prescribe psychotropic medication while patients who belonged to an HMO were significantly less likely to receive a prescription for psychotropic medications.

CONCLUSIONS

The limited effects of system changes on diagnosis rates suggests that changes in policy through better incentives are unlikely to be the key to substantial improvements in diagnosis rates. Although this conclusion appears to fly in the face of both lamentations about the negative consequences of system change and excitement about the potential of such change, it is quite consistent with the results of most studies of economic incentives in medicine.

Prior studies have examined how patients, providers, and health care systems respond to changes in financial incentives. Patients, studies suggest, will double their use of general health care services if they can obtain these services at no charge instead of paying their full cost (Newhouse, 1993). Providers might as much as double the number of patients they see in a week if they move from pure salary payment to pure fee-for-service (Gaynor & Pauly, 1990). Moving from fee-for-service to managed care reduces expenditures by 10-15% (Glied, 2000). These effects are large in percentage terms, but, like all percentage effects, their impact on the absolute magnitude of spending depends crucially on the baseline.

In the case of child mental health diagnosis in primary care, the baseline rate is very low. Fewer than 10% of children with a diagnosable disorder received care in a primary care setting in 1991, according to the MECA study (Leaf et al., 1996). Even doubling the rate of diagnosis in primary care—the largest incentive effect identified in the literature on patient and provider behavior—would only increase that rate to about 15%. If all the children newly diagnosed were children who had not been previously identified in any other setting, this dramatic shift in incentives would only increase the share of all children with a diagnosable disorder treated from 50% to about 56%.

Incentives are indeed powerful, but they build on existing resources and technologies. Once these are in place—once the baseline improves—incentives may generate significant changes from baseline. In medicine, the most important factor moving the baseline is technology. Thus, improving the technology of outpatient diagnosis and treatment is a necessary precondition for using better incentives to generate further improvements.

We find ample evidence that the technologies of diagnosis and treatment are improving. Diagnosis rates both with and without an accompanying prescription have increased, as has the rate of diagnosis in patients who do not present with mental health symptoms. The challenge for researchers working to improve diagnosis in primary care is to develop more technologies that can be easily disseminated into primary care practice. These new technologies may take many forms—from diagnostic algorithms to psychopharmaceuticals to simpler mechanisms for referral to arrangements that facilitate partnerships with other mental health professionals. System incentives should promote experimentation and ensure that successful models are disseminated. Currently, though, incentives are neither the primary culprit in poor diagnosis rates nor a panacea for their improvement.

ACKNOWLEDGMENT

This research was supported, in part, by funding from the Columbia Child Psychiatry Intervention Research Center.

NOTE

1. We use methods similar to those described in Glied (1998). Briefly, the National Ambulatory Medical Care Survey (NAMCS) is an annual, nationally representative, survey of physicians in office-based practice (Tenney, White, & Williamson, 1974). We use data from the NAMCS for the years 1985 and 1989 through 1998. The survey asks randomly sampled physicians to report demographic, diagnostic, treatment, and visit characteristics of about 30 randomly selected visits that take place within a sample week. Physicians describe the most important three reasons for a visit, up to three diagnoses, services provided at the visit, method of payment, and duration of visit. We calculated the average duration of a visit with all child patients without a mental health diagnosis by a provider. Only providers who had seen at least five patients without a mental health diagnosis were included.

   The NAMCS includes information on physician specialty. In the NAMCS, each office visit is associated with up to three *ICD-9-CM* diagnoses. Our classification of mental health diagnoses excludes organic psychotic conditions that do not result from substance abuse, organic nonpsychotic conditions and mental retardation. The NAMCS assigns to each unique drug a 6-digit code, up to six of which are recorded for each physician visit. Each drug compound is assigned a National Drug Code (NDC) directory drug class, which include 626 (sedative, hypnotic), 627 (anxiolytic), 628 (antipsychotic), 630 (antidepressant), 631 (anorexiant), and 632 (miscellaneous psychotropic). NDC codes yield a preliminary list of drugs to which we compared an index of psychiatric agents from the 1999 Tarascon Pocket Pharmacopoeia (Tarascon Publishing, Loma Linda, CA). Also, any recently released drugs with psychiatric indications from the FDA Orange Book were included. This list was reviewed and refined by several practitioners for completeness. Drugs were excluded if, on the basis of primary and secondary indications and practitioners' opinions, a significant portion of their clinical usage was not in the treatment of a diagnosable psychiatric disorder. For an analysis of means and variance, we use STATA (College Station, Texas).

   We adjusted all analyses using population weights so that results reflect the experience of a random sample of patients throughout the country. The sample design of the NAMCS includes multiple patients seen by the same physician. We adjusted for the effect of this intracluster correlation on the statistical significance of the findings. Our calculations also incorporate the effects of stratification on the standard errors of estimates. Since we do not know the strata, we use a method suggested by Potthoff, Woodbury, and Manton (1992) and adjust N for the sample as a whole over all years of data. This correction increases standard errors for the full sample by about 40%. Inflation factors for individual years are generally smaller than 40%.

   The NAMCS collects information on expected payment source for each visit. We used the following hierarchy to assign primary insurance coverage type for each individual: (1) Any private insurance (employer- or union-sponsored insurance, individual nongroup insurance, CHAMPUS/CHAMPVA military coverage); (2) Public insurance only (Medicaid, Medicare, other government programs). We could not distinguish uninsured visits from those that were paid out-of-pocket for other reasons.

REFERENCES

Badger, L. W., deGruy, F. V., Hartman, J., Plant, M. A., Leeper, J., Ficken, R., Maxwell, A., Rand, E., Anderson, R., & Templeton, B. (1994). Psychosocial interest, medical interviews, and the recognition of depression. *Archives of Family Medicine, 3*(10), 899-907.

Brody, D. S., Hahn, S. R., Spitzer, R. L., Kroenke, K., Linzer, M., deGruy, F. V., & Williams, J. B. (1999). Identifying patients with depression in the primary care setting: A more efficient method. *Archives of Internal Medicine, 158*(22), 2469-2475.

Burnam, M. A., & Escarce, J. J. (1999). Equity in managed care for mental disorders. *Health Affairs, 18*(5), 22-31.

Burns, B. J., Teagle, S. E., Schwartz, M., Angold, A., & Holtzman, A. (1999). Managed behavioral health care: A Medicaid carve-out for youth. *Health Affairs, 18*(5), 214-25.

Coffey, R. M., Mark, T., King, E., Harwood, H., McKusick, D., Genuardi, D., Dilonardo, J., & Buck, J. (2000). *National estimates of expenditures for mental health and substance abuse treatment, 1997.* Rockville, MD: U.S. Department of Health and Human Services, Substance Abuse and Mental Health Services Administration.

Costello, E. J. (1986). Primary care pediatrics and child psychopathology: A review of diagnostic, treatment, and referral practices. *Pediatrics, 78,* 771-774.

Costello, E. J., Costello, A. J., Edelbrock, C., Burns, B. J., Dulcan, M. K., Brent, D., & Janiszewski, S. (1988). Psychiatric disorders in pediatric primary care: Prevalence and risk factors. *Archives of General Psychiatry, 45,* 1107-1116.

Cutler, D. M., & McClellan, M. (2001). Is technological change in medicine worth it? *Health Affair, 20*(5), 11-29.

Depression Guideline Panel. (1993). *Depression in Primary Care: Volume 1. Detection and Diagnosis. Clinical Practice Guideline, Number 5* [AHCPR Publication No. 93-0550]. Rockville, MD: U.S. Department of Health and Human Services, Public Health Service, Agency for Health Care Policy and Research.

Eisenberg, L. (1992). Treating depression and anxiety in primary care. Closing the gap between knowledge and practice. *New England Journal of Medicine, 326*(16), 1080-1084.

Feldman, S. (1998). Behavioral health services: Carved out and managed. *American Journal of Managed Care, 4,* SP59-SP67.

Findlay, S. (1999). Managed behavioral health care in 1999: An industry at a crossroads. *Health Affairs, 18*(5), 116-24.

Frank, R. G., Goldman, H. H., & McGuire, T. G. (2001). Will Parity in Coverage Result in Better Mental Health Care? *New England Journal of Medicine, 345*(23), 1701-1704.

Frank, R. G., & McGuire, T. G. (2000). Economics and mental health. In A. Cuyler & J. Newhouse (Eds.), *Handbook of health economics* (Vol. 1A). New York: Elsevier.

Gardner, W., Kelleher, K., Wasserman, R., Childs, G., Nutting, P., Lillienfeld, H., & Pajer, K. (2000). Primary care treatment of pediatric psychosocial problems: A study from pediatric research in office settings and ambulatory sentinel practice network. *Pediatrics, 106*(4), 44.

Gaynor, M., & Pauly, M. V. (1990). Compensation and productive efficiency of partnerships: Evidence from medical group practice: *Journal of Political Economy, 98*(3), 544-73.

Glied, S. (1998). Too little time? The recognition and treatment of mental health problems in primary care. *Health Services Research, 33*(4, Pt. 1), 891-910.

Glied, S. (2000). Managed care. In A. J. Cuyler & J. P. Newhouse (Eds.), *Handbook of Health Economics* (pp. 707-754). Amsterdam: North Holland Press.

Glied, S., Garrett, A. B., Hoven, C., Rubio-Stipec, M., Regier, D., Moore, R. E., Goodman, S., Wu, P., & Bird, H. (1998). Child outpatient mental health service use: Why doesn't insurance matter? *Journal of Mental Health Policy and Economics, 1*, 173-187.

Glied, S., & Graff Zivin, J. (2002). Physician practice in a mixed payment environment. *Journal of Health Economics, 22*, 337-353.

Glied, S., Hoven, C. W., Moore, R. E., Garrett, A. B., & Regier, D. A. (1997). Children's access to mental health care: Does insurance matter? *Health Affairs, 16*(1), 167-74.

Goldberg, D. P., Jenkins, L., Millar, T., & Faragher, E. B. (1993). The ability of trainee general practitioners to identify psychological distress among their patients. *Psychological Medicine, 23*(1), 185-93.

Goldman, L. S., Genel, M., Bezman, R. J., & Slanetz, P. J. (1998). Diagnosis and treatment of attention-deficit/hyperactivity disorder in children and adolescents. *Journal of the American Medical Association, 279*(14), 1100-1107.

Grossman, M. 1972. *The demand for health: A theoretical and empirical investigation.* New York: Columbia University Press.

Horwitz, S., Leaf, P., Leventhal, J., Forsyth, B., & Speechley, K. (1992). Identification and management of psychosocial and developmental problems in community-based, primary care pediatric practices. *Pediatrics, 89*(3), 480-485.

Hughes, D. C., & Luft, H. S. (1998). Managed care and children: An overview. *Future of Children, 8*(2), 25-38.

Jellinek, M., Murphy, J., Little, M., Pagano, M., Comer, D., & Kelleher, K. (1999). Use of the Pediatric Symptom Checklist to screen for psychosocial problems in pediatric primary care. *Archives of Pediatric and Adolescent Medicine, 153*, 254-260.

Keeler, E. B., Manning, W. G., & Wells, K. B. (1988). The demand for episodes of mental health services. *Journal of Health Economics, 7*(4), 369-392.

Kelleher, K. J., Childs, G. E., Wasserman, R. C., McInerny, T. K., Nutting, P. A., & Gardner, W. P. (1997). Insurance status and recognition of psychosocial problems. *Archives of Pediatric and Adolescent Medicine, 151*, 1109-1115.

Kelleher, K. J., McInerny, T. K., Gardner, W. P., Childs, G. E., & Wasserman, R. C. (2000). Increasing identification of psychosocial problems: 1979-1996. *Pediatrics, 105*(6), 1313-1321.

Kennedy, L. (1993). Children receiving SSI payments, December 1992. *Social Security Bulletin, 56*(2), 77-83.

Kessler, L. G., Cleary, P. D., & Burke, J. D. (1985). Psychiatric disorders in primary care. *Archives f General Psychiatry, 42*, 583-587.

Kirby, J. B., Machlin, S. R., & Thorpe, J. M. (2001). Patterns of ambulatory care use: Changes from 1987 to 1996 [MEPS Research Findings No. 16. AHRQ Pub. No. 01-0026]. Rockville, MD: Agency for Healthcare Research and Quality

Klinkman, M. S., Coyne, J. C., Gallo, S., & Schwenk, T. L. (1997). Can case-finding instruments be used to improve physician detection of depression in primary care? *Archives of Family Medicine, 6*(6), 567-573.

Klinkman, M. S., Coyne, J. C., Gallo, S., & Schwenk, T. L. (1998). False positives, false negatives, and the validity of the diagnosis of major depression in primary care. *Archives of Family Medicine, 7*(5), 451-461.

Kroenke, K. (1997). Discovering depression in medical patients: Reasonable expectations. *Annals of Internal Medicine, 126*(6), 463-465.

Lavigne, J. V., Binns, H. J., Christoffel, K. K., Rosenbaum, D., Arend, R., Smith, K., Hayford, J. R., & McGuire, P. A. (1993). Behavioral and emotional problems among preschool children in pediatric primary care: prevalence and pediatricians' recognition. *Pediatrics, 91*(3), 649-655.

Leaf, P. J., Alegria, M., Cohen, P., Goodman, S. H., Horwitz, S. M., Hoven, C. W., Narrow, W. E., Vaden-Kiernan, M., & Regier, D. A. (1996). Mental health service use in the community and schools: Results from the four-community MECA Study. Methods for the Epidemiology of Child and Adolescent Mental Disorders Study. *Journal of the American Academy of Child and Adolescent Psychiatry, 35*(7), 889-897.

Leaf, P. J., Livingston, B. M., Tischler, G. L., Freemand, D. H., Weissman, M. M., & Myers, J. K. (1988). Factors affecting the utilization of specialty and general medical health services. *Medical Care, 26*(1), 9-26.

Lemelin, J., Hotz, S., Swensen, R., & Elmslie, T. (1994). Depression in primary care. Why do we miss the diagnosis? *Canadian Family Physician, 40*, 104-108.

Leon, A. C., Olfson, M., Weissman, M. M., Portera, L., & Sheehan, D. V. (1996). Evaluation of screens for mental disorders in primary care: Methodological issues. *Psychopharmacology Bulletin, 32*(3), 353-361.

Main, D. S., Lutz, L. J., Barrett, J. E., Matthew, J., & Miller, R. S. (1993). The role of primary care clinician attitudes, beliefs, and training in the diagnosis and treatment of depression. *Archives of Family Medicine, 2*(10), 1061-1066.

Marks, J. N., Goldberg, D. P., & Hillier, V. F. (1979). Determinants of the ability of general practitioners to detect psychiatric illness. *Psychological Medicine, 9*(2), 337-353.

Mechanic, D. (1990). Treating mental illness: Generalist versus specialist. *Health Affairs, 9*(4), 61-75.

Mechanic, D., McAlpine, D., & Rosenthal, M. (2001). Are patients' office visits with physicians getting shorter? *New England Journal of Medicine, 344*, 198-204.

Mulrow, C. D., Williams, J. W., Gerety, M. B., Ramirez, G., Montiel, O. M., & Kerber, C. (1995). Case-finding instruments for depression in primary-care settings. *Annals of Internal Medicine, 122*(12), 913-921.

National Institutes of Health. (1999). *Bridging science and service: A report by the National Advisory Mental Health Council's Clinical Treatment and Services Research Workgroup* [NIH 99-4353]. Bethesda, MD: National Institutes of Health, National Institute of Mental Health.

Newhouse, J. P. (1993). *Free for all?: Lessons from the RAND health insurance experiment. The insurance experiment group.* Cambridge, MA. Harvard University Press.

Olfson, M., Marcus, S. C., Druss, B., Elinson, L., Tanielian, T., & Pincus, H. A. (2002). National trends in the outpatient treatment of depression. *Journal of the American Medical Association, 287*, 203-209.

Pincus, H., Tanielian, T., Marcus, S., Olfson, M., Zarin, D., Thompson, J., & Zito, J. (1998). Prescribing trends in psychotropic medications: Primary care, psychiatry, and other medical specialties. *Journal of the American Medical Association, 279*(7), 526-531.

Potthoff, R. F., Woodbury, M. A., & Manton, K. G. (1992). "Equivalence sample size" and "equivalent degrees of freedom" refinements for inference using survey weights under superpopulation models. *Journal of the American Statistical Association, 87*, 383-396.

Reed, M. C. (2000, May). *Why people change their health care providers* [Data Bulletin No. 16]. Washington, DC: Center for Studying Health System Change.

Rogers, W. H., Wells, K. B., Meredith, L. S., Sturm, R., & Burnam, M. H. (1993). Outcomes for adult outpatients with depression under prepaid or fee-for-service financing. *Archives of General Psychiatry, 50*(3), 517-525.

Rosenbach, M., Ellwood, M., Czajka, J., Irvin, C., Coupe, W., & Quinn, B. (2001). *Implementation of the State Children's Health Insurance Program: Momentum is increasing after a modest start.* Mathematica Policy Research Report to HCFA Contract No. 500-96-0016 (03).

Rushton, J., Clark, S., & Freed, G. (2000a). Pediatrician and family physician prescription of selective serotonin reuptake inhibitors. *Pediatrics, 105*(6), 82.

Rushton, J., Clark, S., & Freed, G. (2000b). Primary care role in the management of childhood depression: A comparison of pediatricians and family physicians. *Pediatrics, 105*(4, Suppl), 957-962.

Sharp, L., Pantell, R., Murphy, L., & Lewis, C. (1992). Psychosocial problems during child health supervision visits: Eliciting, then what? *Pediatrics, 89*(4), 619-623.

Social Security Administration. (2000). *Children receiving SSI: December 2000.* Baltimore, MD: Author

Spitzer, R. L., Kroenke, K., & Williams, J. B. W. (1999). Validation and utility of a self-report version of PRIME-MD—The PHQ primary care study. *Journal of the American Medical Association, 282*(18), 1737-1744.

St. Peter, R. F., Reed, M. C., Kemper, P., & Blumenthal, D. (1999, December). The scope of care expected of primary care physicians: Is it greater than it should be? *Center for Studying Health System Change Issue Brief 24.*

Stancin, T., & Palermo, T. (1997). A review of behavioral screening practices in pediatric settings: Do they pass the test? *Journal of Developmental and Behavioral Pediatrics, 18,* 183-194.

Stroul, B. A., Pires, S. A., Armstrong, M. I., & Meyers, J. C. (1998). The impact of managed care on mental health services for children and their families. *Future of Children, 8*(2), 119-133.

Sturm, R., & Klap, R. (1999). Use of psychiatrists, psychologists, and master's-level therapists in managed behavioral health care carve-out plans. *Psychiatric Services, 50*(4), 504-508.

Substance Abuse and Mental Health Services Administration. (2000). *State profiles, 1999, on public sector managed behavioral health care.* Washington, DC: U.S. Department of Health and Human Services.

Sullivan v. Zebley, 110 S. Ct. 885 (1990).

Tenney, J. B., White, K. L., & Williamson, J. W. (1974, April). *National Ambulatory Medical Care Survey: Background and methodolody: United States, 1967-72.* National Center for Health Statistics Reports, Series 2. Data evaluation and methods research, Number 61.

U.S. Department of Health and Human Services. (1999). *Mental health: A report of the Surgeon General.* Rockville, MD: U.S. Department of Health and Human Services, Substance Abuse and Mental Health Services Administration, Center for Mental Health Services, National Institutes of Health, National Institute of Mental Health.

U.S. Food and Drug Administration. (2001). *The pediatric exclusivity provision: January 2001 status report to Congress.* Rockville, MD: Author.

Vitiello, B., & Jensen, P. (1997). Medication development and testing in children and adolescents: Current problems, future directions. *Archives of General Psychiatry, 54*(9), 871-876.

Weissman, M. M., Broadhead, W. E., Olfson, M., Sheehan, D. V., Hoven, C., Conolly, P., Fireman, B. H., Farber, L., Blacklow, R. S., Higgins, E. S., & Leon, A. C. (1998). A diagnostic aid for detecting (*DSM-IV*) mental disorders in primary care. *General Hospital Psychiatry, 20*(1), 1-11.

Wells, K. B., Hays, R. D., Burnam, M. A., Rogers, W., Greenfield, S., & Ware, J. E. (1989). Detection of depressive disorder for patients receiving prepaid or fee-for-service care: Results from the medical outcomes study. *Journal of the American Medical Association, 263*(17), 2298-2300.

Wells, K. B., Manning, W. G., & Valdez, R. B. (1990). The effects of a prepaid group practice on mental health outcomes. *Health Services Research, 25*(4), 615-625.

Williams, J. W., Mulrow, C. D., Kroenke, K., Dhanda, R., Badgett, R. G., Omori, D., & Lee, S. (1999). Case-finding for depression in primary care: A randomized trial. *American Journal of Medicine, 106*(1), 36-43.

Zito, J. M, Safer, D. J., dosReis, S., Gardner, J. F., Boles, M., & Lynch, F. (2000). Trends in the prescribing of psychotropic medications to preschoolers. *Journal of the American Medical Association, 283*(8), 1025-1030.

DISCUSSION SUMMARY
written by Thomas M. Yerkey

The discussion following Dr. Glied's presentation at the KSU Psychology Forum was animated and centered on three issues. First, both physicians and psychologists present at the meeting expressed concerns regarding the conclusions drawn by Dr. Glied. Second, potential changes in the training of physicians based on Dr. Glied's conclusions were discussed. Finally, attendees at Dr. Glied's Kent State University colloquium raised the question of why should resources be spent trying to identify children with psychosocial problems in primary care medical practices when it appears that schools are much more effective at identifying these children? Dr. Glied's responses to questions in each of these areas solidified the importance of economic factors and tools in understanding the identification of children with psychosocial problems.

The first area of discussion centered on concerns that Dr. Glied's results could be interpreted as meaning that physicians choose to identify psychosocial problems when there is financial reward for making the identification. Dr. Glied quickly pointed out that this was not what she intended to communicate in her chapter. Dr. Glied asserted that she employed economic tools in order to track where identification of child psychosocial problems regularly occurred. That a physician in a specific situation identified a child and then requested reimbursement does not indicate physician greed. Instead, it showed the conditions under which physicians will make an identification. Physicians will identify and treat children with psychosocial problems when they are aware of and trained to use an effective, empirically supported, and available treatment for the identified disorder. Thus the frequent identification of ADD and ADHD can be interpreted differently than they often are. It is widely accepted that there is an over diagnosis of ADD and ADHD. Dr. Glied's presentation provides us with a new and useful tool for understanding both the over diagnosis of these disorders and the under diagnosis of other types of psychosocial problems such as child depression, anxiety, or other internalizing type problems. Physicians and mental health professionals are clearly aware that stimulant medications are an effective treatment for the symptoms commonly exhibited by children with ADHD. There is a broad literature that supports the use of stimulants for this purpose. The use of stimulant medications to treat ADD and ADHD also fits the medical/disease model of psychopathology. Obviously, the vast majority of physicians in the United States are trained in the medical model. Last, stimulant medications are very easily obtained by physicians and parents. So, in the cases of ADHD and ADD, there exists a treatment that is known to be effective in minimizing symptoms, that fits the primary training model employed in American medical schools, and that is easily obtained. Dr. Glied asserted that when these factors are in place, physicians do identify and treat a particular type of psychosocial problem. If this assertion is true, then we have an idea of how to proceed if we wish to increase physician identification of other psychosocial diagnoses. It is necessary to develop empirically supported treatments for child psychosocial problems, to educate physicians in how to utilize these treatments or how to direct their patients to resources where they can obtain these treatments, and it is necessary to make these treatments broadly available to physicians and their patients.

The discussion of these issues led to the question of how physician training could be changed to result in increased identification rates. The first step that was suggested was to increase physician education in the areas of psychosocial problems and existing effective treatments. Physician training in identifying and treating psychosocial problems is frequently limited to 1 to 3 classes during medical school. This limited training restricts new physicians exposure to and understanding of not only psychosocial problems and their treatment, but also to understanding approaches and language used by mental healthcare professionals. Discussion between developmental and behavioral pediatrics fellows and psychology graduate students at a recent national conference supports this claim. At a fellows meeting during the 2002 annual meeting of the Society for Developmental and Behavioral Pediatrics in Chicago, developmental and behavioral pediatrics fellows generally agreed that their exposure to psychology, psychological thinking and theory was extremely limited until they began their fellowships. Increasing the training exposure across the disciplines of medicine and psychology as well as other areas of mental healthcare could begin to improve identification rates.

The last point of discussion regarding Dr. Glied's chapter was the concern that identification of child psychosocial problems may be better attempted in our schools since that is where the data indicate most identifications occur presently. Dr. Glied asserted that the schools do play an important role in the identification equation. However, there is a wide consensus among national agencies, physicians, and mental healthcare providers that identification should be a priority in primary care medical practice. Additionally, schools are more likely to identify psychosocial problems that are particularly evident in the school context. Thus, child externalizing problems such as ADHD, oppositional defiant behavior, or aggressive behavior are most frequently identified.

Dr. Glied's chapter provides primary care researchers with a glimpse of how collaboration with other disciplines can enhance the quality of our understanding of data gathered during research. The interpretations produced through an economics based analysis are very different from those usually produced in clinical research. Examining our research from alternate points of view may be uncomfortable, but doing so can only improve the quality of our research and understanding of the data, and this quality, after all, is our goal.

CHAPTER 8

INTERVENTIONS IN PRIMARY CARE

Psychology Privileges for Pediatricians

W. Douglas Tynan
AI duPont Hospital for Children,
Division of Behavioral Health
Wilmington, DE

Pediatricians have long been the first resource for parents who are concerned about their children's behavioral difficulties. Traditionally the role has been to provide advice and guidance, and when problems became more complex, to refer on to a mental health professional (Kelleher, 2001). With the increased penetrance of managed care, the primary care role has become more complicated because of the gatekeeping responsibility, to decide who should access specialty services, including mental health. The professional role in primary care now is to first identify, then to treat or to refer children who have behavioral and emotional problems. The referral process itself can be cumbersome and time consuming, made more complex by the "carve out" nature of many insurance policies for mental health services. Often health insurance cards do not indicate which subcontracted companies will provide mental health coverage, all

Treating Children's Psychosocial Problems in Primary Care, 171–198

that is given is a toll-free telephone number for further information and referral. For the busy primary care provider, the process, whether it is to treat or to refer, is complicated. If one is to refer, the task is then to find an appropriately skilled and trained provider, and if a provider is found, determine if they are included in the patient's network of providers determined by an unknown insurance company. As cited in the Surgeon General's Report on Mental Health (1999), "the system for delivering mental health services to children and families is complex, sometimes to the point of inscrutability."

Served by this system are approximately 20% of all children who have diagnosable emotional or behavioral disorders at some time during their childhood and adolescent stages of life (Costello & Shugart, 1992). Rates of significant behavioral difficulties in children are even higher in families that have additional risk factors such as poor education, low income or single-parent status. Along with these existing high rates, there is further evidence that these problems may well be increasing in frequency (Achenbach & Howell, 1993) in the population. At the same time, access to treatment resources remains available to fewer than one quarter of children who are in need of service, a situation unchanged for the last 20 years or more (Knitzer, 1982; Surgeon General, 1999).

Despite these increased rates of behavioral difficulties and the additional responsibility placed for treatment and referral now placed on primary care physicians, nurse practitioners and physician assistants, primary care providers usually have not received comprehensive training concerning psychosocial problems, which would include basic scientific knowledge on etiology, assessment and treatment. A review of practices (Shonkoff, Dworkin, & Leviton, 1979) revealed a lack of experience and training more than two decades ago, and training models have not substantially changed since then in terms of time allocated for training in these areas. While a more recent survey (Dobos, Dworkin, & Bernstein, 1994) indicates a greater facility in screening for problems in general pediatric settings and initial counseling, there are no outcome data on effectiveness of treatment done in those settings for behavioral problems (Cheng, DeWitt, Savageau, & O'Connor, 1999). For example, pediatric residency training requires only one month of the 36-month residency in pediatrics to be devoted to developmental and behavioral issues (Accreditation Council for Graduate Medical Education, American Medical Association, 1997), despite the fact that these problems have comprised the majority of parent questions and concerns in outpatient settings for quite some time (Glascoe, 2000). In the clinical training of primary care providers, there may be rotations and clinical experiences with providers in the professions and specialties of developmental pediatrics, psychiatry, clinical psychology, social work and psychiatric nursing who may all present differing approaches and conceptualization from differing theories and practices. Usually, there is very little exposure in a systematic way to the risk, and prevention, factors leading to the most commonly diagnosed difficulties, empirically supported assessment and interventions for emotional and behavioral problems. Often, major portions of training involve discussions of particularly difficult cases, while assessment and management of the most common and routine problems is addressed briefly. Coming from this training background then, it is no surprise that primary care providers are hesitant to formally assess and attach diagnostic labels to children. While the *Diagnostic and Statistical Manual of Mental Disorders–Primary Care* (*DSM-PC*) offers a diagnostic system of behavioral difficulties that is more suited to pediatric practice (Drotar, Sturner, & Nobile, 2003), it has yet to be widely implemented in the field. With limited time in office visits, emotional and behavioral issues are often addressed quickly with the only tools available; those are brief advice, medication or referral to a mental health professional. Unfortunately, there are no data on the effectiveness of advice given.

As to other therapies, as the recent Multimodal Treatment Study of Attention Deficit Hyperactivity Disorder demonstrated, medication as it is usually prescribed in community settings is not very effective (Jensen et al., 2001). With regard to referral to mental health services, the data indicate that when such referrals are made, fewer than half of the families keep the appointments (Kelleher, 2001). Thus, the system for children who do have behavior problems which are identified in primary care, as it currently exists, has serious flaws in accessibility, acceptability, and effectiveness.

The accessibility problem is apparently due to the shortage of appropriately trained mental health specialist providers for children, the lack of resources within primary care, and obstacles posed by reimbursement systems. The most recent review by the Surgeon General (2001) on the supply of providers indicates a severe shortage in all three of the traditional mental health professions (psychology, psychiatry, social work) for providers who have had training to treat children. More recently, possibly due to insurance obstacles, there has been a further decrease in access and utilization of psychotherapy services, and an increase in medication (Surgeon General, 2001). Thus, with a decreased number of specialists, and insurance "gates" (which, as we well know, become hurdles when they stay closed) to be kept, an even greater burden has been placed on primary care providers now to provide mental health services in their own setting. Most pediatric and family practice physicians, nurse practitioners and physician assistants do provide counseling and advice for families on behavioral and emotional issues. However, it has not routinely been recognized as intervention, and there has been little formal systematic training in providing these types of services, even for the most common problems.

Thus, to meet the mental health care needs of children, and the educational needs of primary care providers, development of a system of mental health care is recommended here, that would include the delivery of basic mental health services in primary care settings. This would involve additional training of primary care providers so that they can provide both screening and the needed intervention services within their practice for the most common behavior problems. This suggests a range of services including preventative interventions available to all families, and targeted toward at risk families, as well as brief specific interventions done at the primary care site.

A number of studies have indicated (Kazdin, Siegel, & Bass, 1990; Surgeon General, 2001) the most common behavior problems are the disruptive, noncompliant oppositional behaviors, which includes the *DSM-IV* diagnoses of attention deficit hyperactivity disorder, oppositional defiant disorder, conduct disorder, intermittent explosive disorder and adjustment disorder with conduct problems. These comprise more than half (Kazdin, Siegel, & Bass, 1990) and in some settings nearly three quarters (Tynan, Schuman, & Lampert, 1999) of referrals for child mental health.

Given the high frequency and the early onset of these externalizing, disruptive problems, initial interventions for these and related difficulties could be done within the existing framework of providing advice for parents on child rearing, a traditional role for primary care. For those children who do not respond to brief parental advice and other interventions provided in primary care, a more comprehensive structured empirically supported intervention for parenting skills would comprise the next level of intervention. This could be done in the primary care setting, or in a mental health environment. For those whose needs exceed the scope of brief intervention or a structured group program, referral on to mental health specialists is in order.

But even in those cases, referral to mental health specialists usually fail, with over half of the referrals having no result (Kelleher, 2001), with families either not making an appointment, or not showing for an initial visit. There is some limited evidence that a referral is likely to result in treatment if they are in the same suite of offices (Schroeder, this volume), or building, or to a provider the parents have had some contact with already in the primary care setting (Maynard, Tynan, & Werner, 2003). This suggests greater acceptability if the mental health provider is closely affiliated with the primary care provider. A model that emphasizes collaboration between medical and mental health providers could build on that pattern of acceptability of treatment. Regardless of details, the model suggested is one of a seamless transition from one level of care to another, rather than the fragmented system that currently exists. To reach this goal requires rethinking and redesigning professional roles and interactions.

But one may ask why is there such a need for change now, and what are the prevailing pressures to develop newer models of intervention? In 1999, the Surgeon General of the United States released a comprehensive report on mental health for the nation, which included a detailed chapter on children and mental health. In that report, the system for delivery of services was described as complex, "sometimes to the point of inscrutability-a patchwork of providers, interventions and payers" (p. 179). One of the conclusions was that a high proportion of children needing services receive no services, and the fact that this situation has not changed since the 1986 report by the U.S. Office of Technology Assessment which indicated that 70% of children in need do not receive services. These data are similar to Jane Knitzer's (1982) report for the Children's Defense Fund 20 years ago, which gave an estimate that 80% of children requiring services were not receiving them, well before the dawn of managed care. Clearly the policy data from the past 20 years show not that the system has broken. It indicates that the system has never worked well to provide needed services to the majority of children who require them. Thus, the time has come to develop a system that can begin to meet the mental health needs of children, and building it from the base of primary care may be an approach that will yield further success.

The most recent Surgeon General's conference (2001) focused specifically on mental health needs for children, highlighting the crisis in service delivery. Curiously, what appeared to prompted this report, along with a White House Conference on mental health needs in children and a related conference on psychopharmacology in children this past year was not any specific crisis due to general lack of available treatment. Instead, interest was sparked by data (Zito, Safer, dosReis, & Gardner, 2000) and the perception that the rate of use of psychiatric medicines in preschool children had risen dramatically in five years, the perception of too much pharmacological treatment. The primary cause for the concern was that very little research had been done on the treatment effects and side effects of these medicines on preschool children. The public perception that psychiatric medications were being overprescribed for younger and younger children appeared to be confirmed by Zito and colleagues (2000) findings. What made these findings more disturbing was the off-label use of many medications and the combinations of medications used on children as young as 24 months of age. Thus, attempts to more widely treat behavior problems with pharmacology highlighted the overall need for services. Publication of these papers initially sparked interest in appropriate drug testing in pediatric psychopharmacology. In the process of examining the psychopharmacology issue, the broader topic of provision of all mental health services, not just psychopharmacology, for children emerged. As a result, a number of key issues were outlined in the most recent report by the Surgeon General (2001). Included were the following four recommendations, which are directly relevant to the provision of mental health care in primary pediatric and family practice settings:

- Screening and early identification of children who have behavior problems within the health and education systems.
- Increasing access to services.
- Implementing evidence-based treatment and services.
- Providing adequate and appropriate education and training to frontline providers in screening and intervention.

These are the core issues for primary care pediatric providers and the mental health professionals who work closely with them. Schroeder (Chapter 1, this volume) has provided in her chapter a history of pediatric psychology integrated within primary care, and provides an essential foundation on which to build our future models of care. As she states in her chapter, we must reach "beyond our guilds" and professional boundaries if we are to provide care for all of the children who need it, and to address the needs defined in the most recent reports. She also identified needs in practice, the common overlap between Psychology and Pediatrics and the need for collaboration between all service providers for children and adolescents, that is health care, mental health, education, day care, child protection and judicial systems.

Screening

Screening for behavior problems has been a major focus in pediatrics for some time. Indeed, it has been over a quarter century since the "new morbidity" of behavior problems was raised (Haggerty, Roghman, & Pless, 1975) as an issue in pediatric medicine. Nearly 25% of children have disabilities such as speech-language impairments, mental retardation, learning disabilities, and emotional/behavioral disturbance. Although such children are twice as likely to seek health care than children without disabilities are, only half are detected prior to school entrance. The reasons are understandable: Most behavioral and emotional disabilities are subtle and children who have them often appear to be developing normally, especially at younger ages. Often it is the first preschool or kindergarten experience that results in teachers or other parents noticing problematic behaviors. These children tend to have a high frequency of visits to primary care, which indicates that the parents perceive difficulties that are not being addressed and resolved. Often these are the parents and children who are of the greatest concern for their physicians and nurses because the core problems are not sufficiently addressed, and often take up quite a bit of time in the office. The lack of accurate detection and referral is unfortunate because it eliminates the possibilities of early intervention by mental health, education and other therapy services, including speech, occupational and physical therapy. Screening and detection must be linked to intervention services. In order to improve pediatricians' ability to detect children with developmental and emotional/behavioral problems, the American Academy of Pediatrics Committee on Children with Disabilities has recommended the use of standardized screening tests at well visits. However, most pediatricians find the more popular measures too lengthy to give routinely, and studies have consistently shown that pediatricians tend not to use checklists (Costello, 1986). Fortunately, there are now brief screening instruments widely available, such as the Pediatric Symptoms Checklist (PSC) (Jellinek & Murphy, 1999). The PSC and a brief article detailing scoring is available free, on-line for providers (http://www.dbpeds.org/handouts). Screening for developmental problems can be done quickly with instruments such as Parents' Evaluations of Developmental Status (PEDS) (1994), the Child Development Inventories, or the Bayley Infant Neurodevelomental Screen (BINS) (1996). Clearly, advances have been made in making screening realistic and possible in pediatric and family practice offices, but screening without intervention provides no meaningful service. Perrin (1998) in a somewhat provocative editorial has raised this issue, and the need for development and implementation of systems of mental health care that are accessible to primary care providers. Primary care providers are the gatekeepers for a range of services, but as described in the Surgeon General's report, the services are provided within a confusing patchwork of complex overlapping public and private agencies that fall in the domains of mental health providers, educational providers and other allied health care providers. Thus, while we may be making progress on screening, it is at the intervention phase that we lack effective tools. Stancin and Palermo (1997) have noted that while screening in primary care should be clearly defined in terms of goals (e.g., entire clinic population vs. high-risk groups), and applications. Screening without having the capacity to either provide or refer to interventions will only lead to further frustration for primary care providers and the patient families.

Intervention Access and Acceptance

Traditionally, mental health service delivery is thought of as a separate specialty system where children, who have problems, are referred to mental health specialists by primary care. In this model, the primary care providers deliver routine child guidance advice, and refer those children with diagnosable disorders out to specialists. While many think of the system in those terms, the reality is much more diffuse. In terms of service delivery, the primary care providers deliver early screening and intervention, and long-term support for the family. It is in these roles that many levels of care are provided at the pediatric or family practice office. It is the traditional role in pediatrics and family practice to provide counseling, advice and anticipatory guidance on a range of issues, but especially those concerning behavior and development. Primary care providers also provide linkages and information for families to other services. Families often find out about Child Find and other public screening and early intervention programs at their primary care office. Coordination with schools starts early, with the required physical examination before any school program can start, and filling out of necessary forms documenting health, vaccination and other basic screening. The primary care physician, or nurse practitioner plays a central role when behavior problems occur. It is the first place that parents turn to when there are problems, and it should the site of the first level of both assessment and intervention.

Developing Behavioral Levels of Care

To develop a system of care that integrates primary care and mental health care into a continuum of service, the concept of level of care needs to be addressed. Instead of dwelling on a primary care versus specialty care dichotomy, in an alternative model, the primary care providers deliver routine child guidance advice, and preliminary intervention, before referring those children with more complicated problems out to specialists. In terms of service delivery, the primary care providers deliver early screening and intervention, and long-term support for the family. It is in these roles that many levels of care are provided at the pediatric or family practice office. It is the traditional role in pediatrics and family practice to provide counseling, advice and anticipatory guidance on a range of issues, but especially those concerning behavior and development. In developing a system of care, it is essential that we evaluate what services, both prevention and intervention, could be provided in primary care, and how we can possibly improve them, and integrate them with higher level, more complex care. To manage the current level of need, it is essential that we not only develop intervention within primary care, but also use this point of contact with families as a source of preventative help. That would include using some aspects of a public health model to address behavior problems.

Public health models have a history of intervention through the reduction of risk factors for specific diseases and disorders, as well as promoting health. Decreasing risk and increasing protective factors are at the heart of a prevention approach. Research on the development of behavioral and emotional disorders has led to a set of conclusions that lend themselves to a prevention approach. First, providers must appreciate that development is complex and multifaceted, and thus both competence and disorders have many factors (Greenberg, Domitrovich, & Bumburger, 2001). There is no single cause, or risk factor, for the common disorders (e.g. disruptive disorders, affective disorders). Risk factors include community, within family and biological factors in the neighborhood, family, and child. Second, it is doubtful that addressing only one factor, particularly causes that exist within the child, can fully and successfully treat most disorders. There is no one cause for these disorders, and therefore medications will never suffice as a complete treatment. Third, many risk factors (e.g. family conflict, poor parent education), are not specific to one disorder, and may lead to different poor outcomes in different children. Therefore while many of the prevention strategies appear to target one type of disorders, improvement in parenting skills and decrease in family conflicts may reduce rates of a number of problems. If there is a focus on increasing protective factors, it may well lead to an overall lowering of the incidence rate of disorders and improving the competence of children. As a public health model in reducing risk factors, this is a far cry from diagnosing specific children with a single group of related *DSM-IV* diagnoses, and then prescribing medicine as the primary treatment, the model into which many practitioners are drawn.

In their review of effective prevention programs (all in nonmedical settings) that targeted both disruptive and internalizing (anxiety/depression) disorders, Greenberg, Domitrovich and Bumburger (2001) reached several conclusions with certain applicability to prevention in primary care:

> Short-term prevention interventions produce time limited benefits, while multi-year programs yielded enduring effects. Primary care providers typically follow families over years and can provide a longitudinal perspective.

Prevention operates effectively when developmentally appropriate factors are targeted, but intervention needs to start in the preschool or early elementary school years to be effective. Primary care usually has the most contact with families during infancy, toddler and preschool years, long before other systems.

Prevention programs that target risk and protective factors are better than those that target specific behaviors are (e.g., programs that enhance adolescent interaction with parents work better than programs specifically targeting drug use or school behaviors). Primary care is a site where working on improving generic parenting skills fits the mission of most practices.

Interventions need to be aimed at multiple domains, changing institutions and environments as well as individuals. Primary care physicians in most communities are in a unique position to bring influence on other agencies such as schools.

Programs that focus on the child are not as effective as those that both focus on the child and change the home and school environment. Pediatric care is family focused with both parents and child included in nearly all visits.

Prevention programs need to be integrated with systems of treatment. In this way communities and providers in medicine, mental health and education develop common models, language and procedures that maximize effectiveness of programs across areas. Coordination is the key between health, mental health and education.

In Australia, Sanders (1999), has developed a comprehensive integrated five-level system (Triple P) of mental health care that includes both primary care and specialty providers and ranges from educational programs for new parents to intensive wrap around home-based mental health services for children who have severe problems. While Sanders' (1999) program provides a framework, there are also existing programs and therapy approaches in the United State that correspond to each of the levels described in the Triple P program. The following description parallels the Sanders program by suggesting similar approaches that are already available here in the United States. In many ways, at least four of the five levels that Sanders describes are available, and the major issue is coordination, and training to provide several of these services in primary care.

Education and Universal Prevention Level

In this model, the first level of care is that of parent education and guidance. In the United States this is provided to families in a variety of ways, by different professions. Traditionally, this does not involve mental health professionals, but does involve primary care physicians. Education and prevention are also defined as major professional roles and duties of both nurse practitioners and physician assistants. As the numbers of providers in these professions grow, there is an opportunity to develop behavioral prevention and intervention skills for those professions, and thus help meet the needs in primary care. It could well be that the most important providers of mental health services in primary care will be neither physicians, nor psychologists, but other health professionals, specifically physician assistants and nurse practitioners. The goals of early intervention and prevention are to inform parents of normal developmental stages in all areas of functioning in children including cognitive development, emotional processes, milestones for specific goals, and the best way to assist in teaching children to achieve certain goals (e.g. advice on toilet training). Often, the health care provider is consulted on common behavior problems (e.g., fighting between sibling, tantrums) and asked for recommendations regarding these problematic behaviors that occur in almost all children. Education and guidance can be achieved in a number of ways. This includes brochures and pamphlets distributed at the primary care office, face-to-face advice given during routine check ups and visits, or books recommended to the parents. It may also include some one-time classes on parenting provided by local organizations, or within the practice (Schroeder, Chapter 1, this volume). Most frequently parenting advice comes to parents from their own parents, friends, relative and neighbors. In the United States, helping to develop parenting skills as a form of prevention and early intervention is rarely routinely implemented or examined, despite the fact that there is a large amount of data supporting this type of approach. For example, Webster-Stratton (1992) has developed a ten session group therapy program (further on this program below) that utilizes videotape presentation of materials, and has implemented it as a prevention early intervention with a group of Head Start parents (Webster-Stratton, & Hammond, 1997). But this is an extensive education and intervention program, not casual advice giving or role modeling as is practiced by primary care providers. A full 10-session parenting program such as the Webster-Stratton program is a good intervention for families who have children who are at high risk or already have diagnosable problems, but is, perhaps, not practical to implement widely for the general population. For that, shorter approaches would be more useful (Roberts & Brown, this volume).

Video Presentations

To be sure, prevention strategies for behavioral problems have been well researched, but usually not implemented, particularly in primary care settings. It is clear that given the number of children who have these common behavioral problems, and the number of providers available, that the current approach is doomed to failure in terms of addressing the needs of the numbers of children to be served. Less costly prevention and early intervention strategies may go a long way to meeting the needs of the children to be served. The use of effective early intervention strategies can be done in several ways, through broadcast television to homes, or recorded materials made available to parents. To reach large numbers of parents, and to make some intervention that is universally available, we must consider intervention through electronic media. We have not, to date, utilized our electronic media of television for this purpose (Biglan, 1992), despite the fact that evidence from public health indicates that media-based approaches can be effective in increasing awareness and has shown some impact in modifying health related behaviors, such as cigarette smoking (Sorenson, Emmons, Hunt, & Johnson, 1998). While there is considerable thought paid to the use of the media to sell things to families, or to provide entertainment that results in no improvement and, at times, harm, little thought or effort has been placed on using the same media to provide solid, informative parenting advice and education here in the United States. To be sure, no one in the United States has really tried to improve parenting skills though electronic media. While Corporation for Public Broadcasting has diligently worked to develop helpful programming for children, parents and families members have been left out. Despite the great potential of this medium for positive change, when we consider children and families, television remains the "wasteland" described by former Federal Communicatiosn Commision Chairman Newton Minnow over 40 years ago.

Sanders (1999) has developed a promotional campaign including a television-based, prevention-oriented intervention and examined its impact in New Zealand. More than just a television series, the media program consisted of multiple elements. This included brief, 30-second radio and television commercials announcing the program, a one-year series of weekly newspaper columns on parenting issues, a series of 40- and 60-second audio presentations on parenting, printed advertising and tip sheets for parents, a series of press releases to local media outlets asking for support and a coordinators "how to" kit on implementing the program. With these materials in place, a media campaign was developed, centered on a television series "Families" which was shown on a commercial TV network, with 13, 30-minute episodes of an "infotainment," or news magazine approach. It was shown in prime time (7:30 P.M.) from October to December 1995 and was funded by private business donations and New Zealand on Air. The program used the infotainment format popular in New Zealand, and programs with this format attract 25-30% of the viewing audience. The series provided practical information and advice on common problems (e.g. tantrums, sleep problems). A 5- to 7-minute segment on the formal positive parenting program (Triple P) each week allowed regular viewers to complete the entire Triple P program at home through television. Thus viewers could either casually pick up advice segments, or more diligently complete the entire parenting course via television. Promotional messages on radio and newspapers prompted viewers to watch the show and inform them of place to contact to get more information on parenting. Participating families self-reported a reduction in behavior problems, comparable to that seen in families completing the standard Triple P parenting course (Sanders, Montgomery, & Brechman-Toussaint (2000), and overall the program was rated second in its time slot after the first month.

The Sanders program documents quite well that there is a demand and a market for this type of service, but, to date, it has not been attempted in the United States. Certainly, if one watches programs on daytime television, there is certainly a common theme of family strife and misbehaving children and parents, with some moderator trying to give advice. There is an element of this in a number of daytime programs involving a host/moderator and guests. The popularity of newspaper columns on parenting and family advice, the number of books published and sold on this topic all indicate a need to be met in a creative yet clinically sound way. Clearly the demand is there, but our professional organizations have not responded to it, nor developed effective programming. Using the media more effectively to do a better job should be a goal.

Brief Interventions: Psychology Privileges for Physicians

By brief intervention, if it is defined as guidance given in one or two sessions ranging from 20 to 50 minutes in length, there is little or no research done to examine its effectiveness. Historically, pediatricians have written books for parents on these topics including Brazelton (1994), often utilized by practicing pediatricians, but the effectiveness of this approach has been untested. Within psychology, Leach (1997) has published a series of books over the past 25 years offerering advice based on applied developmental psychology priniciples. From a perspective based in behavioral psychology, Christophersen (1975) developed materials for use in a children's hospital pediatric clinic to help primary care physicians in training manage the most common behavior problems of disruptive behavior, feeding and toileting issues, and sleep problems. His chapter (Christophersen, 1982) in a major pediatric book series highlighted the applicability of valid behavioral procedures for many common problems, but the types of interventions and language used were not common in medical centers at the time. All of these recommendations were based on approaches that had been empirically validated at least in single subject intervention designs. In a general pediatric setting, Kanoy and Schroeder (1985) documented the most common behavioral problems seen in pediatric practices and provided efficacy outcome data on brief interventions. Anecdotally, other psychologists working in pediatric settings do report a significant number of families who do consult for one or two sessions around a specific behavioral difficulty, or to answer questions regarding development. Medical practitioners are often asked for advice about specific topics, and some are better prepared than others to meet that need. Christophersen (1998) presented a model of "continuing education" for parents in primary care that normalized the process of seeking advice regarding behavior, and was based on brief interventions delivered periodically during childhood and adolescence. His discussion emphasized the ongoing need for parent education through childhood and mirrors what Greenberg et al. (2001) mention as essential for a good intervention program, that is, ongoing contact over the child's development. As part of that model, based in a children's hospital, texts were developed to guide pediatricians in giving advice (Christophersen, 1994), and materials for parents (Christophersen, 1998).

Another model of brief intervention is the Behavior Change Clinic (BCC) first developed by Kelley at a primary care clinic in a general hospital setting in 1990 (D. Miller, personal communication, 2001). In this clinic, children are seen at their primary care site, but by a psychologist, not the pediatrician. Visits are brief (30 minutes), and focused on a specific behavior problem. Parents are instructed in a particular strategy to cope with the problem and are given a handout on how to implement that strategy at home. They are encouraged to come back for a few follow up visits (four or five), as needed. Those with more severe or pervasive problems are referred on for more lengthy evaluations and treatment. In a variation on this model (D. Miller, personal communication, 2001), children were seen in a psychology clinic based in a children's hospital, providers who were licensed psychologists or trainees. The major difference in this approach is that the families do not go to the primary care site, but are referred to a separate specialty clinic in psychology. Thus the parents have to go to a different office, which can be an obstacle to following through on treatment. As expected, for these specific problems, most of the approaches were behavioral, and based on strategies that had some empirical support in the literature. These include problems such as tantrums, sibling fighting, bed wetting, and defiant behavior, and closely mirror the initial work by Christophersen (1982). However while the behavioral procedures used in the program have an empirical base, the program itself has not been evaluated for effectiveness or acceptability.

In a funded study of providing brief behavioral interventions in primary care, Finney, Riley and Cataldo (1991) found that disruptive behaviors and school problems were the most common complaints, comprising nearly two thirds of the patients. The behavioral interventions, when compared to a standard treatment control group, yielded clinical improvement, high satisfaction and a reduction in utilization of other mental health services.

Sanders (1999) has utilized a brief intervention approach in a rural Australian setting in a manner that integrates it within a continuum of mental health services that includes prevention and more intensive intervention. Perhaps the major contribution that Sanders has made is in training primary care providers in a very structured manner to a level of competence in these behavioral interventions, and then having them implement them effectively and independently. Described in his program as "Level 2" or "Selective Triple P," these interventions involve one or two 20-minute, problem-specific sessions with the primary care provider to review a problem, offer advice and give a handout for that problem. All handouts are written in English at a sixth-grade level, avoid technical language and are culturally and gender sensitive. In addition, there are four brief videotapes to supplement the program (for parents who cannot read). These interventions are designed for behavior problems that are not complicated by severe family dysfunction or major psychiatric disorder in the child. At the core of this program, and of all successful prevention and early intervention programs, is the recognition of the family as the central agent of development of skills and of behavior change; the role of the professional is to assist the family in that process (Sanders, 1999). In general this type of intervention is successful when the parent is seeking help, suggesting a high level of motivation, the problem behavior is well defined and is of mild to moderate severity. It is also predictive of success if the behavior is recent, the family is stable, they have done well with advice in the past and there is no major psychopathology in the child or parents.

General practice physicians participated in a study of their training in these Selective Triple P methods and its impact on their practice (Sanders, Tully, Turner, Maher, & McAuliffe, 2003). Results indicated that post training, physicians were more comfortable with and utilized the behavioral intervention skills far more frequently and had an extremely high level of satisfaction with skills acquired. In terms of types of intervention, those who completed the program were more likely to rehearse a strategy (e.g., actually rehearse a time out, or giving labeled praise), provide a written hand out to the parent, and were less likely to prescribe medication for the problem. An audit of patient visits to doctors who completed the program showed that there was no increase in length or number of consultations for these problems (Sanders, Tully, Turner, Maher, & McAuliffe, 2003). Thus, although treatments were more effective, costs did not increase. Effectiveness in terms of parent perception of improvement is documented in a number of studies that include all elements of the Triple P program (Sanders, Markie-Dadds, Tully, & Bor, 2000).

Distinct from the one or two session intervention, which on the surface, closely resembles how many pediatricians manage behavioral difficulties in practice, is the more structured four session approach, which is described as the "Level Three" or "Primary Care" Triple P program. This approach is more involved and includes four separate 20-minute sessions that includes actively training skills in the parents and selective use of hand outs covering common behavioral or developmental problems. It differs from the Selective Triple P approach in that it builds some generalization strategies to teach the parents how to apply their new skills in novel situations or with other children in the family. In many ways this program is very similar to the "Helping the Noncompliant Child" program of Forehand and McMahon (1981), a four session program by psychologists in a mental health setting that has strong empirical support and long-term outcome data to support it. The first session of Primary Care Triple P is devoted to clarifying the problem, setting goals and establishing a system for the parent to count or monitor behavior. During Session 2, the provider reviews the data, any progress made and the parents' perception of the child. It brings the focus on the problem behavior, so the discussion is more in the nature of "my child has at least two tantrums every day," rather than "my child is out to drive me crazy because he has a chemical imbalance." The second session also involves introduction of some specific positive strategy and a review of any obstacles to that strategy. Session 3 reviews progress and any obstacles to reaching the goals, and at time teaching additional strategies. Essential in all sessions is a high level of praise and reinforcement to parents for their efforts. Session 4 is a final progress review, feedback and termination. The family is instructed to return if no progress is made, and if needed, referral is made to the next level of intervention: the "Level 4" or "Standard Group Triple P."

As with the "Selective" program, "Primary Care" Triple P is not designed for children who have severe problems. It still targets discrete problems that do not have a lengthy history, and which are not complicated by family dysfunction or psychopathology. In general, children involved in both "Selective" and "Primary Care" Triple P probably would not formally meet the criteria for a *DSM-IV* disorder such as oppositional defiant disorder or attention deficit hyperactivity disorder, but would have significant subclinical levels of behavior. Thus if one is taking an overall prevention point of view to reduce risk factors with the goal of reducing the rate of clinical problems in the population, this approach is a reasonable extension. By improving parenting skills at critical points of development, problems are averted. Further, by providing those services in primary care, continuity of care and the access to periodic interventions as needed through development is provided, again meeting the criteria of what works best for prevention.

Parenting Group Interventions

In practice, one of the major differences between medicine and psychology is the idea of group intervention. As a rule, pediatricians rarely do group interventions, or if they do, it is in a less formal setting of an educational format. They do not, as a rule, provide group therapies and bill for them. Thus, a busy pediatric practice might have an educational meeting or gathering for new mothers, or for children about to go to school or some other large group of patients who are about to go through some developmental change. Psychologists, on the other hand, have a rich history of using group interventions to bring about behavior change. In education, almost all instruction or behavior change is done in a group. Public health targets groups, but often reaches groups of people individually through print or electronic media. Usually when we discuss group interventions we are talking about groups in which in there is both instruction by the leader or therapist and some discussion among the participants.

Group interventions to develop and improve parenting skills are targeted both for high-risk individuals and children who have been formally diagnosed with behavior problems. By high risk, for example, a group of young children from a low-income area that has high levels of behavior problems in schools may have a group program offered to their parents. Webster-Stratton & Hammond (1997) utilized such an approach to target a group of Head Start parents to reduce overall the rates of disruptive behaviors in preschool children as a supplement to the cognitive stimulation the children were receiving in the preschool program. The goal was to improve the cognitive skills and behaviors on the children, and improve the parenting environment so that the gains could be maintained. There are a number of empirically-supported, parent group interventions which share a common set of goals as defined by Kazdin (1997), who has classified these approaches under the heading of "Parent Management Training" (PMT). The general view of PMT is that conduct problems are inadvertently developed and sustained in the home by maladaptive parent-child interactions. These interactions include paying attention to disruptive behavior, ineffective commands, harsh inconsistent punishments and failure to attend to appropriate behavior. All PMT programs are designed to alter the interaction pattern so that prosocial rather than coercive behavior is reinforced and supported within the family. In PMT treatment is primarily conducted with the parents who meet with a therapist who teaches them specific techniques to achieve the goals. Parents are trained to identify, define and observe behaviors objectively, and then to carefully deliver reinforcement or negative consequences. Parents are also trained to increase overall the level of positive interactions with their children with play and other positive activities.

Overall, PMT is the best-researched strategy to both prevent and treat child conduct problems. Positive treatment effects have been shown in numerous studies over the past 30 years (Brestan & Eyberg, 1998) but almost exclusively in mental health or university psychology clinic settings. Of the programs evaluated in the Brestan and Eyberg (1998) review, those based on Patterson and Gullioin's (1968) manual *Living with Children* have been found to be superior to control groups and to other non-behavioral psychotherapy treatments. The core features of PMT are to be found in *Living with Children*.

More intriguing as a potential intervention in a primary care site is the videotape modeling program of PMT originally developed by Webster-Stratton (1984), in which therapists utilizing the videotape materials were compared to the typical didactic presentation and tended to do better with the videotape. Webster-Stratton evaluated self-administered videotape programs (1992) for families which, while not as powerful as a therapist administered program, showed some significant effects as a low-cost intervention that could be used within a parent education program within a pediatric practice. Later work by Webster-Stratton and Hammond (1997) with at-risk populations (e.g. children in inner city Head Start Programs) show that these types of group administered parent training programs can significantly reduce behavior problems, when administered in a setting that parents routinely visit (e.g., Head Start centers).

A number of these group parent training programs have been implemented by psychologists in primary care settings (Kanoy, & Schroeder, 1985). In the Sanders (1999) program, this group level of care is provided by mental health specialists in an 8-hour format that includes four hours of group time and follow up phone calls in the rural settings where travel to clinic often is lengthy and difficult. Sanders' outcome data for the 8-hour group program are very similar to the outcomes found in the Webster-Stratton and Patterson programs.

To address the needs of families in rural areas with no access to mental health providers, the Sanders group (Connell, Sanders, & Markie-Dadds, 1997) has also developed a self-administered program (initially developed as a control condition for the therapist administered group) that uses books and skills to be practiced at home, with weekly phone contact with a therapist for guidance. Again, the results are not quite as powerful as an actual group or as the videotape program of Webster-Stratton, but are still in the moderate range (treatment effects of 0.5 or higher) of effectiveness. Thus, even for children not responding to brief interventions, group interventions using structured materials that are well validated, and even automated in the case of videotape or videodisk, could be done in a pediatric setting.

These are two examples of self-administered group treatment programs that have been shown to be effective in mental health and early preschool settings. In a primary care setting, conducting the groups could well fall in the domain of a parent educator, whose profession could be nurse, physician assistant, licensed counselor or psychologist. Thus, even this level of intervention could potentially be readily accessible and acceptable at a primary care site, in hours convenient for parents. This type of program could go a long way to provide initial effective treatment to reduce the intensity and frequency of these behavior problems.

Training Providers

A number of factors already cited has resulted in a call for increased child mental health services. There has been a call for more child psychiatrists (Surgeon General, 2001), and the School Psychology division of the American Psychological Association called for massive increases in funding for services at schools. Twenty years ago Jane Knitzer (1982), in a commissioned paper for the Children's Defense Fund, called for increased training of psychologists and social workers to serve children. While simply to increase the number of providers appears to be the logical solution to the problem, it may not be the most effective. Already it is estimated that two thirds of all visits for "help" with behavior problems occurs in primary care (Glied, 2001). Thus, it may make more sense to first train the people doing most of the work already so that they can be more effective at identification, treatment and referral. Knitzer (2001) emphasizes funds for directly training professionals in skills and competencies for child mental health. Now her broad call is for professionals from health care to day care providers to receive child mental health training. She also emphasizes the importance of collaboration between the systems of care.

At the Surgeon General's conference, Kelleher (2001) suggested that the brevity of pediatric visits (11 to 15 minutes) precluded any meaningful intervention. He noted that when patients are referred for mental health services fewer than 40% went to see a mental health provider. The solutions offered were to link primary care with mental health by having mental health providers on site and to be more effective at screening so referrals would be appropriate. Kelleher (2001) also maintained that training primary care physicians in better management "seemed to have no impact except for those who complete a two year fellowship training." Thus the goals laid down in this conference indicated a high level and lengthy training is needed. But this is in marked contrast to other programs in which health care professionals, educators, and paraprofessionals have been trained to both design and administer behavioral interventions after only 8 to 12 hours of training (e.g., Tynan & Gengo, 1992; Budd, Leibowitz, Riner, Mindell, & Goldfarb, 1981). Programs that train teachers in classroom management that are highly effective in reducing overall rates of behavior problems in elementary and middle schools require less than a week of training (U.S. Department of Education, Office of Special Education and Rehabilitation, 2000). It would appear that the time to train a physician in these strategies should be the same as that for a teacher or nurse.

Indeed, in developing the Triple P program for primary care, Sanders, Tully, Turner, Maher, and McAuliffe, 2003 (2003) use a three-day intensive training program that presents theory, background and rehearsal with a follow up at eight weeks to assess skills. As discussed above, this training produced an increase in measurable skills, a decrease in prescribing of medications, and a high level of professional satisfaction in the physicians. For the patients, there were decreases in behavior problems, but overall medical utilization data were not reported.

Following past success in training teachers, nurses, day care providers and other professionals who work with children in learning basic behavioral strategies, one way to make primary care providers more effective is to teach these strategies in an effective way. Mental health professionals that have higher level of skills in these areas can then serve as consultant and trainer.

Costs

Child mental health treatment is not expensive. At the Surgeon Generals 2001 conference Sherry Glied of Columbia University indicated that children constitute 28% of all people, account for 14% of health care dollars and only 7% of mental health dollars (Glied, 2001). In 1996, a child with a diagnosed and treated mental health problem received $984 worth of services. Of those funds, almost 40% of the money spent on inpatient services, 24% on physician services, 22% on medicines and only 10% of the money spent on nonphysician (psychology and social work), even though they provide the vast majority of psychotherapy services (Glied,

2001). Translating these numbers into system improvements, if we *tripled* psychotherapy services tomorrow, we would only raise child mental health costs by 20%. It is understandable that managed care companies closely monitor inpatient costs, given the track record of inpatient treatment (which has little or no evidence of effectiveness). However, it really makes no financial sense to closely monitor outpatient therapy, while allowing medication visits and medication benefits to go unchecked. (Many plans specify limits to psychotherapy but unlimited medicine visits.) Currently, the money does not flow toward either effective intervention or prevention programs.

Significant issues for primary care services are cost and payment. Primary care groups are either managed (reduced) fee-for-service, or they are capitated, receiving funding per month per patient. If these providers are to deliver mental health services in their setting, they must ask if they can be reimbursed for the counseling, or if there is any increased in their funding by taking on the added responsibility. These are empirical financial questions that need to be answered in a cost effectiveness study. Sanders, Tully, Turner, Maher, and McAuliffe (2003) data on primary care providers trained in Triple P suggested no increase in visits by these families. Likewise, Finney, Riley, and Cataldo (1991) suggest that addressing child mental health needs with brief interventions actually reduces the numbers of visits overall. Thus, families who have children with behavioral difficulties utilize primary care services at a high level already, and the data suggest training the providers to manage these difficulties more effectively may, in fact, decrease utilization with a better outcome for patients. It is an issue that warrants further study with large pediatric practices.

Conclusions

Survey and policy data indicate that we have made little or no progress in meeting the mental health needs of our children in the past 20 years. While nearly 20% of children require some level of services, only 4% receive those services (that is 16% of those who need services receive them). This is not due to cost: children's health care, and, in particular, mental health care costs, are quite low compared to other age groups. Indeed, of the little money that is spent on child mental health, the lion's share goes to inpatient stays, drugs and physicians, with only 10% on outpatient psychotherapy. The other trend that has remained constant is that primary care physician provide the majority of counseling that is done for families.

Despite reported gloom on accessibility of services (Surgeon General, 2001) there are a number of areas where there have been improvements. The first is that we have a much better understanding of which therapies are effective, and the most effective therapies for common problems, are actually the least costly. Brief behavioral interventions and structured parent management therapy are highly effective interventions for the disruptive behaviors that can be delivered in primary care settings. There are now better data on the impact of stimulant medication, and recommendations for improved effectiveness of those therapies in primary care (Jensen et al., 2001). These advances in psychosocial and pharmacological intervention, coupled with impressive gains in the field of screening for behavioral problems in primary care (Jellinek, & Murphy, 1999) suggest that the necessary methods to both assess and treat common behavioral and emotional problems in primary care pediatrics are available. How to implement these into practice is the major obstacle.

To meet the mental health needs of children within the existing framework of care in ways that are effective, accessible, and acceptable, we need to seriously examine implementation within primary care. While training primary care providers in screening has long been suggested, I would suggest systematically training in basic intervention strategies that have been shown to work well. The Sanders (1999) model is one that may well work in the United States, but a drawback may be the time needed for each patient, in primary care. However, the other professions in primary care, specifically nurse practitioners and physician assistants could potentially play a key role in delivering these services. Both of these professions emphasize patient education and prevention, and typically, when appointments are scheduled they are allocated more time to spend with each family than physicians are given. It may well be that in terms of resource allocation, and training the primary mental health care providers of the future may be neither physician, psychologist nor social worker, it may be members of theres newer specialties and professions. We have the models available, what is needed is the organizational and financial structure to support it, and the flexibility to cross professional boundaries (Schroeder, Chapter 1, this volume) and create new systems where none exist now.

REFERENCES

Achenbach, T. J., & Howell, C. T. (1993). Are American children's problems getting worse? A 13-year comparison. *Journal of the American Academy of Child and Adolescent Psychiatry, 32*, 1145-1154.

Accreditation Council for Graduate Medical Education, American Medical Association. (1997). *Pediatric residency review program requirements.* Chicago: American Medical Association

Bayley Infant Neurodevelomental Screen. (1995). San Antonio, TX: The Psychological Corporation.

Biglan, A. (1992). Family practices and the larger social context. *New Zealand Journal of Psychology, 21,* 37-43.

Brazelton, T. B. (1994). *Touchpoints: Your child's emotional and behavioral development.* New York: Perseus.

Brestan, E. V., & Eyberg, S. M. (1998). Effective psychosocial treatments of conduct disordered children and adolescents: 29 years, 82 studies and 5272 kids. *Journal of Clinical Child Psychology, 27,* 180-189.

Budd, K. S., Leibowitz, J. M., Riner, L. S., Mindell, C., & Goldfarb, E. (1981). Home based treatment of severe disruptive behaviors: A reinforcement package for preschool children. *Behavior Modification, 5,* 273-298.

Cheng, T. L., DeWitt, T. G., Savageau, J. A., & O'Connor, K. G. (1999). Determinants of counseling in primary care pediatric practice. *Archives of Pediatric and Adolescent Medicine, 153,* 629-635.

Child Development Inventories. (1996). Behavior Science Systems, Box 580274, Minneapolis, MN 55458

Christophersen, E. R. (1975). *Behavioral change for children.* Unpublished manuscript.

Christophersen, E. R. (1982). Incorporating behavioral pediatrics into primary care. *Pediatric Clinics of North America, 29,* 261-196.

Christophersen, E. R. (1994). *Pediatric compliance: A guide for the primary care physician.* New York: Plenum.

Christophersen, E. R. (1998). *Beyond discipline: Parenting that lasts a lifetime* (2nd ed.). Shawnee Mission, KS: Overland Press.

Connell, S., Snaders, M. R., & Markie-Dadds, C. (1997). Self directed behavioral family intervention for parents of oppositional children in rural and remote areas. *Behavior Modification, 21,* 379-409.

Costello, E. J. (1986). Primary care pediatrics and child psychopathology: A review of diagnostic, treatment and referral practices. *Pediatrics, 78,* 1044-1051.

Costello, E. J., & Shugart, M. A. (1992). Above and below the threshold: Severity of psychiatric symptoms and functional impairment in a pediatric sample. *Pediatrics, 90,* 359-386.

Dobos, A. E., Dworkin, P. H., & Bernstein, B. A. (1994). Pediatricians' approaches to developmental problems: Has the gap narrowed? *Journal of Developmental and Behavioral Pediatrics, 15,* 34-38.

Drotar, D., Sturner, R., & Nobile, C. (2003). Diagnosing and managing behavioral and developmental problems in primary care. In B. Wildman & T. Stancin (Eds.), *Treating children's psychosocial problems in primary care* (pp. 199-224). Greenwich, CT: Information Age.

Finney, J., Riley, A., & Cataldo, M. (1991). Psychology in primary health care: Effects of brief, targeted therapy on children's medical care utilization. *Journal of Pediatric Psychology, 16,* 447-462.

Forehand, R., & McMahon, R. (1981). *Helping the noncompliant child: A clinician's guide to effective parent training.* New York: Guilford Press.

Glascoe, F. P. (2000). Early detection of developmental and behavioral problems. *Pediatrics in Review, 21,* 272-280.

Glied, S. (2001). Systems of care: Financing and organizing service systems. *Report of the surgeon general's conference on children's mental health: A national action agenda* (pp. 45-47). Washington, DC: U.S. Public Health Service, Department of Health and Human Services.

Greenberg, M. T., Domitrovich, C., & Bumbarger, B. (2001). The prevention of mental disorders in school age children: Current state of the field. *Prevention and Treatment, 4,* Article 1.

Haggerty, R. J., Roghman, K. J., & Pless, I. B. (1975). *Child health and the community.* New York: John Wiley Sons.

Jellinek, M. S., & Murphy, J. M. (1999). *Psychosocial problems, screening and the Pediatric Symptoms Checklist.* Available: http://www.dbpeds.org/handouts

Jensen, P. S., Hinshaw, S. P., Swanson, J. M., Greenhill, L. L, Conners, C. K., Arnold, L. E., Abikoff, H. B., Elliott, G., Hechtman, L., Hoza, B., March, J. S., Newcom, J. H., Pelham, W., Severe, J. B., Vitiello, B., Wells, K., & Wigal, T. (2001). Findings from the NIMH Multimodal Treatment Study of ADHD: Implications and applications for primary care providers. *Journal of Developmental and Behavioral Pediatrics 22,* 60-73.

Kanoy, K. W., & Schroeder, C. S. (1985). Suggestions to parents about common behavior problems in a pediatric primary care office: Five years of follow up. *Journal of Pediatric Psychology, 10,* 15-30.

Kazdin, A. E. (1997). Parent management training: Evidence, outcome and issues. *Journal of the American Academy of Child and Adolescent Psychiatry, 36,* 1349-1356.

Kazdin, A. E., Siegel, T. C., & Bass, D. (1990). Drawing upon clinical practice to inform research on child and adolescent psychotherapy: A survey of practitioners. *Professional Psychology: Research & Practice, 21,* 189-198.

Kelleher, K. (2001). Primary care and identification of mental health needs. *Report of the surgeon general's conference on children's mental health: A national action agenda* (pp. 21-22). Washington, DC: U.S. Public Health Service, Department of Health and Human Services.

Knitzer, J. (1982). *Unclaimed children.* Washington DC: Children's Defense Fund.

Knitzer, J. (2001). Discussant: Panel on systems of care and financing. *Report of the surgeon general's conference on children's mental health: A national action agenda* (pp. 50-51). Washington, DC: U.S. Public Health Service, Department of Health and Human Services.

Leach, P. (1997). *Your baby and child: From birth to age five.* New York: Knopf.

Maynard, C., Tynan, W. D., & Werner, A. (2003). *Coordinated evaluations of disruptive behaviors.* Manuscript submitted for publication.

Parents' Evaluations of Developmental Status. (1994). Ellsworth & Vandermeer Press, Ltd. PO Box 68164 Nashville, TN 37206

Patterson, G. R., & Gullion, M. E. (1968). *Living with children: New methods for parents and teachers.* Champaign, IL: Research Press.

Perrin, E. C. (1998). Ethical questions about screening. *Journal of Developmental and Behavioral Pediatrics, 19,* 350-352.

Sanders, M. R. (1999). Triple P-Positive Parenting Program: Towards an empirically validated multilevel parenting and family support strategy for the prevention of behavior and emotional problems in children. *Clinical Child and Family Psychology Review, 2,* 71-90.

Sanders, M. R., Markie-Dadds, C., Tully, L. A., & Bor, W. (2000). The Triple P Positive Parenting Program: A comparison of enhanced, standard and self directed behavioral interventions for parents of children with early onset conduct problems. *Journal of Consulting and Clinical Psychology, 68,* 624-640.

Sanders, M. R., Montgomery, D., & Brechman-Toussaint, M. (2000). The mass media and the prevention of child behavior problems: The evaluation of a television series to promote positive outcomes for parents and their children. *Journal of Child Psychology & Psychiatry and Allied Disciplines, 41,* 939-948.

Sanders, M. R., Tully, L. A., Turner, K. M. T., Maher, C., & McAuliffe, C. (2003, September). Training GPs in parent consultation skills: An evaluation of training for the Triple P Positive Parenting Program. *Austrailian Family Physician, 32*(9), 763-768.

Shonkoff, J. P., Dworkin, P. H., Leviton, A. (1979). Primary care approaches to developmental disabilities. *Pediatrics, 64,* 506-514.

Sorenson, G., Emmons, K., Hunt, M., & Johnson, D. (1998). Implications of the results of community intervention trials. *Annual Review of Public Health, 19,* 379-416.

Stancin, T., & Palermo, T. M. (1997). A review of behavioral screening practices in pediatric settings: Do they pass the test? *Journal of Developmental and Behavioral Pediatrics, 18,* 183-194.

Surgeon General. (1999). Chapter 3: Children and mental health. *Mental health: A report of the surgeon general.* Washington, DC: U.S. Government Printing Office.

Surgeon General. (2001). *Report of the surgeon general's conference on children's mental health: A National action agenda.* Washington, DC: Department of Health and Human Services.

Tynan, W. D., & Gengo, V. (1992). Behavioral staff training in a pediatric hospital: Development of behavioral engineers. *Journal of Developmental and Physical Disabilities, 4,* 299-306.

Tynan, W. D., Schuman, W., & Lampert, N. (1999). Concurrent parent and child therapy groups for externalizing disorders: From the laboratory to the HMO. *Cognitive and Behavioral Practice, 6,* 3-9.

U.S. Department of Education, Office of Special Education and Rehabilitation (2000). *Guidelines for discipline and behavior management.* Available: http://www.ed.gov/offices/OSERS/OSEP/adminbeh.web.pdf

Webster-Stratton, C. (1984). Randomized trial of two parent training programs for families with conduct disordered children. *Journal of Consulting and Clinical Psychology, 52,* 666-678.

Webster-Stratton, C. (1992). *The parents and children videotape series: Programs 1-10.* Seattle WA: Seth Enterprises.

Webster-Stratton, C., & Hammond, M. (1997). Treating children with early onset conduct problems: A comparison of child and parent training interventions. *Journal of Consulting and Clinical Psychology, 65,* 93-109.

Zito, J., Safer, D., dosReis, S., & Gardner, J. (2000). Trends in the prescribing of psychotropic medications to preschoolers. *Journal of the American Medical Association, 283*(8), 1025-1030.

DISCUSSION SUMMARY
written by Thomas M. Yerkey

The discussion following Dr. Tynan's presentation at the forum was animated and enthusiastic. Overall, the forum participants' reaction to the Triple P model was very positive. The participants at the forum were excited that the Triple P training program might provide a usable framework for setting up similar parent education and support programs in the United States. Several ideas and concerns about the potential utility and implementation of a program similar to the Triple P program in the United States arose during this discussion, and the forum participants concentrated on potential ways to address these concerns. Carolyn Schroeder, Ph.D., began the discussion.

Dr. Schroeder commented that in 1973, her original collaborative pediatric practice started out as very similar to the Triple P program and appeared to work well for certain problems. She commented that the Triple P program might provide a way to generalize preventive approaches to child psychosocial problems. The other forum attendees generally shared this enthusiastic response to Dr. Tynan's presentation, but several concerns about the feasibility of this type of program in the United States were brought forward.

First among these concerns was the idea that because of the nationalized healthcare system in Australia, much of what has been accomplished by the Triple P program there may be impossible in this country. The managed care and third party payment system in the United States could cause serious problems for funding a similar program. Without data to support the effectiveness of a similar program in the United States, insurance companies are not likely to be flexible in what kinds of mental healthcare services that they will pay for. Until these issues are addressed, it is unlikely that a program like the Triple P program can be implemented in the United States.

Another concern that was discussed was that state insurance licensing boards frequently license programs that place limits on physician and state ability to provide mental healthcare for children, such as limiting the types of medication or therapy that can be used with a specific problem. This problem has dramatic impact on child mental healthcare in our current system. It is not likely that these insurance companies will look kindly on a new mental healthcare system that is likely to be expensive to implement. Thus, investigation needs to be performed of how a program like

Triple P would interface with managed care and third party payment for medical and mental health services in the United States.

Implementation of a comprehensive treatment model like the Triple P program would require changes in physician training and practice. Forum attendees pointed out that the psychosocial model needed for a comprehensive treatment model to function properly is presently given a great deal of attention in medical school training. However, in practice physicians tend to rely on a much more biological model. This reliance on a biological model is probably due to physicians' tendency to focus on problems that they can address with success. Physicians are quite comfortable prescribing medications for biological problems. Additionally, frequently reported psychosocial problems such as ADHD have effective biological treatments (i.e. stimulant medications). The general thought during this discussion was that physicians are likely to ignore or refer patients with psychosocial problems for which they have no known biologically based treatment. Dr. Joseph Hagan expressed concern that families' psychosocial problems are much more likely to be ignored than to be referred, that in general these families are simply not served. The primary point of this line of discussion was that there is a need for increasing physician understanding and use of biopsychosocial models of child psychosocial problems. This need would have to be met before physician reluctance to treating psychosocial problems can be changed. And, in order for a comprehensive program such as the Australian Triple P program to be successfully implemented in the United States, physicians have to become more comfortable than they presently are in treating psychosocial problems.

Overall, in spite of the participants' expressed interest in the Triple P program and in the idea of physicians' having psychotherapy privileges, the forum participants did not appear to believe that similar programs could be implemented in the United States in the near future. A grassroots movement within the medical community to increase physician willingness to deal with psychosocial problems would be among the first steps toward being able to implement a similar program. Additionally, mental healthcare professionals and physicians will have to be creative in searching out ways to fund this type of program. One of the most important potential sources of funding for research and implementation of a Triple P-like program could be the federal government. Physicians and mental healthcare professionals will also need to be creative in the use of nontraditional treatment modalities such as television programming and internet resources. With appropriate enthusiasm, training, flexibility, and creativity, the Australian Triple P model presented by Dr. Tynan may provide a new model for increasing the treatment of child psychosocial problems in the United States.

While the forum participants found the idea of implementing a program similar to the Triple P program in the United States to be exciting, the concerns that were voiced during the discussion indicated that research is needed before implementation is attempted. Chief among these concerns was answering the question of whether or not American physicians and parents would find the existing Triple P materials, printed and video, helpful. The forum participants generally agreed that the existing printed materials would probably generalize to use in the United States easily, however, there were concerns voiced regarding the cultural specificity of the video and television presentations. If the existing materials are not effective in the United States, then U.S. specific materials, will need to be developed.

CHAPTER 9

DIAGNOSING AND MANAGING BEHAVIORAL AND DEVELOPMENTAL PROBLEMS IN PRIMARY CARE

Current Applications of the *DSM-PC*

Dennis Drotar
Rainbow Babies and Children's Hospital and Case Western Reserve University School of Medicine

Raymond Sturner
Johns Hopkins University

Chantelle Nobile
Case Western Reserve University

USING THE *DSM-PC* TO MANAGE BEHAVIORAL PROBLEMS IN PRIMARY CARE

Primary care practitioners (PCPs), including pediatricians, who practice in the new millennium face extraordinary pressures in managed care environments. Such pressures can affect the quality of care at all levels. In

Treating Children's Psychosocial Problems in Primary Care, 199–224

order to maintain the economic viability of their practice, PCPs need to see increasing numbers of patients, which translates into longer days, spending less time with patients and their families during individual visits, or both. At the same time, modern pediatric practice includes increasing numbers of children with psychosocial problems that are both difficult to detect and time consuming to manage (Kelleher, McInerny, Gardner, Childs, & Wasserman, 2000). Research has consistently noted that large numbers, anywhere from 12% to 25%, of children who are seen in primary care, have significant psychosocial problems (Costello, 1986; Costello et al., 1988; Kelleher & Rickert, 1994). However, only a small subset of these children are identified and referred for treatment (Costello et al., 1988; Lavigne et al., 1993).

The factors that influence the well-documented discrepancy between the prevalence of behavioral and emotional problems and the typical frequency of their recognition and management by pediatricians and other PCPs in primary care settings are multiple and complex. For example, practice-based time constraints undoubtedly affect PCPs' abilities to diagnose and manage behavioral problems. In addition, some PCPs may be reluctant to identify children's behavior problems because they are concerned about labeling children and/or threatening their parents. Problems with access to experienced mental health practitioners and limitations in insurance coverage also influence the recognition of children's behavioral problems (Kelleher & Rickert, 1994).

The diagnosis and management of children's behavioral and emotional problems in the primary care setting requires special skills that differ from those involving physical diagnosis and treatment and are not heavily emphasized in the training of PCPs (Coury, Berger, Stancin, & Tanner, 1999). These include (among others) the ability to utilize specific diagnostic methods, (e.g., interviews, behavior checklists, or screening measures) to make a behavioral diagnosis (Glascoe, 1999; Jellinek, Little, Murphy, & Pagano, 1995; Stancin & Palermo, 1997) and skills to communicate with parents about their children's psychological problems.

Another significant barrier to the diagnosis and management of children's behavioral problems by PCPs, which is the focus of this chapter, involves limitations in the currently available methods of diagnostic categorization of children with behavioral and developmental problems. The primary diagnostic system for the classification of behavioral problems that is currently in use by mental health professionals, the *Diagnostic and Statistical Manual of Mental Disorders*, 4th edition (*DSM-IV*) (American Psychiatric Association, 1994) has several problems that limit its utility for the practice and training of PCPs. For example, the *DSM-IV* describes child and adolescent mental disorders that are both more serious and much less prevalent than the broad spectrum of children's behavioral and developmental problems commonly encountered in primary care. Pediatricians and family practitioners may encounter large numbers of children who present with a very broad spectrum of behavioral and developmental problems that simply do not fit the *DSM-IV* classification system, do not meet threshold for a *DSM-IV* disorder, or both. Consequently, when PCPs encounter such children they may be uncertain about how best to classify children's problems using the *DSM-IV* system. Some may decide not to make a diagnosis of a mental disorder according to *DSM-IV* to avoid mislabeling the child. For these reasons, one would expect that when the rates of PCPs' diagnoses of children's mental disorders are compared to independently assessed prevalence of these disorders according to the *DSM-IV*, they would fall short of optimal recognition, which is in fact what has been found (Costello, 1986; Costello, et al., 1988). On the other hand, if limitations in the applicability of *DSM-IV* are playing a role in underidentification of behavioral problems, one would expect that when PCPs are given an alternative nomenclature, that is, a more comprehensive language with which to describe the range of problems they see in practice, they would identify behavioral problems with greater frequency. In support of this hypothesis, Horwitz, Leaf, Leventhal, Forsythe, and Speechly (1992) found that when pediatricians were given opportunities to use a nomenclature that provided a broader range of choices for diagnosis than the *DSM-IV*, they identified higher rates of behavior problems than is typical for studies that used the *DSM-IV*.

Until very recently, there was no organized, logically coherent alternative to the *DSM-IV* that was available to PCPs to guide their training and practice in the diagnosis of behavioral and developmental problems in children and adolescents. To address this need, an interdisciplinary team organized by the American Academy of Pediatrics (AAP) in collaboration with a number of other professional organizations, developed a method to classify such problems: the *Diagnostic and Statistical Manual for Primary Care (DSM-PC), Child and Adolescent Version* (Wolraich, 1997; Wolraich, Felice, & Drotar, 1996). One guiding assumption behind this effort was that the *DSM-PC* would be more suitable for use by PCPs in diagnosing behavioral problems than the *DSM-IV* or the Zero to Three Diagnosis Classification (0-3 System), which focuses on mental health and developmental disorders among infants and young children (Zero to Three, National Center for Clinical Infant Program, 1994) but was not designed for use by PCPs.

The *DSM-PC* has been available for use by PCPs for more than four years. However, it is not clear how much the *DSM-PC* is currently being used in practice and what specific applications have been implemented. The purpose of this chapter is to describe the *DSM-PC*, some current applications, and recommendations for future use.

Working Assumptions that Guided the Development of the *DSM-PC*

The assumptions that guided the development of the *DSM-PC* (Wolraich, 1997) included the following: (1) children demonstrate symptoms that vary along a continuum from normal variations to severe mental disorders that can be divided into clinically meaningful gradations; (2) the nature of children's environments and exposure to stress have a critical impact on their mental health, and need to be recognized and managed in the context of primary care; (3) a coding system for children's developmental and behavioral problems should be fully compatible with available classification approaches such as the *DSM-IV* and the *International Classification of Diseases* (*ICD-10*); (4) an effective coding system should be clear, concise and usable by PCPs; (5) a coding system should be based on available objective data and professional consensus; and (6) the language used in a coding system should be such that it can be supported, revised based on research findings, or both.

Description of the *DSM-PC*

The *DSM-PC* includes a table of contents, introduction, two major core content areas (Situations and Child Manifestations), and appendices, each of which are briefly described below.

Table of Contents and Introduction

The table of contents for the *DSM-PC* is followed by a detailed list that includes the page number and code number of each diagnosis. A brief introduction then describes the purpose, key assumptions, and organization of the manual. Sample formats for the common behaviors, the concept of the spectrum of behaviors (developmental variations, problems, and disorders), developmental presentations, and differential diagnoses are then described. The introduction also includes guidelines for using the *DSM-PC* such as locating information, a flow chart of steps in coding, and case illustrations of how to use the manual. The introduction also includes a description of relevant issues in assessing the severity of the clinical needs of children and families.

Situations

The Situations section was designed to help practitioners (1) to describe and evaluate the impact of stressful situations that present in primary care and can affect children's mental health, (2) to assess potential consequences of such adverse situations, and (3) to identify factors that may make a child more vulnerable or resilient to the impact of stressful situations to which they are exposed. The following categories of potentially stressful situations that were identified as the most common and/or well-researched are defined in the *DSM-PC*: challenges to primary support group (e.g., marital discord/divorce), changes in caregiving (e.g., physical illness of parent), other functional changes in family (e.g., addition of a sibling), community or social challenges (e.g., acculturation), educational challenges (e.g., parental illiteracy), parent or adolescent occupational challenges, unemployment housing challenges (e.g., homelessness), economic challenges (e.g., poverty/inadequate financial status), inadequate access to health and/or mental health services, legal system or crime problem (e.g., parent or juvenile crime), other environmental situations (e.g., natural disaster), and health-related situations (e.g., chronic or acute health conditions). Information concerning potential risk (e.g., family dysfunction) and protective factors (e.g, intelligence) is also provided to help clinicians evaluate the impact of stressors.

Child Manifestations

The second major content area of the *DSM-PC,* child manifestations or symptoms, is organized into specific sections identified as behavioral clusters. Each of these sections is introduced by a specific presenting symptom that describes concerns in words that are typically used by parents. For example, "my child is not talking" refers to the learning and developmental problems cluster. Practitioners can readily access the manual by referring to the index of presenting complaints.

The 10 behavioral clusters are the following: (1) developmental competency (e.g., learning and developmental problems); (2) impulsivity, hyperactivity, or inattention disorders; (3) negative/antisocial behaviors; (4) substance use/abuse; (5) emotions and moods (e.g., sadness or anxiety); (6) somatic and sleep behaviors; (7) feeding, eating, elimination behaviors; (8) illness-related behaviors; (9) sexual behaviors; and (10) atypical behaviors. Each cluster description has a comparable format that includes the cluster title, presenting complaints, definitions and symptoms, as well as information about epidemiology and etiology. These formats were developed to guide primary care clinicians to consider the following issues for each cluster: (1) the spectrum of severity of a child's presenting problems, (2) common developmental presentations (e.g., infancy, early and middle childhood, and adolescence, and/or (3) differential diagnosis. In order to facilitate a practitioner's ability to make a differential diagnosis, information for each cluster is presented in a specific format.

Spectrum of Problem Severity

Behavioral problems that pertain to each cluster are divided into one of three categories: (1) *Developmental variations* are defined as behaviors that parents may raise as a concern with their child's primary care provider, but are within the range of expected behaviors for the child's age; (2) *Problems* are those behaviors that are serious enough to disrupt the child's functioning with peers, in school, and/or in family, but do not reach sufficient level of symptom severity to warrant the diagnosis of a mental disorder based on the *DSM-IV*; (3) *Disorders* are defined exactly as they are in the *DSM-IV.*

Common Developmental Presentations

To help practitioners recognize how common symptoms (e.g., anxiety) may be expressed among children of different ages, guidelines are provided to facilitate coding of variations, problems, and disorders in four age groups; infancy (birth to 2 years of age), early childhood (3 to 5 years of age), middle childhood (6 to 12 years of age), and adolescence (13 years of age and older).

Differential Diagnosis

Information that is provided in each of the clusters is designed to help PCPs make a differential diagnosis and is divided into two sections: alternative causes and comorbid and associated conditions. The differential diagnosis section describes phenomena that could be alternative causes for specific behaviors including: (1) general medical conditions, (2) substances, legal and illegal, that could cause behavioral manifestations, or (3) mental disorders that may present with similar behavioral symptoms and which, if present, should be coded in place of the disorder in the cluster.

Appendices

The appendices include a list of presenting complaints and page numbers, a section on diagnostic vignettes, which provide informative case material that can be used to practice coding, and a section that summarizes selected *DSM-IV* diagnostic criteria that are likely to be used by PCPs (e.g., attention-deficit hyperactivity disorder, ADHD).

POTENTIAL UTILITY OF THE *DSM-PC* FOR PRACTICE

One of the primary purposes of designing the *DSM-PC* was to develop a manual that would be useful to PCPs in categorizing the problems they commonly see in their practices, especially in two ways: (1) making distinctions among a range of behavioral and developmental problems that vary widely in severity and content, and (2) identifying a wide range of stressful situations that can affect the management of behavioral and developmental problems. Each of these two areas is discussed below.

Making Distinctions Concerning Severity of Behavioral and Developmental Problems

One of the unique features of the *DSM-PC* is that it gives PCPs a way to distinguish among the severity of behavioral/developmental problems seen in children by defining three broad categories: developmental variations, problems, and disorders. *Developmental variations* are those behaviors that parents may raise as a concern to their PCP but are within the range of what is expected for a child of that particular age. The management of symptoms that are classified as developmental variations is most likely to be conducted by pediatricians or family practitioners, and may include assuring parents that their children show age-appropriate behaviors and by providing specific guidance to parents concerning management.

In contrast to developmental variations, *problems* are defined as symptoms that are serious enough to disrupt the child's functioning in any one of a number of contexts, such as the family situation, in peer relations, or at school. Moreover, these problems are often severe enough to cause significant burden or distress for the child or parents. Depending on the level of functional impairment associated with the child's behavioral or developmental problem, degree of distress caused by the problem, or a problem's response to intervention by the PCP, symptoms that are classified as problems may be managed by the PCP or referred to mental health providers.

The above categories provide new options for PCPs to facilitate characterization of a broader spectrum of behavioral and developmental problems but do not replace current *DSM-IV* categories, which are defined as *disorders* in the *DSM-PC*. In this regard, it is important to recognize that some disorders with high prevalence, such as ADHD or enuresis, are commonly managed by PCPs. By including *DSM-IV* categories that are commonly seen in primary care within the text of the manual, the *DSM-PC* encourages PCPs to learn about and use the *DSM-IV*.

Identifying Stressful Situations that Can Affect the Management of Behavioral and Developmental Problems

The Environmental Situations section of the *DSM- PC* was designed to help PCPs categorize stressful situations that might influence the expression and impact of behavioral symptoms and hence shape the kind of intervention that may be provided to children or parents. For example, this would include preventive interventions, including those that focus on helping families manage the impact of stressful situations such as divorce on their children's psychological development. The codes for environmental situations can be used to describe the focus of clinical encounters in which parents, children, or other family members are counseled to manage the impact of stressful situations, such as, parental divorce. Identification of stressful situations can also help PCPs identify potential psychological risk to the child that are associated with environmental stressors and monitor the presence or absence of environmental stressors over time (see Drotar, 1999, for more detail.) Finally, identification of stressful situations can also help PCPs identify factors affecting the clinical management and prognosis of behavioral problems. For example, two children who present with similar behavioral problems but with very different levels of environmental stress might be expected to have different outcomes and potential recommendations for psychosocial treatment: A child who presents with problems with anger and oppositional behavior in a family with chronic marital discord and family violence would be expected to have a very different prognosis than a child with similar behavioral problems whose parents have a supportive relationship with one another.

Promoting a Shared Language for Collaboration and Consultation

Another relevant application of the *DSM-PC* concerns its use in promoting a shared language for collaboration and consultation among pediatricians, other mental health providers, including psychologists, as well as other professionals. The *DSM-PC* includes terms and concepts, (e.g., developmental variation and problems) which can be readily understood and do not require specialized training in a specific professional or theoretical orientation. Consequently, the language of the *DSM-PC* is in many ways ideal for interdisciplinary collaboration concerning clinical care. For example, PCPs can use the *DSM-PC* to inform other professions concerning the nature and severity of a particular presenting problem and to clarify the need for evaluation and management of the child by a wide range of other professionals. Symptoms that reach the level of problem or disorder according to the *DSM-PC* would be much more likely to warrant referral for additional evaluation and/or management by mental health professionals than symptoms that reflect developmental variations

Communicating with Parents About Their Children's Behavioral Problems and About Stressful Situations

The language of the *DSM-PC* translates a wide range of presenting problems into different content categories and levels of severity, which can be used to give parents concrete feedback about their children's problems and the approach to management. For example, in the case of less severe symptoms that nonetheless may be troubling to parents, it may help parents to learn that their children's problems reflect expectable developmental variations. On the other hand, the *DSM-PC* can also be used to help clarify the need for a referral to a mental health professional to parents (e.g., that because the child's symptoms are severe enough to cause distress in the family a referral is needed).

Moreover, many parents ask the question "is my child's problem normal?" and the *DSM-PC* provides information that can help parents appreciate the difference between a developmental variation and something more serious. Parents' experience in responding to specific questions about their child's symptoms that are designed to elicit information to facilitate making a *DSM-PC* diagnosis either in a clinical interview or computerized format (Sturner & Howard, 2000) can also help facilitate their appreciation and recognition of various levels of behavioral and developmental problems. The environmental codes of the *DSM-PC* also may be used to communicate with parents about the potential impact of family and other stressors that may be affecting their children's behavior and need to be considered in management.

APPLYING THE *DSM-PC*: AN EXAMPLE FROM A PRIMARY CARE PRACTICE SETTING

One of the pressing needs in developing the potential of the *DSM-PC* to impact practice involving management of behavioral and developmental problems in primary care is to document examples of its successful application and determine their generalizability to other settings. To address this need, Sturner and Howard (2000) have developed an interesting application of the *DSM-PC* using a parent/child/clinician computer-based program as a component of a comprehensive system known as the Child Health and Development Interactive System (CHADIS). The CHADIS program incorporates several parent questionnaires regarding perception of child's strengths and weaknesses, environmental stresses, and family background adapted from Kemper and Kelleher (1996). In addition, it includes screening measures that combine developmental observation with standardized physical examination procedures. For example, developmental observations during an infant physical examination (McGuinn, Sturner, Howard, & Duggan, 2001) are augmented by an assessment of visual acuity and academic readiness using the Simultaneous Technique for Acuity and Readiness Testing or START (Sturner, Funk & Green, 1994). Hearing, articulation and language are further screened by use of speech signals with the Communication Screening System (Sturner, Layton, Feezor, Craft, & Lewis, 1998).

To facilitate utilization of the *DSM-PC* in the CHADIS application, a computerized version of a parent inventory was developed. The inventory asks parents to identify their level of concern ("very concerned," "somewhat," or "not at all") among a list of general items derived by using the "presenting complaint" section of the *DSM-PC* Child Manifestations section. If more than one concern is identified, the computer asks the parent to prioritize them. The parent is then prompted to respond to an algorithm of questions related to the "chief complaint" that is identified by the parent. The parent continues through the series of questions until: (1) criteria for a diagnostic level is not achieved or (2) all the questions necessary to make a *DSM-PC* diagnosis have been reached. If the parent has indicated additional concerns, he/she is led through algorithms representing successively lower priority concerns, time permitting. Each algorithm only takes a few minutes for the parent to complete and prioritization usually takes less than a minute. The total procedure takes parents between 5 and 20 minutes to complete. When time is limited, the process can be interrupted after an algorithm representing the top concern is repeated. If there are a larger number of significant parental concerns and a detailed review of each is desired, the process can last longer. Based on this information, parents' concerns are translated into hypothesized *DSM-PC* diagnoses of developmental variation, problem or disorder.

A clinical guide in the form of an intelligent medical record has been developed that helps the PCP review the decision tree of responses to double check their reliability and correcting any potential misunderstandings. In most instances, the parents' responses to the questions will be sufficient to make a diagnosis according to the logic of the *DSM-PC*. Additional questions have been included to help the PCP inquire about risk and protective factors that would affect the prognosis and/or management of whatever diagnosis is made.

Furthermore, the clinical guides include highlights or "tips" that describe important considerations for each diagnosis and prompts to review the parents' information with attention to the most important elements in the diagnoses, that is, the level of functional impairment or impact on the family. Once diagnostic impressions based on the *DSM-PC* have been delineated, a related list of management suggestions, appropriate additional clinical tools, and potential resources is automatically generated. Output also includes referral resources in the local area, books for the parent/child related to the problems, games to address areas of weakness, and resources to build on those strengths that have been identified.

Case Example Using CHADIS in Implementing the *DSM-PC*

The mother of Jimmy, a 4-year-old boy, brought her child for his four-year check-up. She was new to the practice and was asked to complete a family history and risk-factor questionnaire at the beginning of the visit. She revealed that Jimmy was an only child and that she was separated from her husband. She also noted that she has felt sad and depressed much of the year. She then filled out the *DSM-PC* questionnaire via a handheld computer terminal.

On the *DSM-PC* CHADIS questions for aggressive/oppositional behaviors early childhood, she endorsed the concern about "not minding/doing the opposite" at the "very concerned" level out of 25 total possible concerns. The mother was then asked about the frequency of and functional impact of each of these behaviors, that is, whether it occurred frequently enough to be a bothersome problem, if it continued after correction, whether it was beginning to interfere with relationships with friends or teachers, if it was leading to a change in routines or if things were being damaged as a result of the behavior. (See Table 9.1 for the questions that she was asked and the algorithm that was used for classification.) Jimmy's mother's answers suggested that all these areas were affected by the problem but also that the problem was of recent onset (1-2 months duration).

Prior to the beginning of the clinical visit, the PCP previewed the "clinician worksheet" of CHADIS and knew that the mother's chief concern about Jimmy was about his noncompliance with her requests and that her responses to questions about this concern were consistent with the *DSM-PC* diagnosis: "Aggressive/Oppositional Problem: Oppositionality." The related diagnosis of oppositional defiant disorder (ODD), was not chosen because Jimmy's presenting behaviors were shorter in duration than those that are necessary to meet criteria for ODD. Other clinical guides prompted the pediatrician to "look for ADHD; consider low cognitive functioning, hearing problems, language and learning disorders; parents who are stressed and/or depressed." It was noted that Jimmy had already passed developmental as well as communication (speech, hearing, and language) screening tests, and there were no concerns in preschool about his academic skills.

Table 9.1. CHADIS *DSM-PC* Questions for Aggressive/Oppositional Behaviors–Early Childhood

1. Does your child **often** do mean things, like (check all that apply):
   a. Hit
   b. Kick
   c. Bite
   d. Grab toys
   e. Say mean things
   f. None of the above

If f is checked, go to 6.
Otherwise, ask:

2. Do your child's friends or teachers get upset when your child is mean?
   a. yes
   b. no
   c. unsure
3. Is your child's mean behavior making people change their day-to-day activities?
   a. yes
   b. no
   c. unsure
4. If your child's mean behavior causing problems at school or in daycare?
   a. yes
   b. no
   c. unsure
5. Does your child damage things when s/he is mean?
   a. yes
   b. no
6. Does your child "not mind" or "do the opposite" often enough to be bothersome to people taking care of him/her?
   a. yes
   b. no

If yes to 2, 3, 4 or 6, continue:
Otherwise, stop.

7. How long has your child been not minding, doing the opposite, or doing these mean things?
   a. less than 6 months
   b. 6 months
   c. more than 6 months

If 7a, stop.
Otherwise ask:

8. Does your child lose his or her temper?
   a. rarely
   b. sometimes
   c. often
9. Does your child argue with adults?
   a. rarely
   b. sometimes
   c. often

Continued

Table 9.1. Continued

10. Does your child actively defy or refuse to follow adult requests or rules?
    a. rarely
    b. sometimes
    c. often

11. Does your child annoy other people on purpose?
    a. rarely
    b. sometimes
    c. often

12. Does your child blame others for his/her mistakes or bad behavior?
    a. rarely
    b. sometimes
    c. often

13. Is your child touchy or easily annoyed by others?
    a. rarely
    b. sometimes
    c. often

14. Is your child often angry and resentful?
    a. rarely
    b. sometimes
    c. often

15. Is your child spiteful (does mean things to get back at someone)?
    a. rarely
    b. sometimes
    c. often

16. Is your child vindictive (wants revenge)?
    a. rarely
    b. sometimes
    c. often

Coding:
If no to 2 through 6, code Aggressive/Oppositional Variation: Aggression V65.44 if cluster Bullies/Hits is endorsed code Aggressive/Oppositional: Oppositionality V65.49 if cluster Not minding/Doing the opposite or Argues/yells/swears is endorsed.
If at least 4 of 8c-16c, code Oppositional Defiant Disorder 313.81.
If none of above coded:
If yes to 2, 3, 4, or 5, code Aggressive/Oppositional Problem: Aggression V71.02
If yes to 6, code Aggressive/Oppositional Problem: Oppositionality V71.02

As summarized in the clinician worksheet, the above information yielded the following impressions: (1) Aggressive/Oppositional Problem: Oppositionality; (2) Environmental stressors including possible maternal depression and parental separation. Based on the above impressions, in this case the PCP chose to refer the parent to a mental health provider for her depression and to discuss behavioral management for Jimmy. This discussion was reinforced by a hardcopy of a report that integrated relevant parent test selections chosen by the PCP including information on how to formalize a "special time" for your child and how to use reinforcers for good behavior, which the PCP demonstrated for Jimmy's mother by rewarding him for components of his cooperation in the office. The PCP also commented on the importance of identifying Jimmy's good behavior, while empathizing with the mother's difficulties managing his behaviors, given the family stresses and the impact of her own sadness and irritability.

Provider and Parent Feedback Concerning the Application of the DSM PC Using CHADIS

The Sturner and Howard (2000) application of the *DSM-PC* is very new, having been used for several months, but has proven feasible in a practice setting that serves families representing a wide spectrum of socioeconomic status. Nearly one third (30%) of families in the practice receive Medicaid. A recent pilot and feasibility study was conducted with group comprised children from this practice and from a group of inner city children who were exposed to cocaine in utero ($N = 27$). Results indicate that parental reactions to participating in visits in which the CHADIS application of the *DSM-PC* was used have been positive. For example, when asked how the use of the computer changed your visit, two thirds of the parents (66%) reported that it had added value to the visit, approximately one fourth (27%) reported no change, and a smaller number (4%) said that it got in the way. The majority of parents (73%) preferred the use of the procedure in a similar way for the next visit with a smaller number reporting either no preference (23%) or a preference against (4%).

Parents reported the following advantages of the approach: "It might raise concerns not thought about otherwise"; "helped organize my thoughts"; "easier, no waiting"; "faster, offers choices better than the paper way"; "doctor would know more about your child and can be better prepared." Disadvantages included the following: "I prefer one-on-one: the doctor is more caring"; "it won't do its job, gives the wrong information"; "time consuming."

The system has been used on a trial basis in a follow-up clinic practice for children exposed to prenatal cocaine. When CHADIS was discontinued, the parents requested it back in the setting. The project has been so popular in the clinical practice setting that several of the parents have volunteered their time to assist the project, including two mothers who are programmers.

The impact of using the CHADIS application of the *DSM-PC* on this practice, including the effectiveness in improving the recognition and efficiency of management of behavioral and developmental problems is now being studied. Because the *DSM-PC* is incorporated routinely into methods of obtaining information and history from parents in a standardized way, one would anticipate that the CHADIS application would increase the numbers of children and adolescents with behavioral and developmental problems who are identified and managed in this practice.

One interesting but as yet unanswered question is the degree to which use of the CHADIS application increases the time that is required by the PCP to manage behavioral and developmental problems and how this might affect the economics of the practice. Routine application of the CHADIS application of the *DSM-PC* (or any consistent application of the *DSM-PC* for that matter) would be expected to increase the time demands of practice. On the other hand, CHADIS is potentially efficient because the clinician and diagnostic worksheets are organized to enable the PCP to focus efforts on presumptive and diagnostic conclusions. For example, PCPs who routinely question parents about their children's behavioral and developmental concerns may actually save some time by systematically gathering information that is supplied by parents. Those PCPs who do not routinely question parents about children's behavior would obviously have to spend more time if they use the CHADIS. Consequently, observational studies are needed to document the impact of this application to practice settings. It is possible that the increased time demands involved in the CHADIS application of the *DSM-PC* would be offset at least to some extent by increased parental satisfaction, assuming that preliminary results of parent satisfaction data reported earlier are sustained.

At this point, the generalizability of the CHADIS system to other settings is not known. However, plans are being made to disseminate the CHADIS application of the *DSM-PC* to pediatricians on a broad scale beginning with faculty in academic centers who provide training for residents in behavior and development. We anticipate the CHADIS application will be of special interest to faculty in pediatric and family practice settings that provide such training, since the associated prompts and guides provide an innovative educational experience at a time of significant motivation for the trainees—the moment of clinical contact. A study of CHADIS' educational impact on pediatric residents at Johns Hopkins is planned for later this year. Pediatric faculty have expressed interest in the CHADIS application because its standardized administration and central data archive capacity can stimulate new opportunities for collaborative research which are based on their existing clinical service and teaching responsibilities.

A survey of academic (mostly in the developmental-behavioral specialty) pediatricians (N = 81) attending national presentation/demonstrations of CHADIS showed a very high level (98%) of interest in becoming a site for the system. We also anticipate that the clinical tools and suggestions for resources for parents that are part of the CHADIS application of the *DSM-PC* may be very appealing to some practitioners. We expect that pediatricians will be in a better position to charge for services they have clearly documented via parents' responses to the questionnaires but the success of such reimbursement remains to be seen. On the other hand, the CHADIS application of the *DSM-PC* (or any other application for that matter) will not remove the barriers to diagnosis and treatment of behavioral and developmental problems that were described earlier, (e.g., time constraints, lack of training in diagnosis and management (Marino, 1997)).

HOW IS THE *DSM-PC* CURRENTLY BEING USED?

The above application describes the use of the *DSM-PC* in one practice setting. One important, but as yet unanswered question is how the *DSM-PC* is currently being used in a range of settings. To provide some preliminary information on this topic, we surveyed two groups, each of whom would be expected to be more knowledgeable about the *DSM-PC* and more likely to use it than the average group of professionals. The two groups were: (1) the Ohio Chapter of the Society for Developmental and Behavioral Pediatrics, (an interdisciplinary group of pediatricians, psychologists and social workers), and (2) an interdisciplinary group who were the faculty trainers for *DSM-PC*. This deliberately biased sampling procedure was employed to assess the frequency of use of the *DSM-PC* among professionals who were most likely to use it and to elicit their responses concerning advantages and disadvantages of the manual. The survey included questions about how often the *DSM-PC* was used, for what activities it was used, what were seen as the most helpful features and what would promote greater utilization of the *DSM-PC*.

The survey was sent to 34 members of the Ohio Chapter of the Society for Developmental and Behavioral Pediatrics and 14 faculty trainers. One survey was sent to individuals who were members of each group. Data were obtained from 22 individuals, including 12 (55%) pediatricians, 8 (36%) psychologists, 1 social worker, and 1 (5%) sociologist. This was a response rate of 42%. The sample was split in terms of who did and did not use the *DSM-PC*: 12 (55%) individuals reported using it and the remaining 10 (45%) individuals reported that they do not use it.

Professionals who reported that they used the *DSM-PC* were divided equally between pediatricians (*N* = 6) and mental health professionals (*N* = 5) and 1 social worker. The frequency of the use of *DSM-PC* ranged widely from monthly or less than once a month (N = 8), to weekly or several times each week (*N* = 3).

Those who reported that they used the *DSM-PC* were also asked to indicate in what areas (i.e., clinical, teaching, or research) they use it. Individuals could list more than one activity. Findings were as follows: teaching (*N* = 10), clinical care (*N* = 7), and research (*N* = 3). Of those who use the *DSM-PC* for clinical care, 3 respondents reported using it with 0-2 clients per week; 1 reported using it with 10 clients per week; and 1 did not indicate the frequency of clinical use. Of those who used the *DSM-PC* for teaching purposes, 9 individuals used it to train medical or pediatric students and residents; 3 used it to train psychology trainees; and 1 individual reported using it with psychiatry fellows.

Professionals who reported using the *DSM-PC* were also asked to describe the advantages and disadvantages of the instrument. Most respondents believed that an advantage of the *DSM-PC* was its conceptualization of behavior problems (*N* = 8). For example, one respondent reported: "[It] allows for a broader conceptualization of the psychosocial context for the child's presenting problem." Others reported that the developmental spectrum and the age-appropriate examples of symptom presentations were very useful (*N* = 4) and the continuum of symptom severity and being able to label subsyndromal conditions was also an advantage (*N* = 7). As one person responded: "the developmental variation, problem, disorder distinction is an advantage. I explain this to parents a lot." Finally, the broad conceptualization of a child's presenting problem within the larger environment and psychosocial context was cited as an advantage by some (*N* = 5).

The primary disadvantage that was reported concerning the *DSM-PC* involved problems with reimbursement from third party payers (*N* = 5). As one person noted: "as far as I can tell, insurance companies do not recognize it." An additional respondent stated: "the V codes are very helpful from a descriptive perspective, but of no help for billing. I stick to the *ICD-9* codes for billing, or be sure I have at least one of those in addition to the V codes".

Additional disadvantages that were described centered primarily on lack of specificity or clarity of concepts outlined within the *DSM-PC* (*N* = 4), and an absence of guides to facilitate its use (*N* = 2). For example, one respondent, who had concerns about the Environmental Situations section, wrote: "I would really hope this could be revised because it should be one of the most useful parts, but the way it is currently arranged and the way circumstances outside the child have been defined most of the important areas I want to code and need to discuss are not included." Another person stated: "examples of symptom presentation occasionally seem confounded with impact/outcome." Finally, one individual reported that there are "not enough different codes for conditions."

Those (*N* =10) who reported that they did not use the *DSM-PC* cited somewhat different problems as reasons for not using it as were noted above, with the exception of problems with reimbursement (*N* = 2). Reasons for not using the *DSM-PC* included: being unaware of the *DSM-PC* (i.e., only recently learned about it; *N* = 2), not having proper training in using it (*N* = 1), not currently seeing clients (*N* = 3), lack of availability of the *DSM-PC* (*N* = 2), and no advantages of the *DSM-PC* over *DSM-IV* (*N* = 1). Those individuals who did not use the *DSM-PC* were predominantly pediatricians (*N* = 6), though 3 psychologists and 1 sociologist also reported not using it.

In responding to the question "what do you think is needed to promote greater utilization of the *DSM-PC*?" most users of the *DSM-PC* felt that gaining greater acceptance (and reimbursement rates) of the *DSM-PC* as a diagnostic system with third party payers was important (*N* = 9). For example, one respondent stated: "reimbursement (or some trust that reimbursement will be coming in the future) for using the system and the clinical work in *DSM-PC* areas" is needed. Another person responded: "for use in primary care, I think it needs to be tied to reimbursement". Furthermore, wider dissemination of the *DSM-PC* among faculty physicians, psychology trainees and community providers with greater support from the AAP was also recommended to promote increased utilization (*N* = 6). For example, one respondent wrote: "greater lobbying effort by the AAP is needed; I don't perceive the academy as having given a high priority to lobbying its member regularly and consistently here the way they do in so many other things."

Finally, some respondents also recommended conducting more research with the *DSM-PC*, particularly regarding its reliability and validity (*N* = 2). One person recommended developing a structured clinical interview for the *DSM-PC*.

Recommendations for Future Directions to Enhance Application of the *DSM-PC*

The *DSM-PC* remains a promising method for the classification of children's behavioral and development problems in pediatric and family practice settings that has yet to live up to its considerable potential. The results of this small-scale survey and our observations suggest that it is not widely used. Salient barriers to the use of the *DSM-PC* include problems with reimbursement and the lack of specific demonstrations of the potential utility of the *DSM-PC* in practice settings. In response to this latter barrier, Sturner and Howard's (2000) application of the *DSM-PC* in the CHADIS system fills an important need.

A concerted effort among many professionals will be needed to promote more widespread use of the *DSM-PC*. Strategies to facilitate greater utilization of the *DSM-PC* include the following:

- continued dissemination of information concerning the *DSM-PC*
- the development of materials to facilitate its use
- promotion of reimbursement for using the *DSM-PC*
- documenting and describing innovative applications of the manual in teaching, practice and research
- greater interdisciplinary use of the *DSM-PC*
- using the *DSM-PC* to target interdisciplinary intervention for children at risk
- research applications

Continued Dissemination of Information Concerning the *DSM-PC*

Many pediatricians and psychologists are still not familiar with the *DSM-PC* and its applicability in practice, teaching, and research. One strategy will be to promote greater professional awareness of the *DSM-PC* by disseminating information in local communities, in meetings of regional and state societies of pediatricians and psychologists, in academic medical centers, and national professional meetings.

Development of Materials to Facilitate Application of the *DSM-PC*

The development of materials that facilitate PCP's abilities to implement the *DSM-PC* in primary care settings (e.g., encounter sheets that list the *DSM-PC* codes) will be important to promote its use. Moreover, a "user's guide" for the *DSM-PC* is very much needed to describe how to best use the manual in practice. Such a guide might include illustrations of common coding dilemmas and approaches to their solution, guidelines for clinical management of various presenting problems and environmental situations, with accompanying handouts. Moreover, it would be useful to include recommendations for specific structured parent interviews and screening instruments to elicit information from parents and children concerning behavioral and developmental problems. One example of a relevant teaching tool is the use of videotapes of parent interviews that illustrate common presenting problems. Practitioners can view these videotapes and use the *DSM-PC* to code the behavioral problems and environmental stressors that they have seen in the interview (Stancin & Drotar, 1998). Another example is the parent interviews that have been developed to implement the CHADIS application of the *DSM-PC*.

Promoting Reimbursement for Using the *DSM-PC*

As noted in the present survey data, the level of reimbursement that pediatricians receive for their work in managing the behavioral and developmental problems that can be coded by the *DSM-PC* is a primary barrier to its use. The level of reimbursement to PCPs for services provided to manage behavioral problems is an important public problem that transcends application of the *DSM-PC* (Rappo, 1997). Nevertheless, an important strategy to promote reimbursement for PCPs' use of the *DSM-PC* will be to educate third party payers concerning the availability of the *DSM-PC* and its potential to facilitate accurate documentation of (1) the following current clinical practice concerning the management of behavioral and developmental problems, and (2) more informed clinical management of such problems, including clearer criteria for referral of behavioral problems to mental health professionals (Rappo, 1997). To best educate insurers, PCPs will need to carefully document their use of the *DSM-PC* as well as the relevant advantages for making decisions about managing children's mental health problems. As more and more PCPs use the *DSM-PC* and develop a track record of use in various practices, more convincing data can eventually be provided to insurance companies. Moreover, case examples and data about how the *DSM-PC* can enhance the efficiency of referrals for children with mental health problems from PCPs and ultimately reduce the costs of mental health care by encouraging earlier, more informed referral, is an important, albeit formidable, future task.

Interdisciplinary Use of The *DSM-PC*

While our report has focused primarily on the use of the *DSM-PC* by PCPs, the *DSM-PC* has potential utility for other professions, especially psychologists who consult with pediatricians who see children and families in primary care settings (Drotar, 1999). For example, our experiences have indicated that the *DSM-PC* can be a very useful tool to train psychologists and mental health professionals who work in pediatric settings to understand the full range of clinical problems and environmental stressors they see in children when providing consultation to PCPs (Drotar, 1995). Because the *DSM-PC* emphasizes the concept of a developmental continuum of behavioral problems, it is also quite compatible with teaching undergraduate and graduate students concepts of child development and developmental psychopathology (Sroufe & Rutter, 1984) and has been used in this way by some faculty.

Using the *DSM-PC* to Target and Monitor Interdisciplinary Community-based Preventive Intervention for Children at Risk

One of the most interesting and important future applications of the *DSM-PC* from a public health standpoint concerns its potential to be used to target and monitor interdisciplinary, community-based preventive intervention for children at risk. Because the *DSM-PC* uses nontechnical language and is not based on profession-specific diagnostic classifications as is the *DSM-IV*, it has the potential to be used by a broad range of professional service providers to organize and target interventions for children at risk of emotional disturbance or who are showing early signs of emotional disturbance.

The *DSM-PC* also provides a method for those who are providing services at the community level to children at risk to categorize the types of environmental situations or stressors that might be expected to affect treatment planning and the child's prognosis as well as be a focus of clinical attention. For example, some children may be given early intervention services to respond to clinically relevant threats to their psychological development that relate to specific environmental stressors (e.g., domestic violence, or problems in caregiving) that can be readily categorized using the *DSM-PC*.

Research Concerning the *DSM-PC*

One of the most important future needs concerns research on various applications of the *DSM-PC* (Drotar, 1999). For example, one of the most important areas for future research concerning the *DSM-PC* is to establish interrater reliability for the key diagnostic distinctions among developmental variations, problems, and disorders. Another research priority is to test the hypothesis, which is a central working assumption of the *DSM-PC*, that training pediatricians to use the *DSM-PC* in primary care will actually result in increased recognition of behavioral and developmental problems.

Because the *DSM-PC* can classify the range of problems that present in primary care, it provides a tool to conduct collaborative descriptive research concerning the incidence and prevalence of problems seen by PCPs and psychologists in primary care as well as in community settings. Data concerning incidence, prevalence, and course of behavioral and developmental problems in young children are very limited, with some exceptions (Lavigne et al., 1993). The *DSM-PC* can also be used to describe the incidence and prevalence of stressful situations to which children are exposed. The *DSM-PC* also can be used to document the patterns of stability versus change in common behavioral and developmental problems and to describe how such problems respond to intervention by PCPs and/or referral to mental health practitioners. Finally, the *DSM-PC* is an ideal instrument with which to document the incidence, prevalence, and management of the large numbers of children who present with behavioral problems that are at the subthreshold level for a diagnosis according to the *DSM-IV* but nonetheless reflect substantial functional impairment (Angold, Costello, Farmer, Burns & Erkanli, 1999). The needs of these children for diagnosis and management by PCPs and mental health professionals represent an important public health problem that has largely been unrecognized (Steinberg, Gadowski, & Wilson, 1999).

ACKNOWLEDGEMENT

The assistance of Susan Wood in processing this manuscript is gratefully acknowledged.

Author's note:

Correspondence may be addressed to the first author at:
The Department of Pediatrics
Rainbow Babies and Children's Hospital
11100 Euclid Avenue
Cleveland, Ohio 44106-6038

REFERENCES

American Psychiatric Association. (1994). *Diagnostic and statistical manual of mental disorders* (4th ed.). Washington, DC: American Psychiatric Press.

Angold, A., Costello, E. J., Farmer, E., Burns, B. J., & Erkanli, A. (1999). Impaired but undiagnosed. *Journal of American Academy of Child and Adolescent Psychiatry, 38*, 129-137.

Costello, E. J. (1986). Primary care pediatrics and child psychopathology: A review of diagnostic, treatment, and referral practices. *Pediatrics, 78*, 1044-1051.

Costello, E. J., Edelbrock, C., Costello, A. J., Dulcan, M. K., Burns, B. J., & Brent, D. (1988). Psychopathology in pediatric primary care: The new hidden morbidity. *Pediatrics, 82*, 415-424.

Coury, D. L., Berger, S. P., Stancin, T., & Tanner, J. L. (1999). Curricular guidelines for residency training in developmental-behavioral pediatrics. *Journal of Developmental and Behavioral Pediatrics Supplement*, 51-54.

Drotar, D. (1995). *Consulting with pediatricians: Psychological perspectives*. New York: Plenum Press.

Drotar, D. (1999). The *Diagnostic and Statistical Manual for Primary Care (DSM-PC) Child and Adolescent Version*: What pediatric psychologists need to know. *Journal of Pediatric Psychology, 24*, 369-380.

Glascoe, F. P. (1999). Using parents concerns to detect and address developmental and behavioral problems. *Journal of the Society of Pediatric Nurses, 4*, 24-35.

Horwitz, S. M., Leaf, P. J., Leventhal, J. M., Forsythe, B., & Speechley, K. N. (1992). Identification and management of psychosocial and developmental problems in community-based, primary care pediatric practices. *Pediatrics, 89*, 480-485.

Jellinek, M., Little, M., Murby, J. M., & Pagano, M. (1995). The pediatric symptom checklist supports a role in a managed care environment. *Archives of Pediatric and Adolescent Medicine, 149*, 740-746.

Kelleher, K. J., McInerny, J. K., Gardner, W. P., Childs, G. E., & Wasserman, R.C. (2000). Increasing identification of psychosocial problems. *Pediatrics, 105*, 1313-1321.

Kelleher, K., & Rickert, V. I. (1994). Management of pediatric mental disorders in primary care. In J. Miranda, A. A. Hohmann, C. C. Attkinson, & D. B. Larson (Eds.), *Mental disorders in primary care* (pp. 320-346). San Francisco: Jossey Bass.

Kemper, K. J., & Kelleher, K. J. (1996). Family psychosocial screening: Instruments and techniques. *Ambulatory Child Health, 1*, 325-339.

Lavigne, J. V., Binns, J. H., Christoffel, K. K., Rosenbaum, D. L., Arendt, R., Smith, K., Hayford, J. R., & McGuire, P. A. (1993). Behavioral and emotional problems among preschool children in pediatric primary care: Prevalence and pediatricians' recognition. *Pediatrics, 91*, 649-655.

Marino, R. V. (1997). *DSM-PC*: Experiences in primary care practice and resident education. *Journal of Developmental Behavioral Pediatrics, 18*, 174-175.

McGuinn, L., Sturner, R. A., Howard, B. J. & Duggan, A. (2001, March). *Can opportunistic observation be made valid by standardizing the infant physical exam and it's observation?* Presented at Maternal and Child Health Bureau Developmental-Behavioral Pediatrics Fellowship Meeting, Baltimore, MD.

Rappo, P. D. (1997). Use of *DSM-PC* and implications for reimbursement. *Journal of Developmental and Behavioral Pediatrics, 18*, 175-177.

Sroufe, L. A., & Rutter, M. C. (1984). The domain of developmental psychopathology. *Child Development, 55*, 17-29.

Stancin, T., & Drotar, D. (1998, May). *Using the DSM-PC: What pediatric psychologists need to know.* Workshop presented at the Great Lake Regional Conference on Child Health Psychology, Louisville, KY.

Stancin, T., & Palermo, T. M. (1997). A review of behavioral screening practices in pediatric settings: Do they pass the test? *Journal of Developmental and Behavioral Pediatrics, 18*, 183-194.

Steinberg, A. G., Gadomski, A., & Wilson, M. D. (1999). *Children's mental health: The changing interface between primary and specialty care*. Philadelphia: Report of the Children's Mental Health Alliance Project.

Sturner, R. A., Funk, S. G., & Green, J. A. (1994). Simultaneous technique for acuity and readiness testing (START): Further concurrent validation of an aid for developmental surveillance. *Pediatrics, 20*, 82-88.

Sturner, R. A., & Howard, B. J. (Eds.). (2000). *The child health and development system.* Millersville, MD: The Center for Promotion of Child Development through Primary Care.

Sturner, R. A., Layton, T. L., Feezor, M. D., Craft, M. B., & Lewis, H. D. (1998). *The communication screening system: Further validation of the speech and language components*. New Orleans, LA: Ambulatory Pediatrics Association.

Wolraich, M. L. (1997). *Diagnostic and Statistical Manual for Primary Care (DSM-PC) Child and Adolescent Version*: Design, intent, and hopes for the future. *Journal of Developmental and Behavioral Pediatrics, 18*, 171-172.

Wolraich, M. L., Felice, M. E., & Drotar, D. (Eds.) (1996). *The classification of child and adolescent mental diagnosis in primary care: Diagnosis and statistical manual for primary care (DSM-PC) child and adolescent version.* Elk Grove, IL: American Academy of Pediatrics.

Zero to Three/National Center for Infant Programs. (1994). *Diagnostic classification: 0-3. Diagnostic classification of mental health and developmental disorders of infancy and early childhood.* Arlington, VA.

DISCUSSION SUMMARY
written by Meghan Barlow

The discussion following Dr. Drotar's talk focused primarily on the utility of the *DSM-PC* for helping in the identification and appropriate treatment of children seen in primary care. More specifically, comments revolved around why the *DSM-PC*, which the participants described very positively and as user-friendly in primary care, is used so infrequently and how it might come to be used more regularly by physicians.

One area that much of the discussion touched on was how the *DSM-PC* could be used (or would potentially be used) in conjunction with current reimbursement systems. The participants were generally concerned that use of the *DSM-PC* would not result in reimbursement for primary care physicians for the time that they would invest in assessing and managing psychosocial problems in their pediatric patients. One of the psychologists noted that general providers may not be motivated to use the *DSM-PC* because it does not translate into reimbursement for them. That is, even though the *DSM-PC* may help primary care physicians assess and diagnose psychosocial problems in children, it has not been integrated into the reimbursement system. Many third party payers do not reimburse primary care physicians for treating psychiatric diagnoses. A foreseeable problem that one physician raised was that insurance companies might ask the question: given the present level of severity and this diagnosis, who would be the *cheapest* professional to treat this child as opposed to who would be the *best* professional to treat this child?

In spite of concerns about the potential financial barriers to widespread use of the *DSM-PC*, participants were enthusiastic with the clinical utility of the *DSM-PC*. One physician emphasized the point that the *DSM-PC* can help physicians focus their assessment of psychosocial problems based on a definition of the problem, rather than on a diagnostic category. That is, in contrast to the *DSM-IV*, the *DSM-PC* would allow primary care physicians to focus on the components of the problem presented, as well as on environmental factors that might affect the problem, rather than focusing solely on diagnostic criteria. Additionally, with environmental stressors and a severity rating, physicians could more readily determine the appropriate course of treatment for their patients. An additional benefit to using the *DSM-PC* discussed by participants was that it provides a common language for practitioners to speak in.

A question of how use of the *DSM-PC* could be encouraged included a suggestion of publishing the *DSM-PC* with the next edition of the DSM. Dr. Drotar stated that this would be a good idea, but that it is unlikely that that would happen.

Some suggestions for funding future research and implementation of using the *DSM-PC* were discussed. One suggestion was to view use of the *DSM-PC* and its potential for targeting the "hidden morbidity" of children with mental health problems who remain undiagnosed and untreated as a public health issue and seek public health funds. Another suggestion was to identify the program as prevention of mental health problems since use of the *DSM-PC* and attention to psychosocial problems in children by primary care physicians would likely identify children at earlier ages and before problems became severe, which would thereby allow investigators and clinicians to pool money from state to state for the implementation of the program. A psychologist pointed out that the *Journal of Child Services* recently published a review of early interventions with parents. He stated that if we know a model is an effective intervention, we are likely to receive funding for implementing the interventions.

The consensus of the group was that the *DSM-PC* was potentially very useful for identifying and managing psychosocial problems in primary care, but that in order for its potential to be realized, reimbursement of services rendered by primary care physicians must be linked to its use. Ideas for linking the *DSM-PC* into existing funding programs and research to help make the case for its utility were discussed.

CHAPTER 10

PATHWAYS TO THERAPY

Medical, Social, and Cultural Determinants of and Barriers to Health Care

Robert J. Johnson
Kent State University

This chapter will discuss medical and social factors that influence access to health care. I will explore characteristics of the physician-patient relationship and medical decision making that influence whether or how parents and physicians recognize the presence of psychosocial problems, and the barriers they face in meeting the need for care. I will also explore the social and cultural models outside of clinical practice and their implications for differential effects on the access to care. Key concepts will include social inequality, social control, risks, cultural values, attitudes toward the efficacy of care, and stigma associated with illness.

This chapter is intended to be a conceptual introduction to the approaches taken by researchers who are attempting to explain who is more or less likely to receive health care. This introduction is intended to be abstract and illustrative of the many approaches to such research in order to reveal the underlying assumptions of the empirical studies. The examples are not meant to be exhaustive or even representative of the research, as some approaches are in greater favor than others. And much

Treating Children's Psychosocial Problems in Primary Care, 225–251

of that research is already more complex than the model components presented here. However, in most of the empirical research on the topic, whether simple or complex, the reader will learn to recognize elements or combinations of the model components presented. By recognizing the common elements, it is hoped, a better understanding of the existing research will result and eventually evolve into more complex combinations in the future. The final model will be one example of a more complex model that can be developed.

This chapter is intended to be a primer in an elaboration strategy for those who previously have not examined these issues from a social problems perspective. As noted above, other research perspectives (including criminal, epidemiological, clinical, etc.) are used and can be appropriate for the study of these problems. However, sometimes these approaches may benefit from a social problems perspective. Often times the research questions may be focused such that only select portions of the most complex social problem models are relevant. Second, others have already recognized the value of expanding "the range of questions that guide treatment research" (Kazdin, 2000) even though "child and adolescent therapy has progressed considerably as reflected in the sheer number of controlled studies, their methodological quality, and identification of empirically supported treatments."

In an effort to expand the range of questions, I will present three different classes of models and discuss the impact that their theoretical constructs have on health care, in general. As often as possible, I will also identify where and when these models can be used in child and adolescent therapy, although often or by necessity examples will be taken from other areas of health and health care as well. First, the chapter will discuss the medical model(s) and the relationship between types of symptoms and types of care. Next, the chapter will address social demographics and social networks of referral based on the social model(s), including basic questions of access to care, inequality, and alternatives to care.

This chapter also will be quite different from most of the others in this volume because it presents the issues using a social problems perspective. "Social problems" is a broad term that covers a great many topics (e.g., drug abuse, prostitution, AIDS risk behaviors, delinquency, mental illness, race relations, etc.), and most of these can also be viewed from an "individual troubles" perspective. When something is seen as an individual trouble, the responses include identifying the source of that person's troubles and proposing a suitable solution that is designed to get that person out of trouble. In essence, the question is "What's wrong with this person and how can we help?" When viewed from a social problems perspective, the responses include determining how many people have that problem, who are they likely to be, what are the possible sources of the problem, maybe questioning why it is even a problem, and finally identifying the ranges of responses and likelihood of particular responses to it. The question of how to help any particular individual may never be asked, although help in some general form is often addressed. Solutions may be identified that simply change the definition of the problem. Of course the ultimate goal of both perspectives is to limit the extent of the social problems and the number and severity of individual troubles in any society. It is also true that a combination of both approaches can be taken, and this actually may be more common in practice, because neither one excludes the possibility of the other. In the next section, I will begin with the traditional medical model that often focuses on the diagnosis and treatment of individual problems.

THE MEDICAL MODEL

The medical model of health care use is perhaps the most widely accepted and often tested model of the pathways to therapy. In its most simplistic form, the medical model posits a causal relationship between illness and care. Once a person becomes ill, they seek care from others. This model can be applied to any form of illness, any type of health care, and at any time in history. And although they may be more or less complex in terms of the number of variables they employ, the essential characteristics of the medical model, as expressed in Figure 10.1, are that illness exists and when it does, care is provided for it.

Though not without legitimate criticism (Gold, 1977; Oleson, 1975; Pescosolido & Kronenfeld 1995), the medical model of health care use is appealing for a number of reasons. As the critics themselves point out, one of the appealing aspects of a medical model approach is that the key elements are already socially constructed realities. Thus social scientists who adopt the medical model often start with clinical definitions of illness symptoms and clinical diagnoses of those illness symptoms, and the assumption that the former leads to the latter in the process of seeking

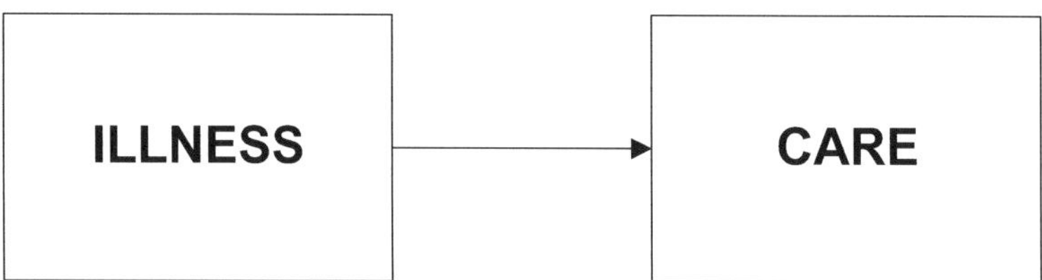

Figure 10.1. The medical model

care. A discussion recently occurred even over the name of the major section in sociology that deals with health issues. The section is called Medical Sociology, and some reflected on the possibility that the name itself showed a bias toward validating the medical model. Pescosolido and Kronenfeld (1995) further explain how the debate over the name of and the reluctance to change it is itself an example of the influence of the medical model on social science and the social scientists themselves.

Another appeal of the medical model approach is that health status, no matter how it is measured or defined, has consistently been shown to be the best predictor of the use of health services (Hulka & Wheat, 1985; Wan, 1989; Wolinsky & Arnold, 1985). As the social science models of health status became more sophisticated and the measurement characteristics of indicators of illness became more reliable, the importance of social factors in these models seemed to decline in influence (Pescosolido & Kronenfeld 1995). Thus, even if one wished to avoid the perception or problems of bias caused by using models that reflected the dominant medical establishment, the bias of leaving out health status surely would be worse. The first step in assessing pathways to health care inevitably continues to involve some assessment of signs, symptoms, or other measures of health status.

A shortfall to this approach is the increasing fear that by focusing on the medical model, social scientists will continue to be dominated by the medical ideologies, and become too complacent with "off the shelf" regression models and the same familiar litany of variables. Notwithstanding the potential bias that may result from ignoring clinical symptoms and diagnoses, or the "tried and true" successes of the medical model in its more sophisticated formulations, some critics seek to challenge or expand the medical model. These changes will be presented when the social and cultural models are presented, and the most serious challenges will be seen to come from the cultural models.

Any investigation of the pathways to therapy using the medical model will inevitably focus on the nature and characteristics of the illness, its diagnosis, and specification of the appropriate therapeutic intervention and regimen. The assumptions for the model to work are that the process involves rational choice, objective signs and symptoms, exhaustive clinical knowledge, competent care, and efficacious treatments. A further assumption is that the illness, its diagnosis, and care are provided in the same setting. The models presented below can apply to different settings: therapy for physical as well as mental illness, for biomedical as well as psychosocial diagnoses, and for medical care as well as mental health therapy. One application of the model will be presented later when I consider the relationship between medical and mental health professionals, where the relationship between diagnosis and care does not occur in the same setting. In this instance, diagnosis is made in a medical setting and referral is made for care in a mental health setting.

In the medical model the pathways to therapy are assumed to be open. As a person begins to suffer the signs and symptoms of illness, they seek competent care and are provided effective therapy. The model is obviously an ideal typology of therapy, but it appeals to clinicians and patients alike. There is also plenty of personal experience bolstered by clinical and scientific evidence that the therapeutic experience works this way, at least more often than not.

Problems with the medical model, it is often believed by its adherents, can be addressed by further focus on and refinement of the concepts of illness and care themselves, or alternatively, the variable degree to which the assumptions of the model can be realized.

The Nature and Characteristics of Illness

For example, lets take a look first at the "illness" dimension of the medical model. Recognizing illness correctly is the first and major aim of the medical model. Much of the history and progress in the treatment of illness derives from the development of an accurate nosology of illness and the objective specification of signs and symptoms that allow accurate diagnoses of specific cases. As a result, the dimensions of illness expand, as depicted in Figure 10.2. With respect to mental disorders, the most influential of these efforts has resulted in clinical guides for mental health professionals, clinical screening protocols for general practitioners and other health professionals (Cappelli et al., 1995), or epidemiological scales for survey research professionals.

The number of illnesses can change over time, in part because new illnesses arise while others are cured. Sometimes, though, discoveries and expanding knowledge simply changes the landscape of the field of nosology. A cursory comparison of the *Diagnostic and Statistical Manual of Mental Disorders*, first edition (*DSM-I*) to the fourth edition (*DSM-IV*) will readily

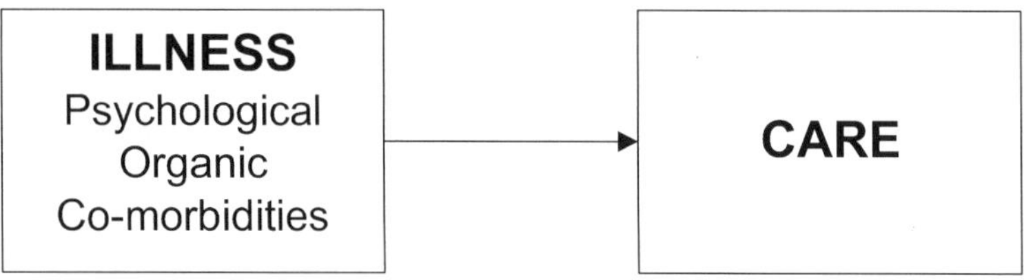

Figure 10.2. The medical model: A focus on the nature and characteristics of illness

demonstrate this phenomenon. In other cases, the number of people to whom the illness label is applied expands. Expanding the definitions of illnesses, as in the case of the emerging new morbidities in pediatric care settings during the past 20 years, or expanding the number of persons to whom they are applied, such as the recent surge in diagnoses of social anxiety disorders, the trend seems to be toward increasing the number of illnesses. This trend is due, in part, to better specifications of the medical model. It is also due, in part, to the process of medicalization as discussed later in the chapter.

The Nature and Characteristics of Care

Recognizing the possibility that different illnesses might require different treatments provides a good opportunity to look second at the "care" dimension of the medical model. The dimensions of care expand, as depicted in Figure 10.3. Psychotherapy, psychopharmacology, institutionalization, surgery and the entire litany of therapeutic approaches to the treatment of illness all derive from the medical model. Some profess the effectiveness of their approach over all or most others for all or most cases of illness, while other therapies are more modest in their claims, such that they are the most effective only for specific types of illness. For an example in child and adolescent therapy, recent empirical reviews are intended to demonstrate how therapists can identify and standardize the treatments of choice, efficacious use of manuals, and matching therapies to illnesses (Hibbs et al., 1997; Kazdin & Kendall, 1998; Kazdin & Weisz, 1998). Perhaps the most interesting and salient from the point of view of what will follow are the reviews of psychosocial treatments for conduct disorder (Kazdin, 1997a) or combinations of treatments and the challenges they present for research and practice (Kazdin, 1996). All these efforts are aimed directly at understanding the relationship between illness and care as it appears in Figure 10.3, the basic medical model.

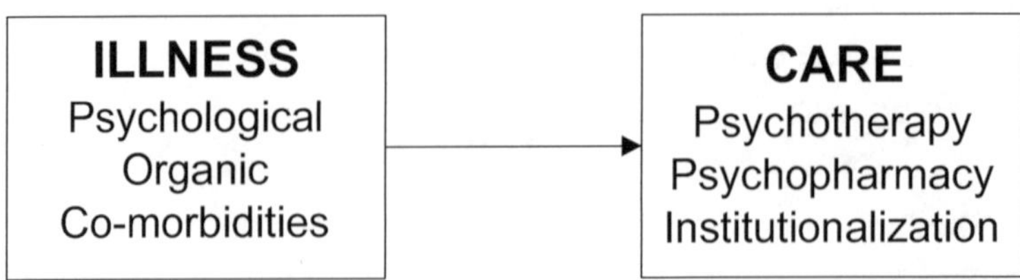

Figure 10.3. The medical model: A focus on the nature and characteristics of care

Efforts to extend the medical model can specify additional medical, social, or cultural constructs. The medical specifications retain the essential characteristics of the medical model. (Social and cultural elaborations will follow.) Questions may arise as to whether or how different illnesses show different relationships between symptoms and care. One such elaboration is to specify the assumptions that are made in the relationship between illness and care. To elaborate one such dimension, we will next examine how medical decision making intervenes in the process. In doing so, research may focus on the diagnosis itself.

Such research is gaining considerable attention. With a specific focus on child and adolescent mental health, concern about the appropriateness of the relationship between illness and care extended even to the arena of public policy and landed on the steps of the White House itself. According to the most recent Report of the Surgeon General's Conference on Children's Mental Health (2000), a new effort was launched to "improve the appropriate diagnosis and treatment of children with emotional and behavioral conditions." Public policy thus seeks to further specify the relationships in the medical model. It is this further specification, and the general form of the model, that I address next.

Diagnosis and Medical Decision Making

Particularly in the first two cases, the many professionals involved in providing care under the medical model are justifiably concerned with accurately identifying the illness. The fact that the medical model is already socially constructed for patients and clinicians alike means that many of the patients' contacts for psychosocial problems are with primary care providers, or in emergency rooms. The social context, educational background, and institutional setting all favor a medical orientation to the problem and its solution. However, often times these concerns are themselves a source of discomfort. Medical students have been noted to comment, "I must first rule out organic disease," or "Psychosocial issues have nothing to do with medical problems," or "If I deal with the psychosocial problems of all my patients, I will be overwhelmed" (Williamson, Beitman, & Katon, 1981). Similar concerns have even been noted among clinicians who are specializing in mental health problems when the diagnosis is particularly difficult. A psychiatric resident asked colleagues, when puzzled about whether there was also an underlying organic cause, "What do you think his diagnosis is? I've got to put some DSM thing down on paper" (Brown, 1987) (Figure 10.4).

Physicians' concern with properly identifying the illness is further enhanced by peers' evaluation of their performance, litigation, and an

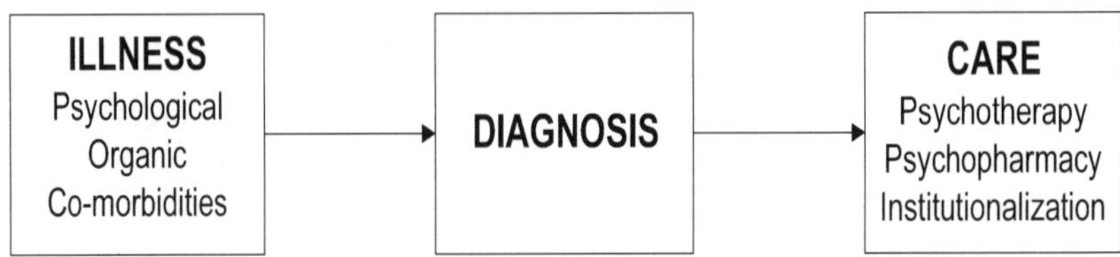

Figure 10.4. The medical model: Diagnoses and medical decision making

awareness of the real negative (sometimes devastating) consequences to the patient for making the wrong diagnosis. When physicians are able to focus on biomedical problems, especially when biomedical treatments are readily available, the rate of diagnosis for that problem increases. Further, the link between that diagnosis and treatment is enhanced. A recent example of this is the increasing diagnosis of social anxiety disorder and the increasing prescribing of a specific antidepressant drug marketed for the disorder (Talbot, 2001). However, it is not the entire explanation for the change, and relieving the stigma associated with the disorder has also been cited as part of the explanation.

In summary, it is clear that many assumptions underlying the medical model are justifiably open to closer scrutiny. Despite the continual need for ongoing scrutiny, though, the medical model is likely to remain secure in its dominant stature for the foreseeable future. And with respect to child and adolescent therapy in particular, Kazdin (2000) is certainly justified in noting the considerable progress that is being made in examining the relationships among these clinical phenomena. It is likely that considerably more progress will be made by in both medicine and child and adolescent therapy by those who are better informed than I on questions that deal precisely with these relationships. The next sections of the chapter, then, shift attention away from the medical model not because of any particular failures or shortcomings, but because there is a wider range of questions that can be asked when conducting research on the relationship between illness and therapy.

THE SOCIAL MODEL

The social model first makes problematic the relationship between illness and care in the medical model: the strength of the association, its sign (positive or negative), its causal order (direction), and whether the models are completely specified (if perhaps some important variables are missing). The problems of strengths of association exist because the observed relationships are never perfect; although illness is often the best predictor of care, and although its effects may be strong, it nonetheless often leaves much of the variation in care unexplained. Even when elaborations are made in the areas of medical decision making, or fitting models where types of illness are more closely aligned with types of care, the relationship is never perfect. The problem of causal direction exists because not only does illness cause care, but sometimes care causes further care, hopefully improved health, but also sometimes greater illness (nosocomial infections, clinical iatrogenesis). The problem of model specification, more precisely underspecification, is that not all the relevant variables are included in the model.

There are many variations on the medical model and each area in social science has one or two of its own favorites. In sociology the most widely tested variant is the behavioral model proposed by Andersen (1968), which places health need as the most proximate cause of health care use (essentially a medical model), but expands on that model by specifying predisposing and enabling characteristics. Adding more variables to the model is an elaboration that permits different interpretations of the illness-care relationship. Health psychology has developed its own models, as has health economics, health geography, and medical anthropology.

Health as Resource and Social Risks to Health

One solution is to continue the elaboration of the model in hopes of better specifying the relationships among the variables, while better measuring them as well. The first obvious elaboration to the model, from a social scientist's perspective, is the specification of the influences of social demographics on illness. Such a model postulates simply that some social groups are more likely to get sick than others. Why this happens is addressed from a variety of perspectives.

The direct effect on symptoms of social demographic variables has been interpreted most often in one of two ways: either from a social inequality perspective, or a social risk or vulnerability perspective.

Social Inequality

The social inequality perspective considers health a valuable resource like any other, and therefore socially disadvantaged groups have limited amounts of this resource, as they do others. The constellation of resource inequality (comprised of such characteristics as education, income, wealth, power) is often related directly to health and illness in these models. Social inequality in health can exist for some disadvantaged groups both because of the dearth of the other resources as well as independent of them. Models that have examined increased illness because of the lack of other resources elaborate on the relationship between social demographic variables and health by specifying these resources as mediating variables. Holding membership in one or more socially disadvantaged groups that increase levels of illness beyond the disadvantage in other resources may consider the effects of oppression and discrimination, biogenetic differences, health risk behaviors, or cultural differences.

Risk Perspective

The risk perspective may overlap with the social inequality perspective when the social disadvantages are believed to cause individuals to take risks (or to forego precautions) in order to overcome or adapt to those disadvantages. The two perspectives can also overlap when the social disadvantages are posited as stress provoking, either exposing individuals to life events or chronic strains that increase the risk of illness or injury. The two perspectives diverge when the social advantages increase the risk of an illness outcome. In such cases, the predictions are completely opposite for social inequality perspectives. However, the increased risks associated with statuses of privilege, which lead to illness and injury, are easily and correctly modeled from a risk perspective.

The social model also challenges the assumptions about the socially constructed medical phenomena, such as illness itself. Illness is problematic in two ways: measurement problems and construct problems. Measurement problems refer not only to reliability, but also to issues of sensitivity and specificity. For example, the strength of the association between illness and care may be weakened by unreliable measures of illness, or measures of illness that are not sufficiently sensitive (allowing too many false negatives), or not sufficiently specific (allowing too many false positives). These measurement phenomena can make medical decision-making, diagnoses, and clinical definitions of illness problematic as well. Attempts to improve measurement are often useful, through the use of reliable scaling and multiple indicators of illness.

Construct problems refer to whether behaviors and/or feelings represent symptoms of an underlying illness, or whether they are merely reflections of underlying differences in cultural values and normative expectations. If a set of feelings, beliefs, behaviors or physical characteristics become defined as illness, the logical consequence is to treat them. And while it is true that all illnesses are states that differ from health, not all differences are illness. When a difference becomes illness, it too becomes problematic in the social model.

While this problem seems similar to the problem of making accurate diagnoses faced in the application of the medical model, there is a fundamental difference. In the social model, the process of defining or legitimizing feelings, beliefs, behaviors, or physical characteristics as illness is known as medicalization. Medicalization occurs when five conditions are met (Conrad, 1976). First, feelings, beliefs, behaviors, or physical characteristics become identified as not merely individual problems but problems for society. Second, other forms of social control do not seem effective or appropriate for addressing the problem. Third, somehow the problem must be socially constructed as a medical problem. Fourth, the problem must be medically constructed as a medical problem. Fifth, the medical establishment must be willing to administer a treatment or therapy for the problem. When all five conditions are met, the professionals/institutions that provide these therapies and treatments take their place among the most influential social control agents/agencies in our society.

Health Care as Resource and Means of Social Control

The model in Figure 10.5 can be easily modified to further explore the role of social demographics in the social model. In Figure 10.6, a direct effect of social demographics on care is added to the model. Often researchers fail to interpret these effects, and simply discuss them in terms of control variables. What follows are interpretations that can be given to these effects.

The direct effect of social demographics on care, independent of symptoms of illness, has been interpreted both as a way to identify inequality in access to care and as evidence of the use of health care as a method of social control. In Figure 10.6, the direct arrow between social demographics and care can be positive or negative. A positive effect for socially advantaged groups (and a negative effect for disadvantaged ones) is taken as an indication of social inequality. A positive effect for socially disadvantaged groups (and a negative effect for advantaged groups) is taken as an indication that care is being used as a form of social control. Each is discussed separately below.

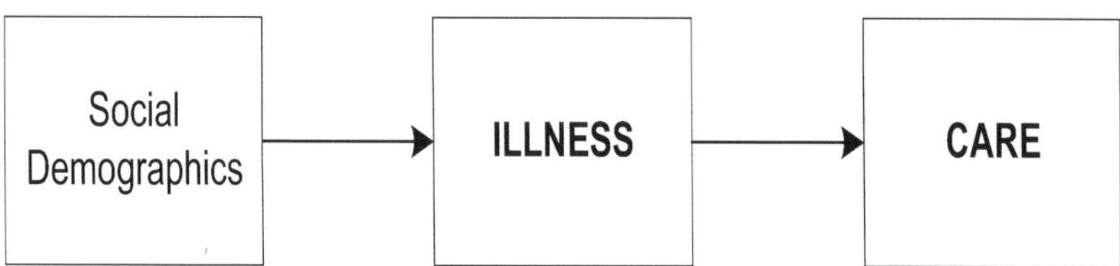

Figure 10.5. The social model: Risks and health inequities

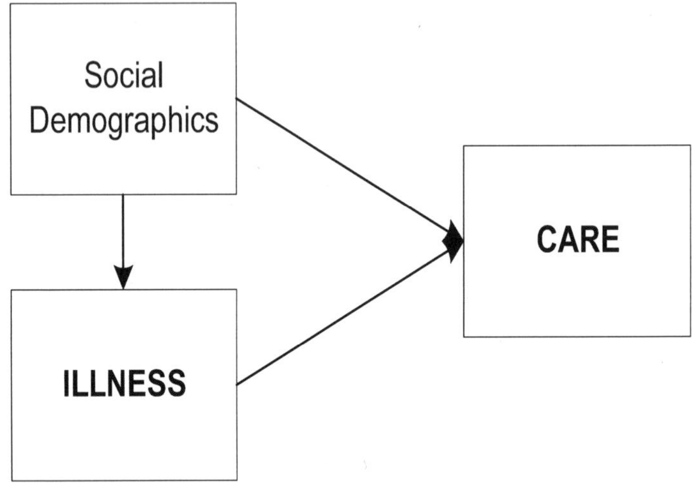

Figure 10.6. The social model: Social inequality and social control

Social Inequality

When the socially disadvantaged groups show lower rates of care, the first explanation is that they may have lower rates of illness. However, in the model above, assume those differentials in rates of illness have been adequately controlled. The net direct effect, then, is often viewed simply as another dimension of inequality. But in this case, health care is the socially valued resource (in addition to health itself) that is being denied to the socially disadvantaged group. Any group that has greater access to health care at any given level of illness obviously receives more of the resource than other groups. The size of the negative effect is the amount of care "taken away" from that group, putting them in a position of unmet need. As levels of illness increase, the differential access to care also means that the disadvantaged groups get less care than expected for reasons other than what the severity of their illness would demand. Another view is that the positive effect is the "excess use" of the resource made by the members of an advantaged group. And finally, the effect also may be viewed at the lowest level of illness as access (+) or barriers (–) to preventive care during periods that the individual is well.

The researcher should be cautious, however, when observing a net direct effect that may indicate social inequality in access to care. An unspecified variable associated with reduced risks for other unmeasured illnesses may be responsible for this effect. The likelihood of this occurring can be reduced when multiple dimensions of health status and multiple indicators of illness are used when testing these models.

Social Control

When socially disadvantaged groups show a higher likelihood of care than can be accounted for by the symptoms, researchers suspect that there is a social control function of the therapy. This is particularly true if the therapy is targeted toward a stigmatizing illness or public health threat. Members of socially advantaged groups may have many alternatives or resources they can utilize to help them avoid the stigmatizing labels of the illness and therapy, if none other than to use their time and resources to rule out false-positive diagnoses. However, members of socially disadvantaged groups may be vulnerable to the stigmatizing labels of the illness or its therapy. The stigma associated with the illness or therapy may in fact be interpreted as yet another risk to which members of socially disadvantaged groups are vulnerable.

As noted above, the researcher should be cautious, when observing a net positive direct effect that may indicate social control function of health care. In this case, an unspecified variable associated with increased risks for other unmeasured illnesses may be responsible for this effect. But again, the likelihood of this occurring can be reduced if multiple dimensions of health status and multiple indicators of illness are used when testing these models.

The Problem of Causal Order

When it comes to the relationship between social advantages and health, the question of causal order can always be raised. Are the wealthy healthy because they can afford care and avoid illness (see Figure 10.7), or are the ill poor because they cannot work and expensive health care saps their resources? The first question reverses the causal order between care and illness (from what was observed in Figures 10.5 and 10.6), and the second question reverses the causal order of both arrows between social demographics and illness from what appears below in Figure 10.8. While a "yes" answer to the second question certainly seems part of the explanation of the total relationship between illness and poverty, I will focus only

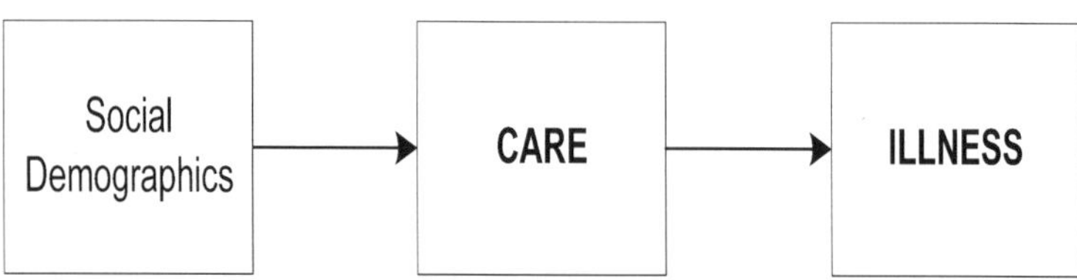

Figure 10.7. The social model: Social inequality and the problem of causal order

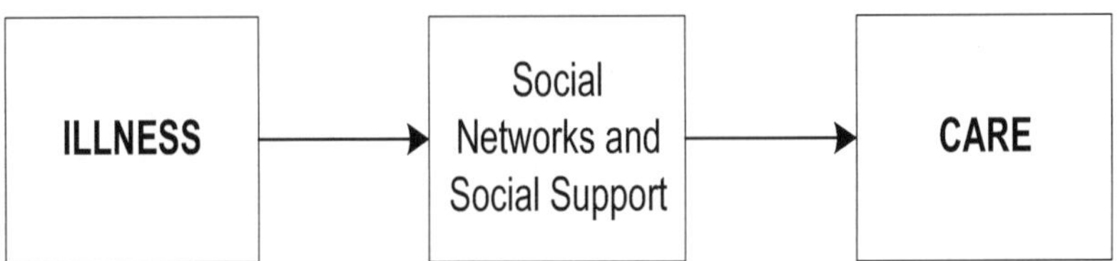

Figure 10.8. The social model: Mediating effects of social networks and social support

on the first question here. Doing so is sufficient to raise the problem of causal order. The first question is especially worth examining because it presents an opportunity to discuss another component of the overall model, because as some readers may have already recognized, Figure 10.7 may be readily interpretable as a preventive care model as well.

Mediating Effects of Social Networks and Social Support

The problem of imperfect relationships between illness and care may be addressed by specification of mediating or intervening variables. These variables can help explain why the observed relationship is smaller than expected. The mediating effects of social networks and social support are twofold. First, members of social networks share attitudes and beliefs about illness and the use of services. These attitudes may be directly sought out or they may be indirectly expressed through established normative structures. In either case, measuring the attitudes that erect barriers to care or facilitate seeking care can be an important elaboration to the medical model. The second way that social networks and social support can mediate the relationship is through direct interaction. Simply put, individuals who fall ill may seek help from informal sources of social support, or they may seek referrals from members of social networks. Seeking advice or help from peers before seeking care obviously mediates the relationship. Alternately, failure to seek advice or referrals leaves those who are ill unaware of available services that other members of their social network might know about.

Attitudes about illness and seeking help also may mediate the relationship. In populations where the relationship between illness and care is weak, it may be explained by attitudes that create barriers to health care. In populations where the relationship between illness and care is stronger, it may be explained by attitudes that support seeking care. These barriers to care and support for care were most clearly specified in the Health Belief Model (Becker, 1974; Rosenstock, 1966). In such models, illness is more distal to care than in the medical models. Individuals must decide for themselves or with help from others whether they are sick and whether they should seek care. Although the Health Belief Model has not seen wide popularity in recent years, the notion that attitudes facilitate or erect barriers to seeking health care is still evident. Recent studies (Esters, Cooker, & Ittenbach, 1998; Kuhl, Horlick, & Morrissey, 1997) continue to examine attitudes related to child and adolescent mental health.

The literature in child and adolescent mental health, with respect to the second mediating mechanism, indeed confirms that some individuals may be more likely to seek informal care or at least seek advice from peers first (Rew, Resnick, & Blum, 1997). Research has been conducted on the question of from whom and when such advice is sought, suggesting that in early adolescents, individuals rely on friends and mothers, while in later adolescence, they rely on parents (though mothers overall more so than fathers) and professionals (Schonert-Reichl & Muller, 1996). Lower levels of social support and help seeking also seem to go hand-in-hand, and social demographics can have an independent impact here as well (Barker & Adelman, 1994; Mata & Magana, 1995; Rickwood & Braithwaite, 1994). The likelihood of seeking help has also been linked to the status of person in the social network from whom help is sought or who is doing the referral, with fathers and mothers referring different problems to different professionals (Raviv, Weitzman, & Raviv, 1992). And finally, some subjects who suffer are simply unaware that services are available (Culp, Clyman, & Culp, 1995), as a result of failure to seek network help or failure of the network to provide it.

Mediating Effects of Forms of Social Inequality

Other forms of social inequality may mediate some of the influence of social demographic variables. Socially disadvantaged groups, for example, may be more likely to have unmet needs when it comes to all forms of health care due to the mediating effects of access to health insurance, type of health insurance or public policies that fail to provide for the health care needs of a population (Figure 10.9). Public opinion about and reaction to HMOs and managed care have recently caused major shifts in public policy, leading to the increased support for a patients bill of rights that could improve access to care and especially referrals to specialists for many people. These relationships need to be closely examined, because the type of insurance may increase overall access to care even while it restricts access to specific types of care. For example, managed care has resulted in greater access to basic behavioral health services for children

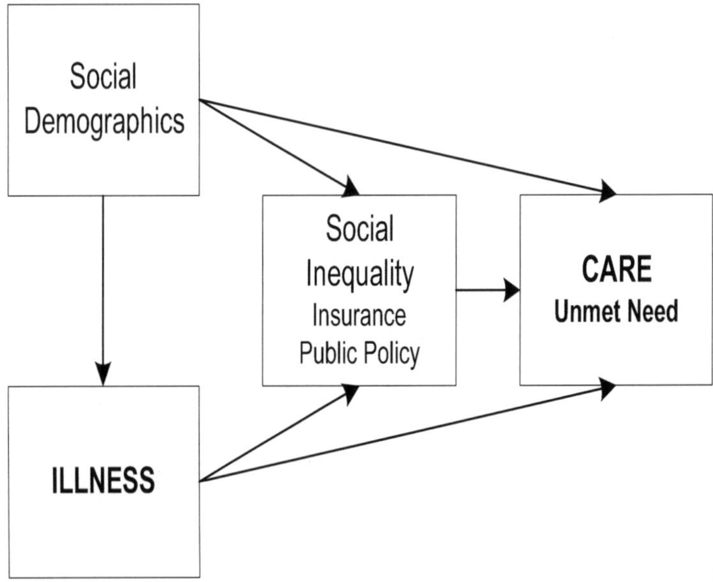

Figure 10.9. The social model: The mediating effects of inequality

and adolescents, though access to inpatient hospital care has been reduced (Stroul, Pires, Armstrong, & Meyers, 1998).

Alternatives to Care and Complementary Care

Seeking care for illness is not always restricted to medical or mental health professionals. As noted above, members of social networks may intervene and mediate the relationship, which also allows for the possibility of referral to alternatives outside the traditional sources of "medical" care. In the figure below, the mediating effect of social networks (as discussed in Figure 10.8 above) and the physician-patient relationship (Figure 10.10 and Figure 10.11) could be specified. They are left out here for clarity in focusing on the other pathways.

The care represents traditional care according to the medical model. The other social responses to or sanctions for illness could include seeking help from or interventions by faith based practitioners, herbalists, the juvenile justice system, school administrators and educators, youth groups, advocacy groups, or other community agencies. A positive relationship between care and other responses or sanctions represents complementary care. A negative relationship here would be an indication of

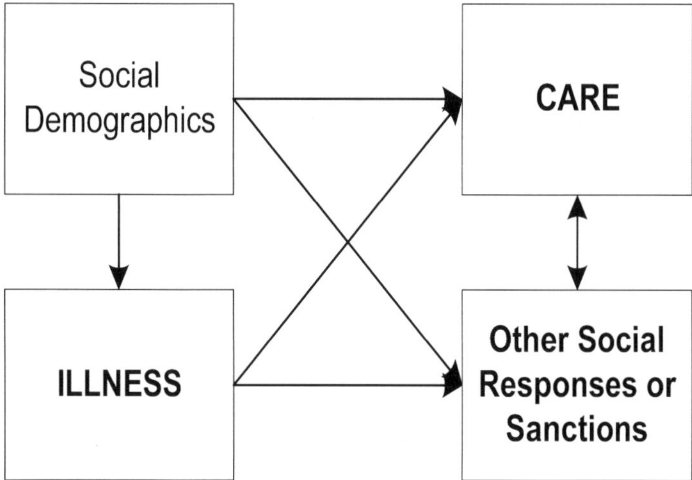

Figure 10.10. The social model: Alternatives to care and complementary care

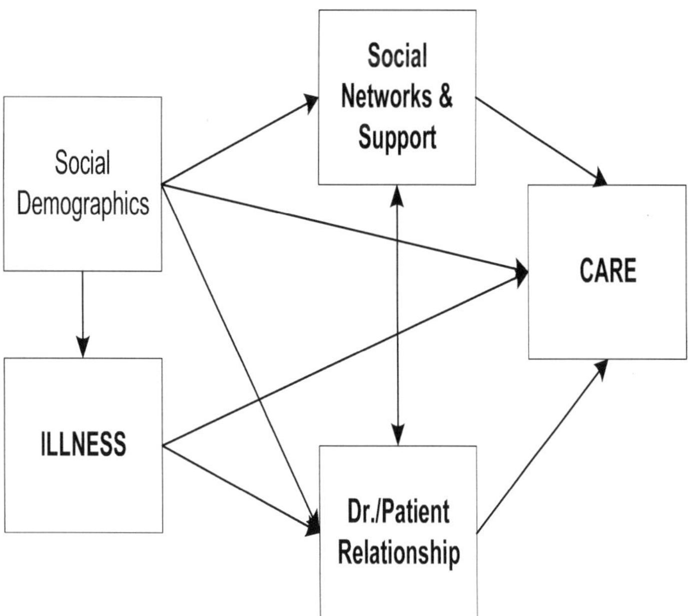

Figure 10.11. The social model: Doctor/patient relationships and other referral networks

alternative to traditional care. The influences of social demographics on illness and care can be interpreted as discussed above. The effects of social demographics on other responses or sanctions are more complex and would depend on the particular outcome. Generally, however, a positive effect for socially disadvantaged groups might be indicative of substitution of traditional care if the other responses or sanctions are alternatives rather than complements to it. A negative effect for socially disadvantaged groups might be interpretable as reduced access to resources, especially if the other responses are complementary to traditional care.

The Doctor/Patient Relationship and Lay Referrals to Care

The examination of the relationship between the physician and the patient is among the deepest roots in medical sociology, going back to the formulations of Parsons (1951).

Szasz and Hollander (1956) expanded the description of the range of relationships between the physician and the patient. Three types of interaction were described, based on the relationship. The first mode was active-passive, a relationship in which the patient relies on the physician. The second type is guidance-cooperation, in which the patient has increased involvement. The physician guides the patient based on information provided by the patient. Ultimately, the patient cooperates in the treatment regimens. The third type of relationship is characterized by mutual participation in which the patient and physician are equal participants. For this to work, both participants must have equal power.

Many other models of physician-patient relationships have been developed since the mid 1950s. They vary by whether the participants have shared beliefs, similar life situations, equal or unequal socioeconomic status, professional socialization of physicians and their beliefs about their own role, barriers to communication, or the effects of differences in sex (Bernstein & Kane, 1981; Campbell, Neikirk, & Hosokawa, 1990; West 1984; Williamson, Beitman, & Katon, 1981). It should not be surprising that male physicians might interact differently with female than male patients, nor that physicians might view lower class patients differently than patients with whom they share a common (upper middle or upper) social class. For these reasons, models are often proposed or advocated that diverge from the types of relationships described in the past. Today, the mutual participation, or "patient-centered," approach is being adopted by bioethicists, relationships in which the wishes of the patients are central to the decisions about care (Tsai, 2001). Whether or how successful such models are remains to be documented.

Another view has been offered in the examination of this relationship. The physician-patient relationship was usually viewed in the context of an adult seeking care from a physician. What happens, though, when the patient is a dependent adult or child? A caregiver is usually present in such circumstances, and the relationship between the physician and the patient likely is altered. Although little research has been done on these encounters, a recent study of both pediatrician and geriatricians indicated that by adding the caregiver, in effect changing the dyad to a triad in medical encounters, predictable changes occurred (Barone, 1999). The caregiver's presence led to a "loss of intimacy, decreased patient participation, and the formation of coalitions between physicians and caregivers." Ironically, forming alliances with the caregiver is a technique advocated by some in family-based therapy (Diamond, Diamond, & Liddle, 2000). And recent clinical techniques such as Parent Management Training (PMT) are the subject of recent investigations (Kazdin, 1997b).

In the model presented in Figure 10.11, a pathway is specified between the doctor/patient relationship and the type of care provided. In the context of patient referral for psychosocial, behavioral, or developmental problems, the nature of this relationship may very likely determine whether or not the physician makes a referral to mental health professionals. The relationship between the physician and patient is influenced by many factors and therefore should be measured in many ways: characteristics of the clinical setting, the practice structure, sociodemographic differences between patient and physician, and differences or similarities in education and training or knowledge about illness. The Internet also promises to intrude on the physician patient relationship as more and more patients will go online to secure information, some of questionable validity (Kassirer, 2000).

THE CULTURAL MODEL

The cultural model of illness and health care has at its roots the concern with (1) a fear of pain and illness (or that which causes it) that increases the likelihood of treatment, (2) stigmatization of illness that decreases the likelihood of treatment, and (3) judgments about the efficacy/cost/efficiency of medical decisions or therapies that influence the likelihood of treatment.

The first concern often is called cultural iatrogenesis. "Each culture gives shape to a unique *Gestalt* of health and to a unique conformation of attitudes toward pain, disease, impairment, and death, each of which designates a class of that human performance that has traditionally been called the art of suffering" (Illich, 1976). When any emotion, behavior, or physical characteristic becomes "insufferable," by whomever is defining it as such, the likelihood of seeking and being provided treatment or therapy increases. However, whenever that same emotion, behavior, or physical characteristic is defined as sufferable still longer (again by whomever is defining it as such), the likelihood of treatment or therapy declines. Illich (1976) spends much of his discussion of cultural iatrogenesis on understanding physical pain (though he includes others such as grief, anguish, fear, etc.), and the difference between cultures that find ways to tolerate such pain and those that spend a great deal of (medical) effort avoiding it or controlling it.

The relationship between illness and diagnosis, between diagnosis and care should both be expected to increase as a result of the recent Report of the Surgeon's General's Conference on Children's Mental Health (U.S. Department of Health and Human Services, 2000). If the increase occurs, it will be clear cultural iatrogenesis at the level of public policy. Consider one of the opening statement that states, "Growing numbers of children are suffering needlessly because their emotional, behavioral, and developmental needs are not being met by those very institutions which were explicitly created to take care of them." The report continues to call for prevention. However, if it is successful in convincing the public of the underdeveloped relationship between illness and eventual care, then cultural values and beliefs will bear on the actions of those involved in the diagnosis and treatment of these illnesses as well.

The "new morbidity" emerged more than 20 years ago in pediatric practices, and today the psychosocial dysfunction in children and adolescents are now the leading cause of disability in childhood and adolescence (Cassidy & Jellinek, 1998). Though stigma and fear still surround childhood and adolescent dysfunction, both the stigma of its psychosocial sources and the fear of it failing to respond to as a disease had to change for it to have attained that status. The work to maintain its status continues in the Surgeon's General's report. The relationship between fear and stigma are even more closely drawn in this report: stigma prevents treatment, and for that we should fear the individual and social consequences of untreated dysfunction.

A good current example of cultural iatrogenesis in clinical form can be found in the *DSM-IV* (American Psychiatric Association, 1994, pp. 537-538), where the diagnostic criteria for gender identity disorder include "persistent discomfort with his or her sex" and "clinically significant distress." Both insufferable conditions must be present in order for the diagnosis to be made. Thus, cross-gender identification is not illness unless and until it becomes insufferable (Figure 10.12).

The second concern is primarily social in its nature and initially social in its consequences. Stigma suppresses the recognition (by self and others)

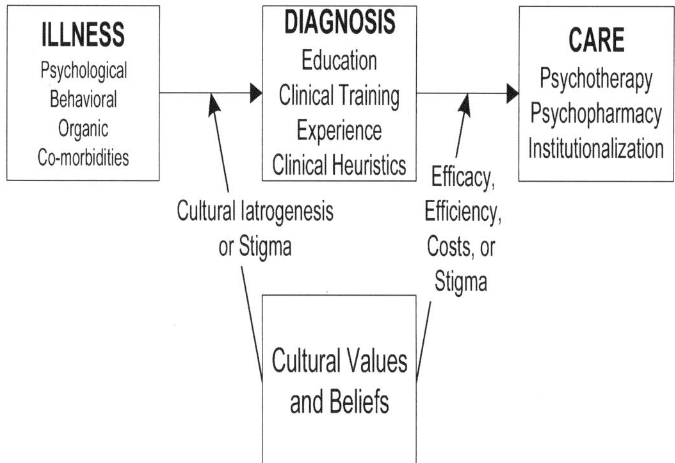

Figure 10.12. The cultural model: Moderating effects of values and beliefs

of emotions, behaviors, or physical characteristics as illness. Thus, on the one hand, any illness that is not stigmatized will easily cause self and others to react by recognizing the illness, and supporting the decision to seek care. On the other hand, any illness that is stigmatized will cause self and others to look for other (nonstigmatizing) explanations and to avoid seeking treatment in fear that the illness will become permanently labeled. With particular reference to child and adolescent mental health, the number one public policy goal today is to "reduce stigma associated with mental illness" (U.S. Department of Health and Human Services, 2000).

The recent Report of the Surgeon's General's Conference on Children's Mental Health (USDHHS, 2000) points to the impact of stigma at the public policy level. "Overriding all of this is the issue of stigma, which continues to surround mental illness." The report implies that the failure of the government to provide sufficient resources for effective prevention and treatment of mental illness is the direct outcome of stigma. Stigma dampens the empirically observed relationship between illness, diagnosis, and treatment. All of the foregoing results in unmet need. The unmet need alluded to in the report is the insufferable current state of these unmet emotional, behavioral, and developmental needs. In other words, this is cultural iatrogenesis.

The third concern stems from the self, members of the social networks of the self, and health care providers and institutions. When any emotion, behavior, or physical characteristic is defined or diagnosed as illness and further is believed to be effectively, easily, and inexpensively treated, the likelihood of treatment increases. Treatment is less likely to occur for illnesses that are believed to be costly, and for which there are believed to be ineffective and difficult treatment regimens.

Toward an Integrated Model of Pathways to Care

An integrated model of the pathways to therapy should combine elements of the medical, social and cultural models. The clinical variables of the medical models (or survey-based proxies for them) can be combined with the sociodemographic (often exogenous) and mediating (explanatory) variables of the social models and the mediating and moderating variables of the cultural models. The resulting bio-psycho-socio-cultural models are bound to be complex, and as such may seem out of reach of either the clinician or researcher. The researcher simply may lack access to clinical samples, and the clinician may see little utility and great costs in expanding the focus of research beyond the clinical setting. It is for this reason that this chapter has developed by examining only components of the overall model, rather than starting with the full model. Once a researcher or clinician identifies which component of the model in which they have an interest, then related components can be added one by one, each elaborating on the former. The important thing is not necessarily how complex the model becomes, or what particular components or forms it takes, but rather that some modeling of these processes begins.

One such elaborated model is presented in Figure 10.13. In the simplest of terms, the model postulates that individuals will vary in their experiences based on their social positions. These social positions influence a host of outcome variables through a series of mediating and moderating factors related to prevention, risks and resources, illness, clinical experiences and characteristics, family and social networks, and cultural attitudes.

The model is one of many possible combinations, but has several key features incorporated in it. Here, multiple indicators of illness, modeled as co-morbidities, can be estimated in the context of a model with multiple indicators of care, modeled as complementary treatment regimens. The alternatives to care are simultaneously modeled with multiple outcomes. Dimensions of social inequality, diagnosis, physician-patient relationships, and social networks/social support mediate the relationship between illness and care. Cultural values and beliefs moderate some of these relationships.

This integrated conceptual model is useful for several reasons: it integrates previously disparate research traditions, it proceeds from a combination of simpler models derived from those traditions, and it allows for

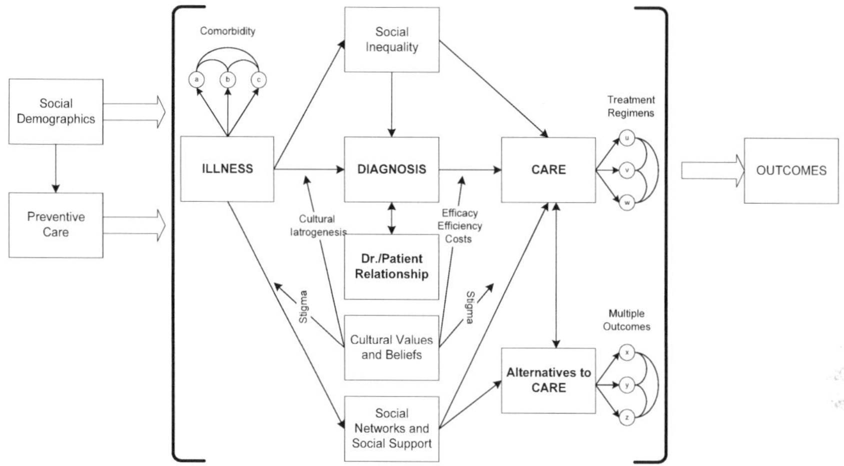

Figure 10.13. Toward an integrated model of pathways to care

testing both prevention (discussed elsewhere in this volume) and outcome processes (see Kazdin, 2000). The model contains both mediating (direct arrows between constructs linked by an intervening construct) and moderating processes (arrow from one construct affecting the relationship between two others). By first recognizing and then closely examining each of the simpler components of the model, the reader can overcome the feelings that complex models are not useful or are not intuitively easy to understand.

REFERENCES

American Psychiatiric Association. (1994). *Diagnostic and statistical manual for mental disorders* (4th ed.). Washington, DC: Author.

Andersen, R. (1968). *A behavioral model of families' use of health services.* Chicago: University of Chicago Press.

Barker, L. A., & Adelman, H. S. (1994). Mental health and help-seeking among ethnic minority adolescents. *Journal of Adolescence, 17*(3), 251-263.

Barone, A. D. (1999). How physicians view caregivers: Simmel in the examination room. *Sociological Perspectives, 42*(4), 673-690.

Becker, M. (1974). *The health belief model and personal health behavior.* San Francisco: Society for Public Health Education.

Berstein, B., & Kane, R. (1981). Physician attitudes towards female patients. *Medical Care, 19*(6), 600-608.

Brown, P. (1987). Diagnostic conflict and contradiction in psychiatry. *Journal of Health and Social Behavior, 28*(1), 37-50.

Campbell, J. D., Neikirk, H. J., & Hosokawa, M. C. (1990). Development of a psychosocial concern index from videotaped interviews of nurse practitioners and family physicians. *Journal of Family Practice 30*(3), 321-326.

Cappelli, M., Clulow, M. K., Goodman, J. T., Davidson, S. I., Feder, S. H., Baron, P., Manion, I. G., & McGrath, P. J. (1995). Identifying depressed and suicidal adolescents in a teen health clinic. *Journal of Adolescent Health, 16*(1), 64-70.

Cassidy, L. J,. & Jellnick, M. S. (1998). Approaches to recognition and management of childhood psychiatric disorders in pediatric primary care. *Pediatric Clinics of North America, 54*(5), 17.

Conrad, P. (1976). *Identifying Hyperactive Children.* Lexington, MA: Lexington Books.

Culp, A. M., Clyman, M. M., & Culp, R. E. (1995). Adolescent depressed mood, reports of suicide attempts, and asking for help. *Adolescence, 30*(120), 827-837.

Diamond, G. M., Diamond, G. S., & Liddle, H. A. (2000). The therapist-parent alliance in family-based therapy for adolescents. *Journal of Clinical Psychology, 56*(8), 1037-1050.

Esters, I. G., Cooker, P. G., & Ittenbach, R. F. (1998). Effects of unit of instruction in mental health on rural adolescents' conceptions of mental illness and attitudes about seeking help. *Adolescence, 33*(130), 469-476.

Gold, M. (1977). A crisis of identity: The case of medical sociology. *Journal of Health and Social Behavior, 8*(1), 16-28.

Hibbs, E. D., Clarke, G., Hechtman, L., Abikoff, H. B., Greenhill, L. L., & Jensen, P. S. (1997). Manual development for the treatment of child and adolescent disorders. *Psychopharmacology Bulletin, 33*(4), 619-629.

Hulka, B. S., & Wheat, J. R. (1985). Patterns of utilizations: The patient's perspective. *Medical Care, 23*, 438-60.

Illich, I. (1976). *The medical nemesis.* New York: Random House.

Kassirer, J. P. (2000). Patients, physicians and the internet. *Health Affairs, 19*(6), 115-123.

Kazdin, A. E. (1996). Combined and multimodal treatments in child and adolescent psychotherapy: Issues, challenges, and research directions. *Clinical Psychology-Science and Practice, 3*(1), 69-100.

Kazdin, A. E. (1997a). Practitioner review: Psychosocial treatments for conduct disorder in children. *Journal of Child Psychology and Psychiatry and Allied Disciplines, 38*(2), 161-178.

Kazdin, A. E. (1997b). Parent management training: Evidence, outcomes, and issues. *Journal of the American Academy of Child and Adolescent Psychiatry, 36*(10), 1349-1356.

Kazdin, A. E. (2000). Developing a research agenda for child and adolescent psychotherapy. *Archives of General Psychiatry, 57*(9), 829-835.

Kazdin, A. E., & Kendall, P. C. (1998). Current progress and future plans for developing effective treatments: Comments and perspectives. *Journal of Clinical Child Psychology, 27*(2), 217-226.

Kazdin, A. E., & Weisz, J. R. (1998). Identifying and developing empirically supported child and adolescent treatments. *Journal of Consulting and Clinical Psychology, 66*(1), 19-36.

Kuhl, J. J., Horlick, L., & Morrissey, R. F. (1997). Measuring barriers to help-seeking behavior in adolescents. *Journal of Youth and Adolescence, 26*(6), 637-650.

Mata, A. G., Jr., & Magana, R. (1995). Inhalant use, social support and help-seeking among rural south Texas community youth. *Free Inquiry in Creative Sociology, 23*(2), 67-76.

Oleson, V. (1975). Convergences and divergences: Anthropology and sociology in health care. *Social Science and Medicine, 9,* 421-25.

Parsons, T. (1951). *The social system.* New York. Free Press.

Pescosolido, B. A., & Kronenfeld, J. J. (1995). Health, illness and healing in an uncertain era: Challenges from and for medical sociology. *Journal of Health and Social Behavior, 3-33.*

Raviv, A. M., Weitzman, E., & Raviv, A. (1992). Parents of adolescents: Help seeking intentions as a function of help sources and parenting issues. *Journal of Adolescence, 15*(2), 115-135.

Rew, L., Resnick, M. D., & Blum, R. W. (1997). An exploration of help-seeking behaviors in female hispanic adolescents. *Family & Community Health, 20*(3), 1-15.

Rickwood, D.J., & Braithwaite, V. A. (1994). Social-psychological factors affecting help-seeking for emotional problems. *Social Science and Medicine, 39*(4), 563-572.

Rosenstock, I. (1966). Why people use health services. *Milbank Memorial Quarterly, 44,* 94-106.

Schonert-Reichl, K. A., & Muller, J. R. (1996). Correlates of help-seeking in adolescence. *Journal of Youth and Adolescence, 25*(6), 705-731.

Stroul, B. A., Pires, S. A., Armstrong, M. I., & Meyers, J. C. (1998). The impact of managed care on mental health services for children and their families. *Future of Children, 8*(2), 119-133.

Szasz, T., & Hollander, M. (1956). A contribution to the philosophy of medicine: The basic models of the doctor-patient relationship. *Journal of the American Medical Association 97,* 585-88.

Talbot, M. (2001, June 24). The shyness syndrome. *New York Times Magazine.*

Tsai, D. F. C. (2001). How should doctors approach patients? A Confucian reflection on personhood. *Journal of Medical Ethics, 27*(1), 44-50.

U.S. Department of Health and Human Services. (2000). *Report of the surgeon general's conference on children's mental health: A national action agenda.* Washington, DC: Author

Wan, T. H. (1989). Antecedents of health services use in the older population. In M. Ory & K. Bond (Eds.), *Aging and the use of formal care.* New York, Routledge.

West, C. (1984). *Routine complications: Troubles with talk between doctors and patients.* Bloomington. Indiana University Press.

Williamson, P., Beitman, B. D., & Katon, W. (1981). Beliefs that foster physician avoidance of psychosocial aspects of health care. *The Journal of Family Practice, 13,* 999-1003.

Wolinsky, F. D., & Arnold, M. (1988). A different on health and health services utilization. *Annual Review of Gerontology and Geriatrics, 8,* 71-101.

DISCUSSION SUMMARY
written by Christine Golden

Dr. Johnson provided the forum with an informative presentation of research models that can be used to understand the pathways to therapy. As a medical sociologist, Dr. Johnson offered forum participants the unique opportunity to examine the importance of placing the research concerning psychosocial problems in primary care within the context of society's influence.

Dr. Johnson used the social problems perspective to frame the research models he presented. He explained that using this perspective to establish research models is different than the individual troubles perspective often used in a clinical approach to research. The social problems perspective looks at issues beyond the individual. It asks how many others have the problem, what is the commonality among those that have the problem, what in society makes the problem, and what is society doing to address the problem? By broadening research designs to include these questions, Dr. Johnson suggested that we will be better able to understand the phenomenon of interest (i.e., the pathways to therapy).

Dr. Johnson began his review of the pathways to therapy by discussing the medical model for forum participants. As he stated in his chapter, "the medical model of health care is perhaps the most widely accepted and often tested model of the pathways to therapy." While familiar with the medical model, forum participants enjoyed listening to Dr. Johnson discuss both the simple and complex issues that can be addressed using it. As he pointed out, using the medical model to understand the pathways to therapy includes a focus on the nature and characteristics of illness, its diagnosis, and specification of the appropriate therapeutic intervention or regimen. In this model, illness leads to care. Therefore, recognizing illness correctly is the first and major aim of the medical model. Since different illnesses may require different treatments and the same illness may be cared for with multiple treatments, there are then multiple outcomes of care within this model. Forum participants were eager to discuss this "abstract concept of care" and continued over the remainder of the forum to delineate amongst themselves the various types of care that a child or adolescent might receive once identified with a psychosocial problem.

The social model was presented next. Dr. Johnson explained that the social model makes the causal relationship between illness and care in the medical model problematic. Different from the medical model, the social model considers the influences of social demographics on illness. It postulates that some social groups are more likely to get sick than others. Dr. Johnson explained that the direct effect social demographics have on symptoms in the social model could be understood according to both the social inequality perspective and the social risk or vulnerability perspective. Forum participants were eager to hear about each as Dr. Johnson shed light on the utility of using more elaborate models in our research designs. In the social inequality perspective, the socially disadvantaged have limited amounts of resources, including the resource of health. Although somewhat overlapping, in the risk perspective, the social disadvantages are believed to cause individuals to take risks in order to overcome or adapt to those disadvantages. Dr. Johnson expanded on these perspectives in his chapter as he discussed alternatives to care and complementary care, as well as the doctor-patient relationship and other referral networks.

Dr. Johnson also discussed the cultural model. In the cultural model, the impact of the fear of pain and illness that increases the likelihood of treatment, the stigmatization of illness that decreases the likelihood of treatment, and judgments about the efficacy, cost, and efficiency of medical decisions that influence the likelihood of treatment are the focus. By focusing on these issues, the moderating effects of values and beliefs on public policy and access to health care become keys topics for exploration. Both kept the Forum participants talking about how to reduce the stigma associated with mental illness.

Ultimately, Dr. Johnson advocated for an integrated model of pathways to care that would combine elements of the medical, social, and cultural models. He discussed how the clinical variables of the medical models could be combined with the socio-demographic and mediating variables of the social models and the mediating and moderating variables of the cultural model. While forum participants and Dr. Johnson agreed that the resulting bio-psycho-social-cultural models are complex, they also agreed on the importance of including some of these processes as modeling begins.

CHAPTER 11

A MODEL OF OBSTACLES TO IDENTIFICATION AND TREATMENT OF PEDIATRIC PSYCHOSOCIAL PROBLEMS

Beth G. Wildman
Kent State University

Terry Stancin
MetroHealth Medical Center & Case Western Reserve University

Epidemiological data indicate that between 15% and 20% of children have behavioral or emotional problems, yet only about 2% are seen by mental health professionals. The majority of these children with psychosocial problems are managed exclusively by their primary care physician (Costello et al., 1988; Earls, 1989). There are data which suggest that the children with psychosocial problems who remain untreated experience behavioral and emotional problems which are as serious as those who receive treatment (Shepherd, Oppenheim, & Mitchell, 1966). In addition, even if one assumes that some of the children identified in epidemiological research have subsyndromal problems, data indicate that subsyndromal problems persist over time and interfere with functioning at school,

Treating Children's Psychosocial Problems in Primary Care, 253–279

with peers, and at home (Costello & Shugart, 1992; Gotlib, Lewinsohn, & Seeley, 1995).

Concern about the underidentification and undertreatment of children with behavioral and emotional problems has received attention in the pediatric, family practice, and psychological literature, particularly over the last 15 years (Goldberg, Roghmann, McInerny, & Burke, 1984; Lynch, Wildman, & Smucker, 1997; Wildman, Kinsman, & Smucker, 2000). Healthy People 2000 and 2010 (Public Health Service, 1991, 2000) have specified improvements in the identification and treatment of children with mental health disorders as a national goal, and the White House and Surgeon General have both held conferences targeting this issue. Most professionals would agree that there is a lack of literature documenting effective interventions for these problems in primary care. However, suggestions and models for referral and collaboration between psychologists and primary care physicians have been in the literature since the 1960s and 1970s (Schroeder, 1996; Wilson, 1964). The most prominent and successful example of collaborative practice between psychologists and primary care physicians is Carolyn Schroeder's work in North Carolina, where she developed a successful collaborative relationship between psychologists and pediatricians in practice (see Chapter 1 in this volume). The Pediatric Symptom checklist was introduced in 1986 (Jellinek, Murphy, & Burns, 1986) as an effective way to screen children for psychosocial problems in outpatient pediatric settings. In spite of effective models for service delivery, effective screening procedures, and an increased focus on physician-patient communication as part of medical training, epidemiological data continue to reflect that most children with psychosocial problems are neither identified nor treated (Costello et al., 1988; Earls, 1989; Street, 1991; U.S. Department of Health and Human Services, 1999).

The present chapter attempts to integrate the data concerning attempts to improve the rate at which children with psychosocial problems are identified and treated with data concerning which children are identified. By integrating information about the children who are identified by physicians and the impact of different interventions to improve the rate with which physicians identify children with psychosocial problems, areas of success and failure can be examined and used to propose a model to guide future research addressing interventions to improve the rates with which children with psychosocial problems are identified and treated.

Psychosocial problems in children have been recognized as an important aspect of child health and both family practice and pediatrics journals have published editorials and articles articulating the commitment of their specialty to attending to these issues. Training in identification and treatment of psychosocial problems in children is part of residency training in both pediatrics and family medicine. The findings that relatively few children with psychosocial problems are identified and treated when effective screening methods and physician training programs exist suggests a need to turn attention toward identifying the reasons why psychosocial issues are not being addressed more frequently in primary care (Wildman, Yerkey, Golden, & Stancin, 2000).

The preponderance of research addressing the problem of lack of identification and treatment of children with psychosocial problems has focused on physicians' failure to identify many of the children with behavioral and emotional problems. This focus seemed, at first, to be an obvious solution to the problem of underidentification, and lent itself to traditional research paradigms that could be used to evaluate interventions and screening instruments. However, the literature suggests that the problem in identification is not due to physician apathy or insensitivity; rather, the problem is much more complex and is related to system factors, which include the health care system, physician, parent, and child factors (Wildman, Yerkey, et al., 2000).

One system obstacle to physicians attending to psychosocial issues in children that has been cited in the literature has been time. The average amount of time that physicians spend with their child patients is less than 15 minutes (MacPhee, 1984). However, a review of guidelines for well-child exams suggests that if physicians followed these guidelines, a health supervision visit would last an hour or more. Physicians must set priorities for their time during any patient encounter. Clearly, primary care physicians cannot assess all aspects of a child's health during the time allotted for visits, and mental health typically does not make it to the top of the priority list for health supervision visits. Sometimes, however, it does. One can excuse physicians for placing assessment and treatment of mental health issues below assessment of physical status, or one can acknowledge that, for most generally healthy children, psychosocial concerns are much more likely than are physical problems, and psychosocial problems are likely to interfere with the child's functioning. In addition, research suggests that a large percentage of parents admit to concern about their child's psychosocial functioning (Hickson, Altemeier, & O'Conner, 1983; Lynch et al., 1997). The focus of the proposed model is to delineate factors which influence whether or not mental health issues are attended to by primary care physicians during both acute and health supervision visits. These factors can be organized into different classes of influence: physician-based factors; parental factors; child factors; and system factors, such as type of medical insurance and access to mental health services.

Intuitively, most people would be likely to assume that factors such as presence of an actual psychosocial problem, physician training, and having health insurance which covers mental health treatment would predict which children were identified and received services. However, previous research has suggested that these factors are not sufficient to explain which children are identified and treated, and which are not (Lynch et al., 1997; Wildman, Kinsman, et al., 2000). In order for research to advise practice, the research concerning the identification and treatment of psychosocial problems in children must expand its focus from intervention studies and the development of user-friendly assessment instruments, such as the Pediatric Symptom Checklist and the *Diagnostic and Statistical Manual of Mental Disorders–Primary Care (DSM-PC)*, to identification of the factors that present obstacles to the primary care physician in placing identification and treatment of psychosocial problems high on their priority list during encounters with their child patients.

In order to impact the problem of poor rates of identification and treatment of children with psychosocial problems, understanding of the factors which influence physician identification and intervention for psychosocial problems is necessary. In addition, lack of empirical data concerning the efficacy of interventions impedes our ability to advise primary care physicians on how to intervene for these problems. Until now, research aimed at helping primary care physicians identify and treat psychosocial problems in children has been primarily focused on the identification of problems, not on their treatment. This research has most likely been predicated on the assumption that once identified, physicians would be able to intervene appropriately. However, there is a lack of clinical practice guidelines for the treatment of psychosocial problems in children seen in primary care.

Data on factors which predict physician identification of psychosocial problems in children suggest that disclosure by mothers to their child's physician of concerns about their child's psychosocial functioning is a good predictor of physician identification of these problems (Wildman, Kinsman, Logue, Dickey, & Smucker, 1997; Wildman, Yerkey, et al., 2000). However, the presence of child behavioral or emotional problems alone is not a good predictor of a mother's disclosure of concerns to her child's physician or physician identification of psychosocial problems in children. The lack of relationship between the presence of child psychosocial problems and both mothers' disclosure of concerns and physician identification of children with clinically significant psychosocial problems has been replicated with both a sample of pediatricians and a sample of family physicians.

The finding that the existence of child psychosocial problems is not a good predictor of physician identification, in conjunction with the general tendency for physicians to fail to utilize effective screening procedures for identification of psychosocial problems suggests the need to examine the obstacles to identification of psychosocial problems by pri-

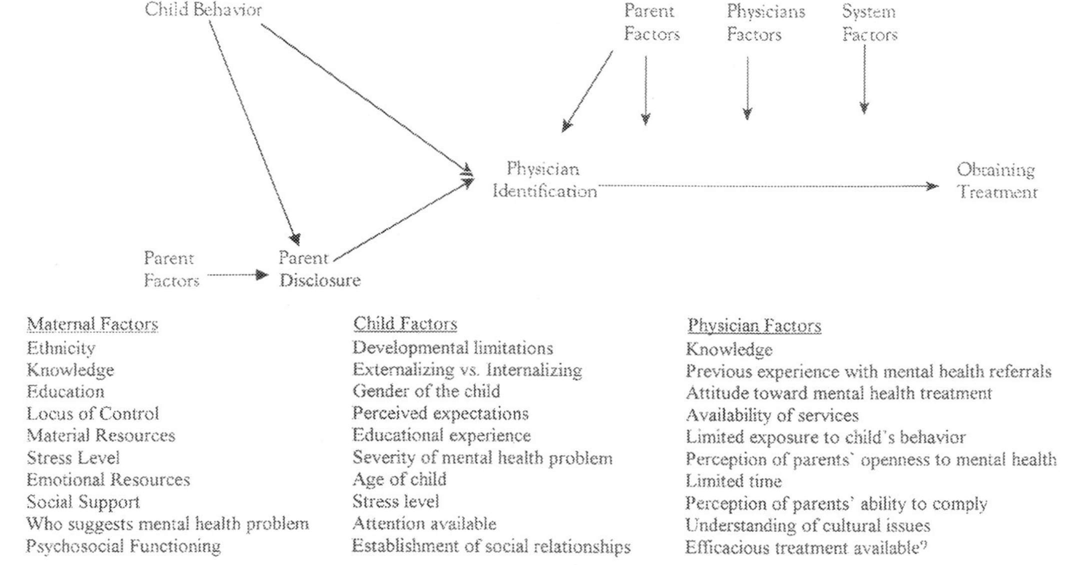

Note: System factors include presence and type of health insurance, mental health resources available in the community.

Figure 11.1. Model of factors affecting disclosure, identification, and treatment of psychosocial problems in children

mary care physicians in a larger context than has previously been considered. That is, improved methods of screening do not seem to be the answer to moving identification of psychosocial problems in children higher on the priority list of pediatricians and family physicians. In order to guide research that may be able to improve the rate with which primary care physicians attend to psychosocial problems in children, a comprehensive model is being proposed here that attempts to delineate possible factors that may influence physicians' practice. Most of these factors have yet to be empirically validated as relevant to identification and treatment of children with psychosocial problems. The proposed model is preliminary and subject to modification as new data are collected. Figure 11.1 illustrates the factors which must be considered in developing a model to understand factors which are likely to influence which children seen by primary care physicians ultimately obtain treatment for these problems.

PHYSICIAN FACTORS

The decision of a physician to use valuable time with a patient to address psychosocial issues is likely to be based on both stable factors of the physician and situational factors in the physician's interaction with the individual child and parent. Stable factors might include: the physician's personal experience with psychosocial problems, the physician's training in assessing and treating psychosocial problems, the physician's knowledge about interventions for psychosocial problems, the physician's perception of the effectiveness of interventions, and the physician's previous experience with addressing psychosocial issues. Situational factors might include the following with respect to an individual child or parent: the physician's perception of whether the parent will react favorably or unfavorably to a discussion of psychosocial issues, the physician's perception of the availability of psychosocial services for their patient, and the physician's perception of the likelihood of the parent following through with interventions.

Gardner et al. (2000), in a study of a large number of children treated by both pediatricians and family physicians, support the contention that physician management of psychosocial problems in children varies with situational factors. Physicians management of child psychosocial behavior problems was related to continuity of care, whether the physician was previously aware of the problem, and the physician's perception of whether the parent would agree with the treatment recommendation.

Stable factors are likely to have an impact on the physician's general approach to psychosocial problems, whereas situational factors are more likely to vary with each patient. Physicians who hold a general negative evaluation of psychosocial interventions and believe that they are not prepared for or effective in addressing these issues are unlikely to vary in their approach to children with psychosocial problems. However, physicians who perceive themselves as competent to address these problems and believe that interventions may be successful may vary in their approach to psychosocial problems as a result of situational factors related to the physician, as well as factors which the parent and child contribute (Ashworth, Williamson, & Montano, 1985; McLennan, Jansen-McWilliams, Comer, Gardner, & Kelleher, 1999).

A physician's sense of competence concerning the assessment and management of psychosocial problems may be related to the physician's training experiences. Both by choice, and availability through the specific residency program at which the physician was trained, residents are exposed to varying amounts of training concerning psychosocial issues. In addition, specialty might affect whether a physician addresses psychosocial issues during a particular encounter. For example, family physicians tend to view all encounters with patients, both well-child and acute care visits, as opportunities to assess psychosocial functioning, while pediatricians tend to view well-child encounters as the appropriate situation to assess psychosocial functioning. Data collected in a family practice setting suggest that physicians are as likely to identify psychosocial problems during acute care visits as they are during well-child visits (Wildman et al., 1997).

Physician attitude concerning mental health issues, as well as physician gender, has been proposed as relevant factors in physician attention to identification and management of psychosocial problems in children. Research concerning physicians' attitude towards mental health issues has yielded only weak support of the relationship between these attitudes, as measured by the Physician Beliefs Scale, and whether physicians addressed mental health issues in their child patients (McLennan et al., 1999). There is some support for differences in types of patients seen by male and female physicians, as well as how male and female physicians view their role in managing psychosocial problems in children (Scholle et al., 2001).

A potentially significant obstacle to physicians attending to psychosocial problems in children may be their perception that there are few resources for referral and few efficacious interventions that can be implemented by primary care physicians. Without effective treatments, little is likely to be gained from identifying a problem. In addition, physicians may correctly perceive parents as unlikely to follow through with referrals to mental health professionals. Kelleher (2000) reported that 60% of children referred by physicians to mental health professionals fail to make a first visit within six months of referral. Of those who do attend a first appointment, only 15-20% will complete six visits.

CHILD FACTORS

The most salient child factor that is likely to influence physician attention to psychosocial issues is the child's behavior. Although data suggest that children who are identified by physicians tend to have clinically significant psychosocial problems (Wildman, Kizilbash, & Smucker, 2000), many children with clinically significant psychosocial problems are not identified by physicians. Wildman, Yerkey, et al. (2000) suggested that parental factors, such as the parents' personal psychosocial distress may mediate whether child psychosocial problems are brought to the attention of physicians. The potential influence of parental psychosocial distress on whether or not children with psychosocial problems are identified and managed by their primary care physician will be discussed in the next section of this chapter, which addresses parent factors that may affect the identification and treatment of children with psychosocial problems.

Although previous research has found only a weak association between child behavior and physician intervention for psychosocial problems, preliminary data suggest that some types of child behavior, such as attention problems, are more likely to be brought to the attention of physicians than are other types of behaviors (Golden, Wildman, & Stancin, 2002). These data are consistent with Achenbach and Edelbrock's (1981) research indicating that parents tend to report externalizing behavior problems in their children more than they do internalizing behavior problems. On the other hand, children are more likely to report internalizing problems than they are externalizing problems (Achenbach & Edelbrock, 1981; Renouf & Kovacs, 1994; Sawyer, Baghurst, & Mathias, 1992; Verhulst & van der Ende, 1991). Since data provided by children are rarely included in epidemiological studies of the incidence of child psychosocial problems, these data may underestimate the incidence of internalizing behavior disorders in children. The results of research targeted at improving the rate with which primary care physicians identify children with psychosocial problems is likely to be affected by whether children as well as parents are used as informants of the child's psychosocial functioning (Kinsman & Wildman, 2001; Wildman, Kinsman, & Smucker, 2000). The likelihood of children receiving mental health services is likely to be heavily influenced by their parent's perceptions of their behavior since children are typically dependent on their parents in order obtain services, and children are rarely empowered to seek services for themselves.

PARENT FACTORS

Parents seem to be the engine that is largely responsible for driving the system of identification of child psychosocial problems. In order for a child to receive mental health services, a responsible adult must take the initiative to arrange for those services. Research suggests that children who receive mental health treatment have symptoms similar to children who do not present for mental health treatment (Shepherd et al., 1966). Parents of children who present for treatment appear to be more distressed than are the parents of children who do not present for treatment (Shepherd et al., 1966). Physician identification of child psychosocial problems is largely influenced by parental disclosure of concerns about their child's psychosocial functioning (Lynch et al., 1997; Wildman et al., 1997). When physicians recognize that parents have disclosed concerns, they are very likely to identify the child as having a psychosocial problem. Wildman et al. (1997) reported that family physicians generally identified psychosocial problems in children when they perceived the mothers as having disclosed concerns to them. Research is needed in order to ascertain whether parents and physicians agree on when parents have disclosed concerns.

If parental disclosure accounts for a large amount of the variance in whether physicians identify psychosocial problems in their child patients, then understanding of when parents disclose becomes a critical question. Logic would suggest that child behavior would be the primary reason why parents disclose concerns about their child's psychosocial status to their child's physician. Although data suggest that parents whose children do not seem to have a psychosocial problem are unlikely to disclose psychosocial concerns, parents of children with psychosocial problems are also unlikely to disclose concerns. Wildman, Yerkey, et al. (2000) reported that child behavior or emotional problems alone do not appear to be good predictors of which parents will disclose concerns about their child's psychosocial functioning to their child's physician.

The finding that the presence of child psychosocial problems is not a good predictor of maternal disclosure of concerns to her child's pediatrician suggests the need to examine other factors which may influence parental disclosure (Wildman, Yerkey, et al., 2000). Golden et al. (2002) have suggested that while overall child psychosocial problems may not be strongly related to maternal disclosure, specific child behaviors may. Golden et al. (2002) have further suggested that specific types of maternal distress may also be related to maternal disclosure of concerns to her child's pediatrician even though general maternal psychosocial distress may not be. Golden et al. found that mothers were more likely to disclose concerns to their child's pediatrician when their child displays behavior problems related to attention problems, such as fidgeting, acting as if driven by a motor, excessive daydreaming, being distracted easily, and trouble concentrating, than when their child displays other externalizing behavior problems or internalizing behavior problems. These data suggest that specific topographies of child behavior may increase the likelihood of parental disclosure. However, even when mothers report attention problems in their children, a large percentage of mothers continue to fail to disclose concerns about their child's behavior to their child's pediatrician. In addition, for the vast majority of children with other types of behavior problems, mothers fail to disclose concerns. These findings have led to the development of a model that views maternal disclosure as a complex behavior that is affected by a large number of factors.

One factor that must be considered in understanding whether mothers disclose concerns about their child's behavior to their child's physician is the mother's propensity toward seeking help for mental health problems, and who mothers are likely to seek help from. One aspect of help-seeking which we have hypothesized as important is the mother's culture. Data suggest that help-seeking varies across cultures, with individuals from certain cultures more likely to seek help than individuals from other cultures. We are currently analyzing data concerning the help-seeking patterns, and factors affecting those patterns for African-American mothers (Rankins, 2001).

In addition to culture, mother's psychosocial distress, and presence of a child psychosocial problem, mothers likelihood of discussing concerns about their child's behavior with their child's physician may be related to the mother's knowledge about normal child development and behavior, mother's education, and whether the family has access to medical insurance for mental health treatment. A related factor for mother's likelihood of attending to and discussing their child's psychosocial problems may be the mother's sense of efficacy, both as a parent and in her ability to comply with treatment suggestions. Fleisher (2003) has suggested that mother's sense of efficacy could be related to whether mothers discuss their concerns about their child's behavior with their child's physician.

The research concerning maternal disclosure of concerns about their child's behavior and emotions has rarely incorporated data about other sources of help mothers may have consulted. Although primary care physicians may be appropriate sources of help concerning child psychosocial problems, little is known concerning who else mothers consult with their concerns about their child's behavior. The availability of family and friends who may be able to provide advice, as well as direct access to mental health professionals may deter parents from consulting with their child's physician about behavioral and emotional concerns. We are beginning to collect data from mothers about whom they consult or would consult if they have concerns about their child's psychosocial functioning. These data are necessary in order to understand whether mothers consult with their child's physician as a first step, or only after other resources have been exhausted. Also, the nature and urgency of a child's psychosocial problem may be related to whom mother's consult. In some cases, an outside source such as their child's school may draw mother's attention to their child's behavior and suggest intervention.

SYSTEM FACTORS

System factors include such factors as whether a child has medical insurance and the type of medical insurance the child has. Some insurance plans make access to mental health treatment easier and less costly than do other plans. In addition, some insurance plans provide financial disincentives to physicians for making referrals to mental health professionals. Few insurance plans reimburse primary care physicians for time spent addressing psychosocial problems in children. These factors suggest that the presence and type of medical insurance may affect whether and how physicians address psychosocial problems in their child patients. However, McInerny, Szilagyi, Childs, Wasserman, and Kelleher (2000) reported no differences in how primary care physicians managed their child patients as a function of whether the children were insured or not. Physicians counseled, medicated, and referred children with and without medical insurance at approximately the same rates. There is a lack of data, however, on parental compliance with physician treatment suggestions, and how parental compliance is affected by availability of medical insurance.

INTERVENTION MODELS AND ISSUES

Understanding of the factors that influence identification and treatment of children with psychosocial problems is a long way off. Until we have a better understanding of the obstacles to the identification and effective management of children with psychosocial problems within the primary care context, clinical practice guidelines that are likely to be widely implemented are unlikely. Clearly, leaving the large number of children with psychosocial problems unidentified and untreated is an unacceptable alternative while waiting for research to provide effective solutions to this pervasive and severe problem which affects nearly one fifth of children and adversely affects their functioning at school, with peers, and with family. Since data indicate that these problems persist over time and do not appear to remit, solutions need to be found which can begin to address this problem.

In general, primary care physicians have not implemented routine screening in their practices. When children are identified, some management is likely. However, much of the management tends to be in the form of support and advice. There are no data to support that these interventions are effective. Without effective interventions, there is little to advise practice for primary care physicians. Alternative service delivery models have been suggested that routinely incorporate mental health specialists into the primary care medical setting (Schroeder, Chapter 1, this volume). The integration of mental health providers into primary care practice may provide a solution to some of the problems, at least in settings where this collaborative practice model is economically feasible. Mental health professionals could provide the type of evaluation and intervention that has received empirical support for effectiveness.

Sound clinical practice dictates that screening should be done within the context of a clinical evaluation that includes a thorough history, direct observation, physical examination and other diagnostic tests. Obviously, a screening procedure must be psychometrically sound, acceptable to parents, accurate, cost effective, and fit into the practice setting.

How can screening methods be incorporated practically in a pediatric office setting? If parent report methods are used, then several options may be considered for incorporating measures: (1) Scales and questionnaires can be mailed to parents in advance and brought to appointments. (2) Parents could complete questionnaires in the waiting room before a visit, aided by office staff when needed. (3) Questionnaires could be completed via interview, which would be most appropriate for parents with poor reading or English skills. (4) Brief measures could be incorporated into routine intake forms. Inclusion of items within a comprehensive intake questionnaire may grant more acceptability to sensitive or difficult items. (5) Computer-assisted screens may be reasonable in some settings. Screening strategies selected should fit both office practice and family needs.

However, Stancin and Palermo (1997) reviewed the topic of behavioral screening in primary care settings in terms of meeting basic scientific criteria for implementation. They concluded that although standardized screening methods have been shown to increase the rate of identification of children with behavioral problems in primary care settings, comparative studies had not been conducted yet in order to recommend any one method over the others. Some brief measures had empirical support for pediatric use as a mass screening instrument (e.g., the Pediatric Symptom Checklist) whereas other more lengthy measures (e.g., Child Behavior

Checklist) were deemed appropriate when a multidimensional focus is desired. The authors cautioned that there is little evidence to demonstrate that the routine use of screening measures would be sufficient to lead to improved evaluation, interventions, and outcomes for children. They concluded that increasing the repertoire of treatment options and resources available to pediatricians, and integrating psychological services with primary care services, would be necessary to result in greater recognition and intervention for behavioral difficulties.

Integration of Identification with Treatment

Many questions remain regarding how to increase physician recognition and management of child behavioral concerns. Whether solutions lie in increased use of screening methods, improved education of providers, or alternative strategies remains to be investigated. There are complex ethical issues that may be raised in the context of screening for children's problematic behavior and family problems. These include questions related to the physician's responsibility after a problem is identified, consequences of labeling, and insuring quality standards for interventions that result from identification. It is not clear what the expectations are for the primary care physician in terms of evaluation and treatment. Although behavioral pediatricians and other mental health professionals view identification and treatment of child behavioral dysfunction as a responsibility, what is the actual motivation for a primary care physician to do so? Do primary care physicians want to participate in more case identification? At this time there are many disincentives to primary care pediatricians for assuming this burden (e.g., lack of reimbursement for services).

Changes in health care financing, especially managed medical care, have resulted in dramatic changes in how primary care physicians practice medicine, including how they make mental health referrals. In fact, Garrison and colleagues found that insurance status was one of the few factors related to pediatrician decisions about referring a child to a mental health specialist. Indeed, under a capitated plan, a primary care physician may have financial disincentives for recognizing a problem that requires referral to a behavioral specialist. In many managed care plans, medical care and mental health care are controlled by separate and unrelated companies, with mental health services considered as a carve out. Determining what mental health provider a child may see because of insurance restrictions can be a daunting task for the most informed and motivated primary care physicians. Lack of control of mental health referrals is likely to frustrate and to undermine further the motivation of primary care providers to identify behavioral dysfunction in children.

Collaborative Care Models

Once a behavior problem is recognized, the provider must decide whether to make a referral to a behavioral specialist and how to best accomplish that task. The problem of finding adequate treatment resources for children with behavior problems haunts many primary care providers. Behavioral resources available to primary care physicians vary enormously. Most primary care physicians need more help with management of children with behavioral problems than with identification, and thus search for a collaborative relationship with one or more mental health professionals in their community.

In the current model of care, primary care providers are responsible for screening for disturbance and then referring to other specialists for treatment. However, once a referral is made, communication between mental health professional and the primary care physician is often limited or nonexistent. Primary care physicians rarely obtain information about mental health evaluations, treatments or progress, and often complain that they lose track of what happens to the child. An efficient model of care would provide for screening of mental health problems and treatment that is done in the same place. This integrated and coordinated approach has been called collaborative care (Perrin, 1999). Practices that integrate mental health professionals, such as psychologists, with primary care pediatricians have been described as a model for facilitating psychological services for children. By working collaboratively with a mental health professional in the office, the primary care physician has ready access to a provider who can address behavioral concerns both effectively and efficiently. Because recognition may by linked to availability of treatment resources, it is reasonable that more behavioral concerns may be identified when there are onsite mental health professionals or behavioral pediatricians to assist in the treatment of behavioral issues. The behavioral screening program at MetroHealth Medical Center is an example of how a collaborative care model can facilitate mental health services (Riekert, Stancin, Palermo, & Drotar, 1999). This service is self-supported by professional fee reimbursement and would be viable in more traditional community practices as well as in academic settings.

The high prevalence of psychosocial problems in pediatric primary care populations, coupled with the insufficient detection and assessment of these concerns, underscore the need for integrating psychological services into primary care settings (see Schroeder, this volume). In response to these needs, a psychosocial behavioral assessment service was developed and implemented by Terry Stancin, PhD in the ambulatory pediatric clinic of MetroHealth Medical Center, a large county hospital serving a predominately urban low-income population in the Cleveland, Ohio area (Stancin, 2000). The goals of the behavioral assessment service were to provide primary care providers (PCPs) with interpretation and integration of a set of standardized parent and teacher behavioral rating scales and to suggest further assessment and treatment options. This section describes this service as an example of one program developed to address the unmet mental health needs in a high-risk population and summarizes outcome data.

The Setting

MetroHealth Medical Center is a public general hospital serving primarily economically disadvantaged families of the Cleveland, Ohio area. The pediatric clinic provides primary and acute ambulatory care to more than 55,000 mostly inner-city children each year. The majority of families receive public assistance including managed care Medicaid. The population served is ethnically and culturally diverse, and children are at high risk for having psychosocial problems. Pediatric psychologists (who have been integrated into the clinic as consultants and teachers since 1986) and other child mental health professionals at the hospital were unable to meet the enormous mental health needs of this population by traditional, individualized mental health services. Because community mental health resources for children were also limited, frequently PCPs were, and continue to be, in the role of mental health provider for these children. Increasing numbers of families were requesting services for child behavior problems from the PCPs, who needed a cost-efficient means of evaluation.

Key Features of the Behavioral Assessment Service

In response to this need an assessment service program was established in 1993 for children identified by PCPs as being at risk for having a behavior problem. When a PCP wishes to obtain the assessment on a child being seen in the MetroHealth Pediatric Clinic, he or she discusses the option with the family and describes the process. PCPs distribute to parents a packet containing several parent and teacher-completed rating scales that are then mailed back to the psychology staff. The assessment packet includes the Achenbach Child Behavior Checklists (Achenbach, 1991a, 1991b) and several other standardized rating scales for parents and teachers. Without seeing the child, psychology staff (which includes graduate student trainees in pediatric psychology) score, review and interpret materials, and provide PCPs with a brief written summary of results and suggestions for further evaluation and possible interventions. Turnaround time for results is dependent on how quickly parents and teachers return forms and also upon seasonal demand. Usually, reports are completed within two weeks of receipt of caregiver forms. PCPs use the report as they choose to provide feedback to families and for making treatment decisions. Initially, the service was available for children ages 4-18 years, but more recently it has been extended downward to age 1.5 years with comparable age appropriate instruments.

It is important to note that the assessment is only provided when requested by the PCP. Therefore, this service is considered to provide brief psychological assessments, rather than screening results (Stancin & Palermo, 1997), since most children served come into the office with a parent already expressing a behavioral concern. A bill for this service is generated, although reimbursement is variable. It is also important to note that this service integrates both parent and teacher data in ways that many PCPs would otherwise find difficult to manage in the typical office practice.

The following example adapted from Riekert, Stancin, Palermo, and Drotar (1999) describes how PCPs might access the screening service. During a routine well-child visit, Mrs. Smith expresses concerns to the PCP that her son, Billy (age 8) is aggressive towards siblings, refuses to complete his homework, and frequently tells lies. She considers him to have a high activity level and says that he is easily distracted. Billy is a healthy child whose parents recently divorced. The PCP initiates the assessment service with a referral question related to whether the symptoms might be associated with attention deficit hyperactivity disorder (ADHD) and provides Mrs. Smith a packet of standardized parent and teacher rating scales. These questionnaires are completed by Mrs. Smith and by Billy's teacher after the visit and returned by mail to the pediatric psychology staff for scoring, interpretation, and written recommendations for the PCP. In the above example, the parent-completed Child Behavior Checklist (CBCL) results indicated clinically significant scores on the anxious/depressed, delinquent behavior, and aggressive subscales, whereas the only Teacher Report Form (TRF) scores to fall in the clinically significant range is the aggressive behaviors subscale score, with borderline scores on the anxious/depressed subscale. The teacher comments that Billy is sociable and does well academically, but sometimes he seems sad and angry. In this case, data were not suggestive of an ADHD diagnosis. Suggestions included on the assessment report included further exploration of Billy's adjustment to the divorce and other family issues by a mental health provider. After receiving the report, the PCP referred the family to a local mental health facility for intervention deciding against prescribing a stimulant medication. As can be seen from the example, the goal of the assessment service was to provide PCPs with assistance in making treatment decisions concerning children's behavioral problems.

WHAT HAVE WE LEARNED FROM THE METROHEALTH BEHAVIORAL ASSESSMENT SERVICE?

The following summarizes results of several program evaluation studies that include:

- Descriptive information on a large sample of consecutively referred children (Reikert et al., 1999; Stancin, Riekert, Palermo, & Whitwell, 1999)
- Service utilization and impact as noted in medical charts one year following assessments (Reikert et al., 1999)
- PCP evaluation of the effectiveness and utility of the service (Stancin et al., 1999)
- Impact of the assessment service on mental health care utilization and parental satisfaction at long-term follow-up (Walders et al., 2000)

An examination of representative samples of the children on whom both parent and teacher data were available by the assessment suggests that a majority of the referred children were elementary school age boys (mean age is 8 years). The ethnic diversity of the referred children reflects the hospital population which includes mostly Caucasians, African Americans, and Latinos (Riekert et al., 1999; Stancin et al., 1999).

Lesson #1: Children Identified for the Service Had Clinically Significant Behavioral Problems

While it is certainly the case that pediatricians see mild behavior problems, data from MetroHealth suggest that they are also addressing concerns reflecting very significant problems. An examination of mean scores on clinical subscales of the CBCL and TRF indicates that there is a high rate of psychopathology in this referred population. In particular, there is a high rate of externalizing behavior problems with the mean *T* scores on these subscales greater than 70. On the CBCL, 70% of the children had a *T* score greater than or equal to 65 on Total problems. Over 60% of the parents and 35% of the teachers reported scores above the clinical cutoff ($T = 70$) on two or more clinical scales of the CBCL and TRF, respectively (Riekert et al., 1999). Only 21% of the parents and 39% of the teachers reported clinical scales within normal limits ($T < 70$) on the CBCL and TRF, respectively. Moreover, results from the CBCL and TRF suggest that a large percentage of children who received the brief assessment service were reported to have multiple behavioral problems (Riekert et al., 1999). Important research questions not answered by available data pertain to how this select referred population from a pediatric primary clinic compares with other settings in terms of severity of problems being managed (or collaboratively managed).

Lesson #2: Primary Care Providers Like the Service and Find it to Be Useful

Primary care providers completed an anonymous written survey to evaluate their perceptions of the utility of the service (Stancin et al., 1999). The survey contained questions about the PCP's use of and satisfaction with the service, and decision-making process when dealing with mental health issues. All respondents reported that they had used the service for their patients during the previous year, and nearly 40% were frequent customers, indicating that they received results on five or more children in the past year.

The PCPs were asked to check all reasons for which they might use the service. The top reason was to gather more data on children when there were concerns about a possible diagnosis of ADHD (92%). A large number of PCPs also reported that they hoped the service would help confirm clinical impressions (70%), determine a need for a mental health referral (64%), provide information for a differential diagnosis (52%), or to evaluate treatment effectiveness (46%).

Most of the PCPs in our study were pleased with the screening service. They reported general satisfaction (77.3%) and found the service was helpful for making treatment decisions (87.5%). They noted that recommendations were helpful (83.3%). However, PCPs were the least satisfied with the speed with which they were given feedback on results (58.3%).

Results suggested that PCPs find the brief assessment results most useful when deciding about prescribing psychotropic medication. This results was somewhat surprising because the assessment service was conceptualized as a way to physicians could identify which children had behavioral symptoms that were serious enough to warrant a fuller mental health evaluation or to triage them for appropriate services.

Two studies led the program researchers to conclude that PCPs did not use the service to screen for mental health referrals. In the first study, medical charts on a subset of children who had been assessed were examined (Riekert et al., 1999). Chart notes indicated that most PCPs documented waiting to prescribe stimulants until after the assessment report and most were looking especially close at the teacher ratings of attention problems. However, of the 42% of children who were referred for mental health services, only half were done so *after* the PCP received the report. Interestingly, children referred to mental health services were more likely to have parent-rated internalizing problems above clinical criteria. Of some concern from this medical chart study was that only a third of the children evaluated actually had documented mental health services beyond the brief assessment provided.

In a second related study, PCPs were asked when they made treatment decisions regarding children with behavior problems (Stancin et al., 1999). Most PCPs (83%) indicated that they "always or often" wait for written results of the screening before prescribing psychotropic medications (usually stimulants). However, only 35% of the PCPs reported they always or often waited for written results when making decisions about making a mental health referral. Similar results were obtained using open-ended questions asking how the PCPs decide about treatments for children with behavioral problems. Most PCPs (71%) made specific reference to the assessment results regarding when they prescribed stimulants whereas less than 17% of PCPs referred to the service when describing how they determined need for a mental health referral for patients.

Taken together, results suggest that PCPs in this setting appreciate the contribution of parent and teacher rating scale results when prescribing psychotropic medication. Other studies are needed to understand the process by which PCPs decide to make referrals for mental health problems. It is likely that PCPs use a complex set of data from multiple sources besides rating scales when making treatment decisions (e.g., family history, family distress, family motivation, treatment acceptability to families, available mental health resources, and medical insurance constraints).

Lesson #3: Parents Continue to Express Behavioral Concerns at Long-term Follow-up

Walders et al. (2000) contacted 84 parents by telephone one to five years after their assessment at MetroHealth. Parents rated the child's current behavioral functioning using the Pediatric Symptom Checklist (Jellinek, Murphy, & Burns, 1986), their use of mental health services, and their perception of the helpfulness of the original behavioral assessments. Attempts were made to contact all 232 children assessed by the service from 1993-1996, but many families (64%) could not be reached because of lack of known whereabouts. At the time of the initial assessment, 62% of the children in this sample had CBCL Total $T > 65$. At follow-up, 43% of the children had PSC > 28, which is generally considered as screening positive for problems and 83% parents described their child currently as having a behavior problem. However, 53% parents indicated that the behavior problems had improved and 63% said that school performance improved since the original assessments had been conducted.

These results suggested that the children assessed with the MetroHealth program had persistent behavioral problems as reported by parents at long-term follow-up. Although a slight majority of parents noted some improvement in behavior and school performance, additional research is needed to examine whether the assessment facilitated these improvements.

Lesson #4: Pediatric Psychologists Need to Work Closely with PCPs to Ensure Mental Health Follow up of Identified Behavioral Problems

Data from this collection of outcome studies suggest that pediatricians often require assistance in order to link children with services, and that screening or assessment alone is of limited usefulness. The parent follow-up study indicated that less than half of the parents recalled discussing the assessment results with their pediatrician or receiving a mental health referral following the assessment (Walders et al., 2000). However, most parents said that they followed through with the referral when suggested by the PCP. It was interesting to note that most parents who had the opportunity to discuss the assessment results with their PCP found them to be helpful (Walders et al., 2000).

There are several ways that psychologists can facilitate mental health services for children following the brief assessment. Because medication is often the only treatment PCPs think they have to offer to families, it is not surprising that they use results to guide medication decisions. It would be helpful to also assist PCPs with other referral or treatment protocols or additional training in behavioral interventions (e.g., see Tynan, this volume). In particular, results suggest that the pediatric psychologist should assume an active role in facilitating physician/family communication about results and linking children to appropriate services. Ideally, follow up psychological services could be provided in the primary care site. One result of the outcome studies was that the MetroHealth pediatric psychology division began offering an optional assessment interview for some patients in order to provide additional training opportunities for our pediatric residents and to assist with linking families to needed services. Future studies are need to evaluate the effectiveness of interventions to assist PCPs in communicating behavioral assessment results and providing mental health treatment or referral recommendations to families.

SUMMARY AND CLINICAL IMPLICATIONS

This chapter presented the basis for developing a conceptual model to help understand potential obstacles to identification and effective management of child behavioral and emotional problems in primary care. The primary purpose of the model is to form a foundation to address the problem of underidentification. In order to effectively address this problem, further research is needed to identify the variables which influence the process of parent disclosure, physician identification, physician intervention, parent compliance with treatment, and effectiveness of treatment. Understanding of the variables contributing to this process is likely to lead to effective ways of improving outcomes for children. However, understanding of the factors and changes in practice are not likely to occur in the near future. In the interim, MetroHealth Medical Center has helped to bridge the gap between research and practice by developing a consultation service.

MetroHealth Medical Center has developed a brief, multi-informant Behavioral Assessment Service that is offered to pediatricians as a way of gathering parent and teacher behavior rating scale data on children who are at risk for having behavioral problems. PCPs are satisfied with the service and find it to be useful in the clinical management of their patients, especially regarding use of stimulant medication. Children in this large inner-city pediatric clinic are at risk for significant and often persistent behavior problems, and PCPs are unduly stressed by their overwhelming mental health needs. The service offers PCPs welcome, inexpensive, and ethically minded linkages to treatments for their patients who might otherwise never receive attention from mental health professionals. However, psychologists need to work closely with PCPs to ensure mental health follow up of identified behavioral problems.

REFERENCES

Achenbach, T. M. (1991a). *Manual for the Child Behavior Checklist/4 - 18 and 1999 profile.* Burlington: University of Vermont Department of Psychiatry.

Achenbach, T. M. (1991b). *Manual for the Teacher's Report Form and 1999 profile.* Burlington: University of Vermont Department of Psychiatry.

Achenbach, T. M., & Edelbrock, C. S. (1981). Behavior problems and competencies reported by parents of normal and disturbed children aged four through sixteen. *Monographs of the Society for Research in Child Development, 46* (1, serial number 188).

Ashworth, C. D., Williamson, P., & Montano, D. (1985). A scale to measure physician beliefs about psychosocial aspects of patient care. *Social Science & Medicine, 19,* 1235-1238.

Costello, E. J., Edelbrock, C., Costello, A. J., Dulcan, M. K., Burns, B. J., & Brent, D. (1988). Psychopathology in pediatric primary care: The new hidden morbidity. *Pediatrics, 83,* 415-424.

Costello, E. J., & Shugart, M. A. (1992). Above and below the threshold: Severity of psychiatric symptoms and functional impairment in a pediatric sample. *Pediatrics, 90,* 359-386.

Earls, F. (1989). Epidemiology and child psychiatry: Entering the second phase. *American Journal of Orthopsychiatry, 59,* 279-283.

Fleisher, C. L. (2003). *Mothers' help-seeking regarding their child's behavior and emotions: The role of parenting subefficacy.* Unpublished doctoral dissertation, Kent State University, Ohio.

Gardner, W., Kelleher, K.J., Wasserman, R., Childs, G., Nutting, P., Lillienfeld, H., & Pajer, K. (2000). Primary care treatment of pediatric psychosocial problems: A study from pediatric research in office settings and ambulatory sentinel practice network. *Pediatrics, 4,* 44.

Garrison, W. T., Bailey, E. D., Garb, J., Ecker, B., Spencer, P., & Sigelman, D. (1992). Interactions between parents and pediatric primary care physcians about children's mental health. *Hospital & Community Psychiatry, 43,* 489-493.

Goldberg, I. D., Roghmann, K. J., McInerny, T. K., & Burke, J. D., Jr. (1984). Mental health problems among children seen in pediatric practice. *Pediatrics, 73,* 278-293.

Golden, C., Wildman, B. G., & Stancin, T. (2002). *Mother's disclosure to pediatricians of child psychosocial problems: Relationship to child behaviors and maternal depression symptoms.* Manuscript in preparation.

Gotlib, I. H., Lewinsohn, P. M., Seeley, J. R. (1995). Symptom versus a diagnosis of depression: Differences in psychosocial functioning. *Journal of Consulting and Clinical Psychology, 63,* 90-100.

Hickson, G. B., Altemeier, W. A., & O'Connor, S. O. (1983). Concerns of mothers seeking care in private pediatric offices: Opportunities for expanding services. *Pediatrics*, *72*, 619-624.

Jellinek, M. J., Murphy, J., & Burns, B. (1986). Brief psychosocial screen in outpatient pediatric practice. *Journal of Pediatrics, 109,* 371-378.

Kelleher, K. J. (2000, September 21). Interview on "All Things Considered," National Public Radio.

Kinsman, A. M., & Wildman, B. G. (2001). Mother and child perception of child functioning: Relationship to maternal distress. *Family Process, 40,* 163-172.

Lynch, T. L., Wildman, B. G., & Smucker, W. D. (1997). Parental disclosure of child psychosocial concerns: Relationship to physician identification and management. *Journal of Family Practice, 44,* 273-280.

MacPhee, D. (1984). The pediatrician as a source of information about child development. *Journal of Pediatric Psychology, 9,* 87-99.

McInerny, T. K., Szilagyi, P. G., Childs, G. E., Wasserman, R. C., & Kelleher, K. J. (2000). Uninsured children with psychosocial problems: Primary care management. *Pediatrics, 4,* 930-6.

McLennan, J. D., Jansen-McWilliams, L., Comer, D. M., Gardner, W. P., & Kelleher, K. J. (1999). The Physician Belief Scale and psychosocial problems in children: A report from the Pediatric Research in Office Settings and the Ambulatory Sentinel Practice Network. *Journal of Developmental and Behavioral Pediatrics, 20,* 24-30.

Perrin, E. C. (1999). The promise of collaborative care. *Journal of Developmental Behavioral Pediatrics, 20,* 57-62.

Public Health Service. (1991). Healthy people 2000: National health promotion and disease prevention objectives (Vol. 3, DHHS publication No. 91-50212). Washington, DC: U.S. Department of Health and Human Services.

Public Health Service. (2000). Healthy people 2010: National health promotion and disease prevention objectives (DHHS publication No. 017-001-00547-9). Washington, DC: U.S. Department of Health and Human Services.

Rankins, J. L. (2001). *Help-seeking for child psychosocial problems among African-American mothers.* Manuscipt in preparation.

Renouf, A. G., & Kovacs, M. (1994). Concordance between mothers' reports and children's self-reports of depressive symptoms: A longitudinal study. *Journal of the American Academy of Child and Adolescent Psychiatry, 33,* 208-216.

Riekert, K. A., Stancin, T., Palermo, T. M., & Drotar, D. (1999). A psychological behavioral screening service: Use, feasibility and impact in a primary care setting. *Journal of Pediatric Psychology, 24,* 405 - 414.

Sawyer, M. G., Baghurst, P., & Mathias, J. (1992). Differences between informants' reports describing emotional and behavioral problems in community and clinic-referred children: A research note. *Journal of Child Psychology and Psychiatry, 33,* 441-449.

Scholle, S. H., Gardner, W., Harman, J., Madlon-Kay, D. J., Pascoe, J., & Kelleher, K. (2001). Physician gender and psychosocial care for children: Attitudes, practice characteristics, identification, and treatment. *Medical Care, 39,* 26-38.

Schroeder, C. S. (1996). Psychologists and pediatricians in collaborative practice. In R. J. Resnick & R. H. Kozensky (Eds.), *Health psychology through the lifespan: Practice and research opportunities.* Washington, DC.: American Psychological Association.

Shepherd, M., Oppenheim, A. N., & Mitchell, S. (1966). Childhood behavior disorders and the child-guidance clinic: An epidemiological study. *Journal of Clinical Psychology and Psychiatry,* 7, 39-52.

Stancin, T. (2000, August). *Brief, multi-informant assessments in a pediatric primary care setting.* Paper presented at the American Psychological Association Symposium: Prevention and Early Intervention in Primary Care Contexts, Washington, DC.

Stancin, T., & Palermo, T. M. (1997). A review of behavioral screening practices in pediatric settings: Do they pass the test? *Journal of Developmental and Behavioral Pediatrics, 18*, 183-194.

Stancin, T., Riekert, K. A., Palermo, T. M., & Whitwell, J. (1999, September). *What do PCPs think about behavioral screening in primary care?* Paper presented at the annual scientific meeting of the Society for Developmental-Behavioral Pediatrics, Seattle, WA.

Street, R. L. (1991). Information-giving in medical consultations: The influence of patients' communicative styles and personal characteristics. *Social Science and Medicine, 31*, 541-548.

U.S. Department of Health and Human Services. (1990). *Mental health: A report of the Surgeon General.* Rockville, MD: U.S. Department of Health and Human Services, Substance Abuse and Mental Health Services Administration, Center for Mental Health Services, National Institutes of Health, National Institute of Mental Health.

Verhulst, F. C., & van der Ende, J. (1991). Assessment of child psychopathology: Relationships between different methods, different informants and clinical judgment of severity. *Acta Psychiatrica Scandinavia, 84*, 155-159.

Walders, N., Stancin, T., Riekert, K., Whitwell, J., Palermo, T., & Quintus, K. (2000, March). *Brief behavioral assessments in a pediatric primary care clinic: Parental views at long-term follow-up.* Poster presented at The Millennium Conference of the Great Lakes Society of Pediatric Psychology: Practice, Research, and Policy Concerning Intervention with Pediatric Populations, Cleveland, Ohio.

Wildman, B. G., Kinsman, A. M., Logue, E., Dickey, D. J., & Smucker, W. D. (1997). Presentation and management of childhood psychosocial problems. *Journal of Family Practice, 44*, 77-84.

Wildman, B. G., Kinsman, A. M., & Smucker, W. D. (2000). Use of child reports of daily functioning to facilitate identification of psychosocial problems in children. *Archives of Family Medicine, 9*, 612-616.

Wildman, B. G., Kizilbash, A. H., & Smucker, W. D., (1999). Factors related to physicians' attention to parents' concerns about the psychosocial functioning of their child. *Archives of Family Medicine, 8*, 440-444.

Wildman, B. G., Yerkey, T. M., Golden, C., & Stancin, T. (2000, September). A model addressing difficulties in identifying psychosocial problems. Paper presented at Society for Developmental and Behavioral Pediatrics, Providence, Rhode Island.

Wilson, J. L. (1964). The pediatric psychologist: A role model. *American Psychologist, 22*, 323-325.

DISCUSSION SUMMARY
written by Courtney Fleisher

In their presentation and chapter, Drs. Beth Wildman and Terry Stancin highlighted the MetroHealth Hospital pediatric ambulatory care clinic's psychosocial assessment service as an example of a program attempting to address the unmet mental health needs in high risk populations. The outcome data on the effectiveness of this program were summarized, and lessons learned from these data are elucidated. In addition, the authors highlighted the complexity of the issue of identification and treatment of children's psychosocial issues in primary care settings. They reviewed research regarding the key influences of physician-based, parental, child, and system factors in addressing mental health issues in primary care and proposed that the process is more complex than the way it has been studied to date. Participants agreed that accessing mental health care for children in primary care is multifaceted, and implications for research and clinical practice were discussed.

RESEARCH

This presentation sparked discussion focused around the crucial piece of the proposed model of how the presence of a psychosocial problem is communicated to the physician. Dr. Wildman emphasized the importance of the mother's disclosure as the physician has only a small sampling of the child's behavior in a highly circumscribed setting. The question was raised, however, of what constitutes an operational definition of disclosure. Dr. Wildman conveyed the importance of both the physician's and the parent's report that disclosure occurred, but she cautioned that these concordance rates have not been explored in the literature. Participants discussed that parents may be attempting to communicate problems to physicians using subtle language that physicians do not accurately perceive. Furthermore, it was noted that some parents do not verbalize their concerns at all, making identification an even greater challenge for the physician. Participants suggested the need for research that ascertains the rate of agreement between parents and physicians that disclosure occurred, as well as research to identify subtle cues parents may use to communicate that their children are experiencing psychosocial problems. The argument was made that in order to learn about both the verbal and nonverbal cues, research samples should include all parents who have concerns about the psychosocial functioning of their children, rather than just the families in which the parent verbalizes concern. Dr. Wildman indicated that it would be interesting to conduct a study wherein appointments are videotaped and both physicians and parents view the tapes and identify when they saw communication regarding concern about psychosocial functioning being conveyed.

Regarding Dr. Stancin's research evaluating her practice's behavioral screening process, participants particularly applauded her follow-up data conducted with the parents of the children involved in the behavioral screening process. Although Dr. Stancin reported that the data were not physician-parent matched, participants iterated the importance of publishing these data as they shed light on the effectiveness of the intervention on the part of the physician. In sum, while a significant number of the parents reported improvement in the child, a significant minority of the children were still significantly impaired. A significant majority of the parents did not recall having discussed the results of the screening with the primary care physician, although the majority of those parents that did recall discussing the results found the feedback to be very helpful.

CLINICAL PRACTICE

Two questions surrounding poor parent-physician communication about child psychosocial functioning were the focus of discussion relevant to clinical practice: (1) what are the barriers to clear communication between parents and physicians surrounding child psychosocial functioning, and (2) what can be done about it now?

An example of missed communication was presented to the participants wherein a mother may state, "Johnny's been a handful," but no further discussion or action results from the comment. Parents may not know how to communicate more specific information about their child's psychosocial functioning without targeted questioning by a professional.

Discussion yielded hypotheses about why communication is so poor. One belief was that mental health issues are not viewed as being "real illness." A physician participant noted about the above example that the mother's statement would be assumed to be insignificant, but with a similarly vague statement related to a medical issue, the same assumption would not be made. Parents' disclosure behavior may be extinguished due to the lack of response to, or reinforcement for, their efforts. It is also possible that parents and physicians just do not have the same vocabulary for discussion surrounding mental health problems. Obviously conveyance of information is difficult when people are communicating without knowing each other's language.

Several ideas were proposed to help ameliorate the poor communication problem. First, one physician participant drew a parallel with the concept stemming from the American Academy of Pediatrics' Bright Futures program, that "trigger comments," like Bright Futures' "trigger problems," need to be identified so that physicians have ideas about what they need to attend to. Second, the idea of having parents complete screening inventories to help cue physicians to problems was raised. Some participants voiced concern about this solution because of its implications for continuing care. Again, from a behavioral point of view, physicians validating parental discussion of psychosocial issues results in the increased likelihood of future disclosure. Additionally, the point was reinforced that although good screening tools are available, they are not being used. Third, participants emphasized the importance of having physicians question children directly in order to include them in the process of identification. Finally, participants noted that the outcome generated through screening such as that done in Dr. Stancin's clinic is good fodder for discussion. When objective data are available for physicians to provide feedback to the parent, the presentation of this information reinforces the process of disclosure and continued discussion surrounding psychosocial issues. Therefore, participants agreed that, like with results from physical tests, physicians should take every opportunity to provide feedback to parents when assessments have been used with a family.

In conclusion, participants were pleased with the proposed, more complex model of investigating challenges to identification of child psychosocial problems in primary care settings. Participants encouraged continuing data collection to evaluate and test this model in order to advance the goal of improved care for psychosocial problems for children. In addition, they were excited about the implications of an in-house assessment referral system like that occurring in Dr. Stancin's clinic. Participants encouraged further publication regarding the effectiveness of this system as well as dissemination of the concepts for the purposes of intervention in specialty and training clinics.

ABOUT THE CONTRIBUTORS

Meghan Barlow holds a B.A. from Denison University in Granville, Ohio and is currently enrolled in the Clinical Psychology doctoral program at Kent State University with a child and family concentration. Her research interests include the identification and treatment of childhood psychosocial problems.

Keri J. Brown is a graduate of Denison University and a Ph.D. candidate in the Clinical Child Psychology Program at the University of Kansas. She is completing an internship in pediatric psychology at the Columbus Children's Hospital in Columbus, Ohio. Her research interests include the prevention of unintentional injuries and psychosocial outcomes for children who are medically compromised. Her clinical interests include adherence, pain management, and coping issues related to pediatric chronic illness.

Dennis Drotar, Ph.D., is Professor of Pediatrics, Psychology, and Psychiatry at Case Western Reserve University and Chief of the Division of Behavioral Pediatrics and Psychology at Rainbow Babies and Children's Hospital. He is also director of the graduate level research training program in the Department of Psychology at Case Western Reserve University. His primary research interest concerns factors that influence the psychological outcomes of children and adolescents with chronic physical illness including methods of psychosocial interventions with this population.

Courtney Landau Fleisher, completed her bachelor's degree in psychology at Bates College in Lewiston, ME. She graduated from KSU with a

Ph.D. in clinical psychology. Presently, Dr. Fleisher has a postdoctoral position at Children's Hospital of Philadelphia.

M. Alex Geertsma, Ph.D., is Chairman of the Department of Pediatrics and Director of the Children's Health Center at St. Mary's Hospital, Waterbury, Connecticut. He holds academic clinical positions at both Yale University and the University of Connecticut Schools of Medicine. Among memberships in various professional organizations, he is an active member of the American Academy of Pediatrics, the Ambulatory Pediatric Association, and the Society for Developmental and Behavioral Pediatrics. He is involved in advocacy for children's behavioral health services via the American Academy of Pediatrics and the Society for Developmental and Behavioral Pediatrics. He represented the Society for Developmental and Behavioral Pediatrics at the 1999 American Academy of Pediatrics' Consensus Meeting on Children's Mental Health Financing held in Washington, D.C. He served in the same capacity at the U.S. Surgeon General's 2000 Conference on Children's Mental Health.

Sherry Glied, Ph.D., is Professor and Chair of the Department of Health Policy and Management of Columbia University's Mailman School of Public Health. She holds a BA in economics from Yale University, an MA in economics from the University of Toronto, and a Ph.D. in economics from Harvard University. In 1992-1993, she served as a Senior Economist to the President's Council of Economic Advisers, under both President Bush and President Clinton. Professor Glied's principal areas of research are in health policy reform and mental health care policy. She is a member of the MacArthur Foundation's Network on Mental Health Policy Research.

Christine Golden is currently pursuing her Ph.D. in Clinical Psychology with a child and family concentration at Kent State University. She graduated from The Catholic University of America, Washington, DC with a BA in Psychology in 1997 and a MA in 1998.

Joseph F. Hagan, Jr., M.D., is Clinical Professor of Pediatrics at the University of Vermont College of Medicine and Chair of the American Academy of Pediatrics' Committee on Psychosocial Aspects of Family Health. Dr Hagan practices primary care pediatrics in Burlington, Vermont.

Robert J. Johnson, Ph.D., is professor and chair of Sociology at Kent State University where he specializes in medical sociology, life course and aging studies, and the social psychology of the self. His research interests involve the social and psychological correlates of physical health, the social and physical correlates of mental health, and models of the use of health care services. Professor Johnson's recent publications have appeared in the *Journal of Health and Social Behavior, The Gerontologist,* and the *Journal of Aging and Health.* Currently, he is investigating a cohort of older adults to determine the impact of the circumstances surrounding the end of life on receiving informal help.

Adam Neufeld holds a B.S. degree in neuroscience from Brown University. In 2000-2001, he worked as a researcher in the Department of Health Policy and Management at the Mailman School of Public Health, Columbia University. He is currently attending Harvard Law School.

Chantelle C. Nobile is a graduate of Tufts University and a Ph.D. candidate in the Pediatric Psychology Program at Case Western Reserve University. Her research interests include the impact of poverty on children's health as well as primary prevention and intervention strategies to be implemented in primary care settings. Her clinical interests include pain management and behavioral interventions for coping with daily stresses.

Peter Rappo, Ph.D., is a primary care pediatrician with 25 years of practice experience. He did his pediatric training at the Boston Floating Hospital and has a particular interest in the care of children with special health care needs. He is a founding member of the Pilgrim Health Care IPA board and chairs their pediatric care committee. He has served the AAP at the state, district, and national level, and is the immediate past chair of the Committee on Practice for that organization. He is an assistant clinical professor of Pediatrics at Harvard University. He also was on the original working group that created the primary care version of the *DSM-IV.*

Michael C. Roberts, Ph.D., is Director of the Clinical Child Psychology Program at the University of Kansas. He graduated from Purdue University in clinical psychology with a specialization in clinical child psychology and interned at the University of Oklahoma Health Sciences Center. He has served as editor for the *Journal of Pediatric Psychology, Children's Health Care,* and *Children's Services: Social Policy, Research, and Practice.* He has authored and coedited several books, including *Handbook of Clinical Child Psychology, Handbook of Pediatric Psychology, Model Programs in Service Delivery in Child and Family Mental Health, Prevention of Problems in Childhood,* and, most recently, *Helping Children Cope with Disasters and Terrorism.* His research interests have been focused on prevention, especially injury control, psychotherapeutic outcomes research and program evaluation in clinical child and pediatric psychology.

Carolyn S. Schroeder, Ph.D., received her Ph.D. from the University of Pittsburgh in 1966. She has held academic appointments in the Departments of Psychology, Psychiatry, and Pediatrics at the University of North Carolina-Chapel Hill. She is currently affiliated with the Clinical Child Psychology program at the University of Kansas. Her clinical and research interests have focused on the psychologists' role in the primary care setting and she was affiliated with Chapel Hill Pediatrics, a private community practice, for over 25 years.

Terri Stancin, Ph.D., is a Professor of Pediatrics, Psychiatry, and Psychology at Case Western Reserve University School of Medicine. She is the Head of the Division of Pediatric Psychology at MetroHealth Medical Center in Cleveland, Ohio, where she is a practicing pediatric psychologist. Dr. Stancin has directed much of her teaching, research, and clinical efforts at enhancing mental health services for children and adolescents in pediatric primary care settings. She is nationally known for her expertise regarding behavioral screening and assessment strategies in primary care settings, and for training pediatric residents in developmental and behavioral pediatrics.

Raymond Sturner, M.D., is an Associate Professor of Pediatrics at The Johns Hopkins University School of Medicine where he directs the fellowship training program in Developmental and Behavioral Pediatrics. He is also Codirector of the Center for Promotion of Child Development through Primary Care. Dr. Sturner formally directed the Duke Child Development Unit at Duke University. Dr. Sturner completed a fellowship in Developmental and Behavioral Pediatrics at Yale University after completing his general pediatric training at the Childrens Hospital of Philadelphia and the University of Colorado.

W. Douglas Tynan, Ph.D., is a Clinical Associate Professor of Pediatrics at Jefferson Medical College and the AI duPont Hospital for Children in Wilmington, Delaware where he directs the ADHD treatment program and the Primary Care consultation program. He received a master of science in child development from the University of Connecticut and a Ph.D. in clinical psychology from Binghamton University.

Beth Wildman, Ph.D., received her bachelors degree in psychology from the State University of New York at Stony Brook. She received both her M.A. and her Ph.D. in psychology from the University of North Carolina at Greensboro. She completed an internship in clinical psychology at the Virginia Treatment Center for Children in Richmond, VA. She joined the faculty at Kent State University in 1982, where she teaches courses in clinical research methods, behavior therapy and assessment, and child psychotherapy. Her current research focus is on factors affecting and barriers impeding management and outcomes of psychosocial problems in children seen in primary care medical settings.

Thomas M. Yerkey received his B.A. at The University of Akron in 1998. He is currently a graduate student in the Department of Psychology at Kent State University, where he completed his masters thesis in the area of primary care and mental health in children and is currently working on his dissertation in the same area.

INDEX

9 781593 110840